The Emergence of

AIDS

The Impact on Immunology, Microbiology, and Public Health

Edited by
Kenneth H. Mayer, MD
and H.F. Pizer

Cover art by Cheng-Chieh Chuang, MD

Table of Contents

DEDICATIONS

This book is dedicated to the memories of my father, Paul Mayer, who taught me the importance of humanistic values and the satisfaction of taking on new challenges, and my uncle, Dr. Norbert Freinkel, who showed me how fulfilling a career in biomedical research can be, and to Fred Mandel, Dr. Ira Gold, Duncan Erley, Jonathan Shuster, Mark Pfetsch, Dr. Sandy Reder, Dr. Nick Rango, and the myriads of other friends and patients who died too young because of HIV, robbing the world of the full expression of their many talents. – Kenneth H. Mayer

The book is dedicated to my wife, Christine, my daughter, Katie, and my mother, Estelle Y. Pizer, b. March 17, 1916; d. November 26, 1999. – H.F. Pizer

Common Acronyms

ACTG	AIDS Clinical Trials Group
AIDS	Acquired Immunodeficiency Syndrome
AZT	Azidothymidine
CDC	Centers for Disease Control and Prevention
DHHS	Department of Health and Human Services
DNA	Deoxyribonucleic Acid
FDA	Food and Drug Administration
HAART	Highly Active Antiretroviral Therapy
HIV	Human Immunodeficiency Virus
HTLV	Human T Lymphotropic Virus
IDU	Intravenous Drug User
IOM	Institute of Medicine
MACS	Multicenter AIDS Cohort Study
MSM	Men Having Sex with Men
NIAAA	National Institute on Alcohol Abuse and Alcoholism
NIAID	National Institute of Allergy and Infectious Diseases
NIDA	National Institute on Drug Abuse
NIH	National Institutes of Health
NIMH	National Institute of Mental Health
PCP	*Pneumocystis carinii* Pneumonia
PHS	Public Health Service
RNA	Ribonucleic Acid
UNAIDS	United Nations Program on AIDS/HIV
WHO	World Health Organization
ZDV	Zidovudine

ACKNOWLEDGEMENTS

Without the clerical and administrative assistance of Nancy Lapham, Michelle Anatone, Doreen Salgueiro, Lola Wright, and Dennis Thomas, this book would not have been possible. I would like to thank my many colleagues over the past 2 decades at Fenway Community Health, particularly Dr. Stephen Boswell, Martha Moon, Robert Goldstein, and Tom Lasalvia; and in the Brown University AIDS Program, particularly Drs. Valerie Stone, Charles Carpenter, Timothy Flanigan, Sally Zierler, Susan Cu-Uvin, and Anne DeGroot, for their ongoing intellectual engagement in helping me understanding this evolving epidemic, and for their wonderful clinical care and advocacy they have provided. I would be remiss if I didn't acknowledge my academic colleagues and collaborators, particularly Drs. George Seage, Deborah Anderson, Marshall Posner, Lisa Cavacini, Richard D'Aquila, and Raphael Dolin, and especially Dr. Stephen Zinner, who has been both an insightful mentor and considerate friend. Most important, I would like to acknowledge the generous and heroic contributions of all the persons living with HIV whom I have had the privilege to know, who have shared the details of their intimate lives, and their bodily fluids and tissues, with biomedical and behavioral researchers so that we can soon live in a world without AIDS.

Kenneth H. Mayer

[Cover art by Cheng-Chieh Chuang, MD] Dr. Chuang was born in Taiwan and grew up in Argentina. He is a graduate of Brown University and Yale School of Medicine, and completed the Brown University Family Medicine residency program. He is currently working in Provincetown, Massachusetts, and divides his time between providing primary care for disenfranchised people and working on his art, which includes a variety of media, and series that have ranged from flowers to landscapes to illustrations for children's books.

Editors

Kenneth H. Mayer, MD is Professor of Medicine & Community Health at Brown University, Director of the Brown University AIDS Program, Chief of the Infectious Disease Division at Memorial Hospital of Rhode Island, and Medical Research Director of Fenway Community Health in Boston. He is also an Adjunct Professor at the Harvard School of Public Health and serves on the National Board of Directors of the American Foundation for AIDS Research and the Gay and Lesbian Medical Association. His research interests focus on the natural history, behavioral epidemiology, transmission variables, and public policy aspects of the epidemic. He serves on several editorial boards, has been appointed Special Topics Editor for HIV/AIDS for *Clinical Infectious Diseases,* and has published more than 200 articles and other publications about HIV/AIDS. Most recently, Dr. Mayer has worked as a member of the consortia within the NIH's HIV Prevention Trials Network and HIV Vaccine Trials Network (HIVNET) and has led CDC-funded studies of HIV vaccine trials and postexposure prophylaxis against HIV infection.

H.F. Pizer, PA is President of Health Care Strategies, Inc., a consulting firm in Cambridge, Massachusetts, and previously founded and headed another consulting company, New England Medical Claims Analysts, which provided health care cost containment services. He has also served as President of the Massachusetts Association of Physician Assistants. As a medical writer, he has written or coauthored 11 books on health for the general public, including *The AIDS Fact Book* with Kenneth Mayer, MD. His books have been translated into at least 6 foreign languages, including Japanese and Chinese.

Contributors

Ronald Bayer, PhD, is a Professor at Columbia University School of Public Health, where he has taught for 10 years. Before teaching at Columbia, Dr. Bayer conducted research at the Hastings Center on ethical and policy issues raised by the AIDS epidemic. He has examined ethical and policy issues raised by the AIDS epidemic since 1982.

Madhav P. Bhatta, MPH is a doctoral student in Epidemiology at the University of Alabama at Birmingham and a Graduate Assistant in the Sparkman Center for International Public Health Education. He has public health experience in both Nepal (his home country) and in Thailand. His work in the Sparkman Center includes program and proposal review and development of international education projects in resource-poor overseas settings.

Victor G. DeGruttola, DSc, is Professor of Biostatistics and Director of the Statistical and Data Analysis Center (Adult Division) of the AIDS Clinical Trial Group at the Harvard School of Public Health. He holds degrees in bioengineering from Harvard University and in epidemiology and biostatistics from the Harvard School of Public Health. His principal research interest is the development of innovative study designs and analytical methods for the evaluation of new therapies for HIV-related disease.

Myron E. Essex, DVM, PhD is the Chairman of the Harvard AIDS Institute, the Mary Woodard Lasker Professor of Health Sciences at Harvard University, and Chairman of the Department of Immunology and Infectious Disease at the Harvard School of Public Health. He was one of the first investigators to suggest that AIDS was caused by a retrovirus. He and his colleagues later described many of the major viral antigens of the HIV virus critical for blood bank screening and current vaccine design.

Paul E. Farmer, MD, PhD, an infectious disease specialist and anthropologist, divides his time between Harvard Medical School, where he serves as Professor of Social Medicine and directs the Program in Infectious Disease and Social Change, and the Clinique Bon Sauveur in central Haiti, where he serves as Medical Director. In 1993, he received a MacArthur award in recognition of his work, which he donated in its entirety to

Partners In Health, a Boston-based public charity he cofounded that seeks to improve the health of the poor in this hemisphere.

Jennifer J. Furin, MD, PhD is a physician-anthropologist who divides her time between completing her residency in internal medicine at the Brigham and Women's Hospital (Boston, Massachusetts) and directing a project
to treat multidrug resistant tuberculosis in Lima, Peru. She also directs clinical services of the Program in Infectious Disease and Social Change at Harvard Medical School.

Phyllis J. Kanki, DVM, ScD is Professor of Immunology and Infectious Disease at the Harvard School of Public Health. She has directed the collaborative AIDS research program between scientists at Harvard and University Cheikh Anta Diop in Dakar, Senegal, for the past 15 years. Her research interests include HIV pathogenesis, molecular epidemiology, and intervention studies. Her work has described major biological differences and interactions between HIV-1 and HIV-2 that may be important for AIDS vaccine development.

Nancy Krieger, PhD, is Associate Professor of Public Health in the Department of Health and Social Behavior at the Harvard School of Public Health and Associate Director of the Harvard Center for Society and Health. She is a social epidemiologist who investigates social inequal-ities in health involving social class, racial and gender discrimination, and the history and politics of epidemiology and public health. She also examines theories used to explain population patterns of health, disease, and well-being.

Sibylle Kristensen, MSPH, MPH is program director of the AIDS International Training and Research Program at the University of Alabama at Birmingham, which is supported by the Fogarty International Center of the NIH. Born and raised in former Zaire, she has degrees in both International Health and in Epidemiology. She has worked on HIV control in developing countries, hepatitis in Alabama, and disease surveillance in Pakistan.

Jeffrey Laurence, MD, is Associate Professor of Medicine and Director of the Laboratory for AIDS Virus Research at Weill Medical College of Cornell University. He is also an Associate Attending in Medicine at New York Presbyterian Hospital and is Chief Scientist for Programs at the

American Foundation for AIDS Research. His research now focuses on the role of HIV in microvascular endothelial cell damage and advanced atherosclerosis in AIDS.

Carola Marte, MD, PhD, is Senior Medical Advisor and HIV Program Director at Community Healthcare Network in New York City. She practices in underserved communities, has established onsite HIV and gynecological services for methadone treatment clinics in New York City, and works closely with government and community-based agencies on policy issues concerning health care for the poor, HIV, and women's health. Her research has focused on cervical disease in HIV-infected women.

Theresa M. McGovern, JD, is the founder of the HIV Law Project, a nonprofit organization providing legal representation and advocacy services to low-income HIV-infected people and underserved groups. She served as lead counsel in *SP v Sullivan,* the 1990 class action lawsuit alleging race and sex discrimination on the part of the Social Security Administration in its reliance on the CDC definition of AIDS as the standard for dispersing benefits. She is now on faculty at Columbia University School of Public Health.

Jean McGuire, PhD is Assistant Commissioner at the Massachusetts Department of Health, where she directs the HIV/AIDS Bureau. She also served as Director of the AIDS Action Council in Washington, DC and was instrumental in gaining passage of the Ryan White CARE Act and of the Americans with Disabilities Act. Her research has focused on ethical issues in HIV clinical trials.

David G. Ostrow, MD, PhD is Professor of Psychiatry and Behavioral Neurosciences at Loyola University Medical School and Chief of the Addiction Medicine Program at Loyola University Medical Systems. He serves as Consultant Intervention Scientist for a multisite intervention study of HIV infection in IDUs. He focuses most of his work on HIV/AIDS and substance abuse, the development of new interventions for drug-using MSM, the causal mechanisms linking substance abuse and sexual transmission, and the impact of HAART on attitudes and risk behaviors of men at-risk for HIV infection.

Sten H. Vermund, MD, PhD is Professor of Epidemiology and International Health, Medicine, and Pediatrics at the University of Alabama at Birmingham. As an infectious disease epidemiologist, he has worked on diseases of particular interest in developing nations as well as on inner city and rural health issues in the United States. At UAB, he directs the Sparkman Center for International Public Health Education in the School of Public Health and the Division of Geographic Medicine in the School of Medicine. As president of a nongovernmental organization, the Gorgas Memorial Institute for Tropical and Preventive Medicine, he works on training projects in Latin America and the Caribbean.

David A. Walton is a research associate in the Program in Infectious Disease and Social Change at Harvard Medical School. He has worked in AIDS and tuberculosis treatment and prevention in rural Haiti and plans a career in infectious disease.

Sally Zierler, DrPH, is Professor of Medical Science and Women's Studies at Brown University School of Medicine. She was trained as an epidemiologist at the Harvard School of Public Health. Her research has focused on the health of women throughout the life course, especially in relation to the biologic response of social inequalities based on gender, race, class, and sexuality.

Preface

Hindsight is always 20-20. In the early 1980s, the AIDS epidemic had not been foreseen by most public health officials, laboratory researchers, or theoreticians who were trying to understand the sexual revolution. The recognition of its true potential impact on a global scale could not have been possible. However, the lack of urgency in the initial response— clearly related to the affected populations (eg, gays and drug users)—should not have occurred and must never be allowed to repeat.

One of my first electives as a medical student was with Dr. Jeremiah Stamler, a cardiovascular epidemiologist who recognized how social choices directly affected public health. In addition to gaining a broader perspective on society and disease, I learned from Dr. Stamler and his team some of the principles of analyzing large databases from long-term cohort studies. At the same time I began to analyze epidemiological data, I attended meetings of gay medical students who wanted to help improve the health of the community in the near Northside communities of Chicago. The goal of this program was be to attract hard-to-reach persons for screening of asymptomatic sexually transmitted diseases, which at the time were rampant among sexually active gay men.

The Howard Brown Clinic provided me with a unique opportunity to interview individuals who were engaging in multiple sexual activities and to learn how to screen for sexually transmitted diseases. The most common diseases of that era were gonorrhea and syphilis, which were easily treated with shots of penicillin or short courses of tetracycline. Most individuals in the gay community and other sexually active individuals naively thought that although sexually transmitted diseases were embarrassing, they were invariably treatable. Many felt that such diseases were merely the price paid for being free to explore one's sexuality and to develop instant intimacy with new partners.

In fact, one common sexually transmitted infectious disease among men who had sex with men subsequently had very important public health implications for the AIDS epidemic: hepatitis B. In the early 1970s, epidemiologic studies suggested that the virus was readily transmitted through blood transfusions and other contact with blood-contaminated equipment, such as the sharing of injection paraphernalia among drug

addicts. It took several more years to recognize the efficacy of the transmission of hepatitis B via sexual contact, particularly through anal
intercourse. Once appropriate serodiagnostic tests for hepatitis were developed, population-based screening suggested that the virus was particularly
widespread among men who had sex with men, with the majority being
unaware that they had hepatitis. In addition to educating young physicians and other health care workers about the dynamics of sexually
transmitted diseases in the gay community, community health centers and
public health programs oriented toward men who had sex with men
created a research infrastructure that would soon prove invaluable.

Linkages between national public health officials (most notably the
Centers for Disease Control and Prevention), city public health depart-
ments, and members of the gay and lesbian community used hepatitis B
as the model for implementing interventions related to the HIV epidemic.
Community health programs oriented toward gay and lesbian health
problems sprang up in most major US cities, including the Whitman-
Walker Clinic in Washington, DC and the Fenway Community Health
Center in Boston.

The Fenway was founded as a freestanding community health center
in 1975 by a group of community activists. Rather than force disenfranchised persons to travel to a teaching hospital, the Fenway offered
college students, older adults, and gays and lesbians alike a local and
more welcoming option. When I began my residency, I contacted the
Fenway about volunteering but was told that many of the patients were
becoming disaffected with the care they received due to the lack of
continuity. By 1980, I had moved on to an infectious disease fellowship
and developed a specialty clinic to address the increasingly complex
medical conditions that patients presented with at the Fenway.

In those early days of AIDS, several institutions enhanced the awareness of young public health workers about newly emerging epidemics,
thereby creating a national public health community. For example, the
Morbidity and Mortality Weekly Report simultaneously alerted thousands
of physicians, nurses, public health workers, city health department
administrators, state and territorial public health officials, and researchers
at the Centers for Disease Control and Prevention about the new puzzle
called AIDS. Today an Emerging Infections Network on the Internet facili-
tates discussions of new outbreaks in real time. However, even the
weekly delivery via surface mail of internally reviewed data provided
enough common elements to suggest the emergence of a multisite

epidemic. At Fenway Community Health Center, we recognized that this epidemic could greatly impact the gay community, and our infectious disease clinic proved essential.

The specialty of infectious disease came of age with the discovery of newer antibiotics and refinement in the ability to isolate pathogens. In 1982, a late-breaking session at the Infectious Disease Society of America annual meeting dedicated some time to discussion of a newly emerging epidemic among gay and bisexual men, which had also recently been described among injection drug users, called "Gay-Related Immune Deficiency Syndrome" (GRID). Some speakers related hypotheses about the "burn-out of the immune system" and the mutation of known organisms, such as cytomegalovirus, to more virulent forms. Others felt the epidemic was due to a unique etiologic agent. Based on what we observed in patients and their partners at the Fenway (eg, generalized lymphadenopathy, night sweats, unexplained anemia, thrush, and other subacute signs of compromised immunity), I leaned toward a new transmissible agent. Fortunately, the Centers for Disease Control and Prevention were not afraid to go to socially unacceptable epidemic sites (eg, gay bath houses) to collect data and answer key questions. Had the relationships formed to address hepatitis B not been available, progress on the identification of HIV and the understanding of AIDS would have been slower.

Knowledge gained provides the basis for what can be known in the future. In the case of the AIDS epidemic, awareness in the public health community that a competent health care infrastructure existed for gay men and injection drug users and that the model provided by hepatitis B could be useful helped create a conceptual framework that likewise advanced scientific investigation. Conversely, the very work needed to identify the etiologic agent, to screen for transmission, and to develop effective therapy radically transformed other disciplines of clinical medicine, molecular virology and immunology, and public health policies and practice. Ultimately, this book focuses on the evolution of a global pandemic, the lessons learned about AIDS, and the lessons learned from AIDS.

Kenneth H. Mayer, MD
Chief, Infectious Disease Division
Memorial Hospital of Rhode Island
Professor of Medicine and Community Health
Brown University School of Medicine
Director, Brown University AIDS Program

Learning From AIDS

This is a book of lessons learned. It helps complete a circle begun in 1981, when Kenneth Mayer and I began working on *The AIDS Fact Book,* the first book for the general public about the new and frightening AIDS epidemic. At that time, HIV had not been isolated. In the public forum, more conjecture and anxiety could be found than fact upon which to make good health decisions. As the book cover declared, our goal was to "Conquer Fear With The Facts."

Although frequently reported with much uninformed speculation, AIDS quickly became an important story in the mass media. I remember a lawyer-friend calling to ask me if she should share a summer rental in the Hamptons with a gay friend. She was worried about using the same swimming pool. Even medical professionals jumped to unsubstantiated conclusions. During a telephone satellite interview broadcast in Australia, I was stunned by a public health physician who felt no qualms about voicing all sorts of erroneous, prejudiced ideas about homosexuals.

Now we come to this book. After 20 years of research and clinical work in the field, we felt it was time to start pulling together what has been learned from the epidemic. Much of what has been written to date focuses on its continuing tragedy, especially in the Third World. We decided to begin accounting for the ways in which HIV/AIDS transformed an array of distinct albeit related disciplines in health, medicine, science, politics, advocacy, and the law.

Our contributors have devoted much of their professional lives to working in the AIDS arena. We are indebted to them for taking the time to explore what AIDS has done to change and advance their disciplines. They bring to the book their medical, scientific, epidemiologic, public health, and legal expertise and individual lessons learned from their efforts to understand the AIDS pandemic.

We begin with "The Past and Future of HIV," in which Phyllis Kanki and Max Essex present the fascinating history of HIV and mark its enormous impact on studying the natural history of viruses and the disease they cause. As a result of studying AIDS, we better understand how viruses undergo their own selection processes, moving from nonhuman to human hosts and forming subtypes in humans that display different degrees of expression and pathogenicity. The natural history of HIV teaches us that considerable variability exists in how both animals and humans respond to viral challenge. Studying subhuman primates that resist illness altogether and infected individuals who do not become ill or who progress slowly over time holds promise for helping to develop new prevention and treatment options.

Next, Jeffrey Laurence ("The Virus Versus the Immune System") describes the many ways in which HIV research taught us how viruses broadly affect the human immune system. He points out that viruses are more than potentially lethal pathogens: they can also be useful tools for investigating normal immune function, developing immunotherapeutics, and advancing our understanding of the clever tricks viruses employ for subverting detection and eradication. HIV is teaching us to temper somewhat current expectations for high-intensity antiviral drug therapy. HIV research shows we will need new tools for handling viruses that lie latent in safe harbors, where current therapy could take 100 years to eliminate dormant cells.

In "How Infectious Is Infectious," Ken Mayer reviews a body of HIV-related research that has advanced a wide array of disciplines related to infectious disease. He reviews major lessons learned in the understanding of viral-mediated immunopathogenesis, virulence, and patterns of disease dissemination. He points out that techniques developed for quantifying HIV replication and monitoring its effects on the immune system are now applied to other chronic viral infections. Thanks to HIV and hepatitis B, we have also learned to act when occupational or general exposure to infectious diseases occurs. Perhaps of special note to our audience in the public health community is the manner in which the epidemic transformed the delivery of chronic care, including that offered by infectious disease specialists, who in the past had been relegated to providing "acute" consultations. Often the caregivers were, like the patients, outside the medical mainstream. The epidemic raised awareness that people living with HIV/AIDS need access to a broad range of medical, mental health, and social services. While this concept is not wholly unique to AIDS, the challenges raised by this epidemic have offered an important lesson for dealing with other chronic diseases.

In "The Response of Quantitative Scientists to Challenges Posed by the AIDS Epidemic," Victor DeGruttola discusses the often-overlooked advances in statistics catalyzed by the HIV/AIDS epidemic. He reminds us that early in the epidemic inadequate quantitative assessment, based on "statistical naiveté," lulled policy makers into a false sense of complacency. The latency period between infection and symptoms was erroneously thought to be only 1 to 2 years, that only promiscuous homosexuals and intravenous drug users were at risk, and that the blood supply was essentially safe. It was not until 1986 that statisticians and epidemiologists started to provide accurate projections for the real threat of AIDS. The risk was greater than previously thought, and lives may have been lost as a result. HIV and AIDS forced statisticians and epidemiologists to develop methods for studying the natural history of disease, projecting incidence, modeling transmission patterns, designing surveys, and studying the efficacy of programs for screening and testing that in the future may be applied elsewhere to improve health and save lives.

David Ostrow's contribution, "Sex and Drugs and the Virus," notes that the AIDS epidemic in drug users and men who have sex with men is not distinct and that, except for needle sharing, researchers too often ignore the role of substance abuse in spreading the virus. He argues that using "party drugs" during sex interferes with safer sex practices while suppressing cognitive inhibitions generally. A critical public health lesson to be learned, he warns, is that the increased risk resulting from the desire to use drugs to enhance sex is not unique to HIV. If behavioral interventions focus only on infectious agents—and not the sex and drug taking behaviors through which they are transmitted—it will be no surprise should new epidemics come along to replace AIDS. Hepatitis C is already one such candidate. Others are surely on the horizon.

We move on to Sally Zierler and Nancy Krieger's contribution, "Social Inequality and HIV Infection in Women," which examines the social factors that lie at the heart of a woman's risk of acquiring HIV infection. In the United States, women with HIV most often live in neighborhoods burdened by poverty, drug use, crime, and discrimination. They are more likely to be African American or Hispanic than white. What we observe in America can be applied to the epidemiology of AIDS and other causes of morbidity and mortality worldwide: health status and social justice are inextricably linked. From how we collect data to how we offer health education and disease prevention, success depends on strategies that hold accountable the social and economic realities of women at risk. Discovering new treatments or vaccines does these women little good if they lack access to them.

Indeed, Carola Marte and Terry McGovern ("Gender Equity in HIV/AIDS Clinical Trials") reflect on the role of gender, socioeconomic status, and ethnicity in determining who has access to the most advanced health care. They observe that until recently, women were restricted in their access to clinical trials and hence to potentially beneficial new treatments and effective medical follow up. For example, the recognition that cervical dysplasia and cancer were related to HIV infection did not occur until 1993. Gradually, thanks to AIDS advocacy efforts, more women were enrolled in clinical trials, thereby correcting a disparity in delivering services that had been characteristic of the health care system as a whole.

Sten Vermund, Sibylle Kristensen, and Madhav Bhatta remind us that AIDS is a sexually transmitted disease and review the history of combating STDs to help us understand what is needed to inhibit the spread of HIV. In "HIV as an STD," they make clear the direct relationship between public health efforts to control STDs and the rise and fall of their incidence and impact on society. Partnerships between federal and state governments that promote education, testing, case reporting, and condom prophylaxis work. Even before the realization that AIDS was caused by a virus, basic STD protocols could have helped control the epidemic. Governments that do not heed this history are risking lives and future prosperity.

In "The Changing Face of AIDS: Implications for Policy and Practice," Paul Farmer, David Walton, and Jennifer Furin continue the discussion of the social implications of AIDS through an international epidemiologic overview. Today's AIDS, they argue, is a disease of social inequality rather than of risky behaviors or membership in a specific group. In the United States, an AIDS patient often enters the hospital without private insurance, taking neither antiviral therapies nor appropriate prophylaxis for opportunistic infections. In developing countries, struggles to maintain subsistence living contribute to disease transmission where no resources exist for its treatment. As Farmer and his colleagues point out, we may have the tools for preventing many AIDS deaths, but we lack the will to use them.

Ronald Bayer's contribution, "Privacy and the Public Health: Conflict and Change in the AIDS Epidemic," recounts how AIDS forced public health experts, policy makers, and advocates to reexamine medical privacy. Initially, AIDS activists and public health experts generally agreed that strict assurances on privacy would protect individuals from being ostracized and encourage them to come in voluntarily for testing. However, as the epidemic spread and effective treatment became available, these views changed. The debate reached a climax in the area of perinatal testing, leading to a relaxation of the strictest of privacy standards in favor of testing and reporting programs to promote prevention and treatment.

Of special interest to our APHA readers is Jean McGuire's piece on "Inclusion, Representation, and Parity: The Making of a Public Health Response to HIV." She discusses ways in which the epidemic forced public health systems to revise traditional protocols. Antidiscrimination assurances in primary and secondary prevention were instituted, ecological and harm reduction were emphasized, palliative care and social support were advanced, alternative and complementary therapies were incorporated, and medication adherence programs were accentuated. She reminds us these public health systems began to change following political activism on the part of the gay community, which demanded that the people affected by AIDS have a significant stake in developing policy and programs. Including activists in policy making was often uncomfortable for mainstream public health officials, but by 1988, antidiscrimination protections were seen by the public health community as a necessary centerpiece of AIDS control efforts, offering protection in housing, employment, and access to public accommodations and obtaining health-related services. Indeed, the AIDS epidemic taught public health officials to think outside the medical box.

We hope this book highlights lessons learned that may advance worthwhile strategies for combating HIV and AIDS. We are indebted to our colleagues and friends who gave their time and expertise to this effort.

H.F. Pizer
Cambridge, Massachusetts

Section I: Scientific Gains

Although medically and socially devastating, HIV and AIDS have had much to teach us, as illustrated in these first 4 chapters. Searching for the cause of AIDS led to dozens of discoveries that would otherwise have been delayed for years, particularly those related to the intricate workings of the human immune system. The very advances in laboratory technique required to study HIV and AIDS offer dividends far beyond the epidemic at hand. Insights gained and models developed by epidemiologists—and recognition of the key role of epidemiologists by clinicians and scientists—will improve efficiency in characterizing future pandemics. Perhaps most importantly, the AIDS epidemic has forced us to accept the absolute need for integration and cooperation of research efforts. Surely none of us wishes for a "next time," but at least we are better prepared.

Section 1: Scientific Gains

CHAPTER 1

The Past and Future of HIV

Phyllis J. Kanki, Myron E. Essex

E ntering the new millennium, we can evaluate the 20-year history of the HIV pandemic and our response to it. Indeed, by the early 1980s, this unique viral pathogen had already inflicted significant damage on populations of specific risk groups in the United States and Europe as well as less well characterized populations in sub-Saharan Africa. By the mid-1980s, HIV as the cause of AIDS had been described, and we were beginning to appreciate the diversity and complexity of HIVs and their closely related viruses from nonhuman primate species.

Although discussions of how various HIVs and related simian immun-odeficiency viruses (SIVs) evolved were often fueled by more politically motivated assignations of blame, the scientific rationale for such inquiries should not be minimized. We now appreciate that HIV and SIV are members of a large and diverse immunodeficiency virus family. Studies of these viral infections in both humans and monkeys have demonstrated unique biological relationships, sometimes resulting in AIDS (as with HIV-1), sometimes resulting in a more indolent disease course (as with HIV-2 and some SIVs). Understanding how human or monkey hosts evolved to resist the lethal effects of HIV or related viruses may provide valuable clues for developing effective vaccines and drugs.

An Infectious Etiology for AIDS

Despite the major technological advances in biomedical research in the 20th century, the discovery of the etiologic agent of AIDS was painfully slow. Unlike the previous epidemics of the century, such as the 1918 influenza epidemic or that of paralytic polio, AIDS was a unique clinical entity without a known causative agent. If a "new" disease appears, the cause must also be "new." If a new disease is infectious, as was the case with AIDS, the causative agent may have existed previously in one of several possible circumstances.

First, the etiologic agent may represent a more virulent mutation of an organism that previously either infected the same population without causing disease or produced a distinctly different disease profile. Second, the organism may have emerged from an isolated population of people who had developed a relative resistance to the lethality of the agent. Third, the organism may have been introduced to humans from another species. This third explanation seems to best fit our current understanding of the origin of HIV. HIV-2 and various SIVs from African monkeys are close, almost indistinguishable genetic relatives, and it appears that this may also be the case with HIV-1.

AIDS was first recognized as a new and distinct clinical entity in 1981.[1-3] The first cases were recognized because of an unusual clustering of diseases such as Kaposi's sarcoma and *Pneumocystis carinii* pneumonia (PCP) in young homosexual men. Although such syndromes were occasionally observed in distinct subgroups of the population—such as older men of Mediterranean origin in the case of Kaposi's sarcoma or severely immunosuppressed cancer patients in the case of PCP—the occurrence of these diseases in previously healthy young people was unprecedented. Since most of the first cases of this newly defined clinical syndrome involved homosexual men, lifestyle practices were first implicated and investigated.

However, AIDS cases were soon reported in other populations as well, including IDUs[4] and hemophiliacs.[5-7] Although these groups were not exposed to amyl or butyl nitrate "poppers" or to frequent contact with sperm rectally (see Chapter 5 for an in-depth review of poppers and the sex-drug connection), they, like male homosexuals, may have been exposed to frequent immunostimulatory doses of foreign proteins and tissue antigens. Asymptomatic hemophiliacs and IDUs were often found to have inverted T lymphocyte helper:suppressor ratios (ie, less than 1:1 ratio of helper to suppressor cells) similar to some healthy homosexual men and also to many AIDS patients. For patients not infected with HIV, the distorted T cell ratios were more often due to an increase in the number of T suppressor cells rather than the absolute decrease in T helper cells seen in AIDS patients and HIV carriers with progressing disease. The increase in T suppressor cells was presumably due to frequent antigenic stimulation, while the decrease in T helper cells was the more direct effect of the HIV infection.

Three new categories of AIDS patients were soon observed: blood transfusion recipients,[8,9] adults from Central Africa,[10-12] and infants born to mothers who had AIDS or were IDUs.[13-15] The transfusion-associated cases had received blood donated from an AIDS patient at least 3 years before they began showing symptoms.[8,9]

Based on the disparate populations afflicted with this new malady and the emerging epidemiology of the disease, the possible infectious etiology for AIDS was considered.[16] Multiple studies were initiated to determine the possible role of various microorganisms, especially viruses in causing AIDS. These studies measured and compared seroprevalence rates for suspect viruses in AIDS patients and controls.[17] The short list of candidate viruses included: cytomegalovirus, which was already associated with immunosuppression in kidney transplant patients; Epstein-Barr virus, which was a lymphotropic virus; and hepatitis B, which was known to occur at elevated rates in both homosexual men and recipients of blood or blood products. However, based on the unique clinical syndrome and unusual epidemiology of AIDS, if one of these viruses were to be etiologically involved, it would presumably have been a newly mutated or recombinant genetic variant.

At the same time, our group,[18] Gallo and his colleagues,[19] and Montagnier and his colleagues[20] postulated that a variant T lymphotropic retrovirus (HTLV) might be the etiologic agent of AIDS. Indeed, the HTLV, discovered by Gallo and his colleagues in 1980, was the only human virus known to infect T helper lymphocytes at that time.[21] This seemed reasonable since it was already clear that T helper lymphocytes were selectively depleted by the causative agent in clinical AIDS.[13,22-24] In addition, HTLV was known to transmit through the same routes as the etiologic agent of AIDS: sexual contact (with transmission apparently more efficient from males), by blood, and from mother to baby.[25] Finally, HTLV-I was also known to induce immunosuppression.[27]

AIDS patient blood samples were repeatedly cultured in an attempt to find a virus related to HTLV-I or HTLV-II.[28] Although antibodies cross-reactive with HTLV-I and HTLV-related genomic sequences were found in a minority of AIDS patients,[18-20] the reactivity was weak, suggesting either that AIDS patients were also infected with an HTLV or that a distant, weakly reactive virus was the causative agent. Soon after, Gallo and his colleagues obtained proof that AIDS was linked to an HTLV.[29-32] Further characterization of the agent—now termed HIV-1—revealed that it was the same as the isolate detected earlier by Montagnier and his colleagues.[20] Despite controversy over the names and identity of certain isolates, this new and unique human pathogen was clearly not only a distant genetic relative of the known HTLV virus but may have been recently introduced to humans from a primate reservoir.

Origins of Human Retroviruses

Although cancer research in the 1970s had focused on animal retroviruses that caused leukemia and lymphoma, it was not until 1980 that the first human retrovirus—HTLV-I—was described.[21,33-35] HTLV-I occurred at elevated rates in regions such as southwestern Japan, the Caribbean basin, northern South America, and Africa and at lower rates in most of North America and Europe. Gallo suggested that this virus originated in Africa and was spread through slaves taken to southwestern Japan by Portuguese traders.[36] Miyoshi and his colleagues then identified a virus closely related to HTLV-I in Asian monkeys.[37] This virus, designated simian T-cell leukemia virus (STLV), was later found in African monkeys and apes[38] and was associated with lymphoma and lymphoproliferative diseases in captive macaques.[39]

Seroepidemiologic studies in Old World primates from both Asia and Africa revealed that more than 30 species of monkeys and apes had significant infection with an STLV.[40] However, the STLV viruses from Japanese macaques and related Asian species of monkeys were not as closely related to HTLV-I as were STLVs isolated from African primates such as chimpanzees and African green monkeys.[41] Thus, all isolates of HTLV-I—whether from Japanese, Caribbean, or African people—were highly related to STLVs from African primates but not to STLVs from Asian primates.

As a group, the HTLV-I/STLV viruses are quite similar from one isolate to another, while the HIV-1 viruses and the HIV-2/SIV group of viruses vary significantly from one isolate to another.[42,43] This is consistent with the lower replication and mutation rate of the HTLV/STLV viruses in vivo. Presumably, the rate of genetic drift seen in retroviruses is related to their rate of replication. Because HTLV-I is apparently transmitted both between individuals and within the body in a cell-associated manner, the sheer quantity of virus produced is thought to be low, leading to a lower degree of genetic and evolutionary diversity. The high prevalence rates of STLV infection in so many species of Old World monkeys also indicate that STLV only rarely causes lymphoma or other disease under natural circumstances. Although it is unclear why STLV and HTLV-I are so limited in their pathogenicity, evolutionary pressure within the monkey species may have selected for a virus that was not highly virulent. An STLV of low virulence might then have been transmitted to humans, where it remained a virus of limited virulence.

HIVs, as lentiviruses within the retrovirus family, are better able to circumvent the rigid retrovirus requirements for cell division. Regulatory genes not found in simpler retroviruses (eg, HTLV, STLV) allow a rapid increase in replication rate. Unlike HTLV, HIV-1 can replicate to high titers and can be detected as free virus in serum or plasma. In addition, plasma viral levels are predictive of disease course.[44] This replication potential, along with a reverse transcriptase that is substantially more error-prone, helps explain why genomic variation among HIVs is substantially greater than for other retroviruses.[a] These properties would predict a very different and more rapid evolutionary development course for HIV-1, which appears to be the case.

Although the HTLV-I/STLV viruses rarely cause lethal disease in people or in monkeys, the HIV-1 viruses cause AIDS or a related disease in a very high proportion of infected people.[45] The pathogenicity of SIVs appears to depend more heavily on the host species. SIVs appear to be nonvirulent in their natural African monkey hosts but induce a fatal immunosuppression in abnormal monkey hosts, such as various Asian macaque species.[45,46] HIV-2 is less virulent than HIV-1 but is associated with some cases of AIDS.[47-49] The lower replication rate and degree of genetic variability of HIV-2 compared with HIV-1 may play an important role in its reduced pathogenicity.[50-52]

Origin of HIV-1

After HIV-1 was recognized as the cause of AIDS, it was also recognized that this virus was new, at least to inhabitants of the Western Hemisphere. This raised the question of whether HIV-1 was also new in Old World human populations, such as Africa, or whether it recently entered humans from another species. If HIV-1 had been present in populations of people in Africa to the point of evolutionary equilibrium, as seen with HTLV-I, it probably would have been limited to isolated population groups. In this situation, selection for host immunity as well as selection of an avirulent virus might have been favored. However, early clinical studies did not indicate differences in the pathogenicity of the virus-host interactions in Africa compared with the United States or Europe.

HIV-1 or a related virus was likely present in human populations in central Africa at the same time or even before AIDS was diagnosed in the United States. In the early 1980s, Africans residing in Europe were presenting with similar clinical signs and symptoms of AIDS.[10] Serum samples collected from Africans at earlier periods were also examined for the presence of antibodies reactive with HIV-1. In some cases, the examination of stored samples suggested elevated rates of infection in Africa during the mid-1960s to 1970s. Subsequently, it was revealed that most of those surveys were conducted with first-stage tests that were imperfect. In addition, the reactors were mostly false positives, due either to contamination of the HIV antigen or to "sticky sera" containing antibodies that reacted nonspecifically because the sera had been repeatedly frozen and thawed and maintained under poor conditions.[61]

While examining sera taken from Africa in the period 1955 to 1965, we found one antibody-positive sample that was clearly positive in a specific manner.[62] When tested by radioimmunoprecipitation, this sample contained high titers of antibodies that were reactive with virtually all the major antigens of HIV-1 detectable by this technique.[b] This sample represented only a rare positive reactor in a high-risk group of individuals suffering from tuberculosis and AIDS-like illness in a region that subsequently had high rates of infection with HIV-1. However, only 1% or fewer of the individuals who tested positive were from what is now classified as a region of moderate- to high-prevalence (Kinshasa, Zaire), which suggests that the virus was then only rarely present in places that would now be classified as within the "AIDS belt" of Africa.

HIV-1 had probably moved to the cities in this region of Africa only recently. We could speculate that the virus had either moved from subhuman primates to people prior to the mid-1950s or had been introduced to the cities through the migration of a few resistant carriers from a previously isolated group of people. However, if HIV-1 had been present in rural areas, we might expect to find that Africans demonstrate greater resistance to infection and disease development, owing to genetic selection and evolution of the human species. In prospective studies conducted to date, Africans infected with HIV-1 appear to develop clinical AIDS and other signs and symptoms of HIV disease as rapidly as individuals in the United States or Europe.[49,63] Furthermore, the degree of genomic variation seen in African isolates of HIV-1 was greater than that seen for viruses from Europe or the United States.

A virus that could be a progenitor of HIV-1 was isolated from a chimpanzee in central Africa.[64] This finding, combined with the knowledge that all HIV-1 viruses tested appear to be avirulent when inoculated into chimpanzees, is also compatible with a subhuman primate origin for HIV-1. Some African isolates of HIV-1 appear to be as close to the chimpanzee isolate as to other prototype strains of HIV-1.[65,66] These findings appear to have been confirmed by more detailed genetic analysis of a virus from a chimpanzee housed in the United States, although the exact history and pedigree of this animal is unclear.[67]

Distribution of HIV-1 Subtypes

HIV-1 virus isolates from North America and Europe showed distinct genetic variability compared with the variability in viruses from African patients.[53,68,69] This variability was more dramatic than the recognized genetic variability between viral isolates from a single geographic region (ie, interisolate variability).[70,71] In turn, this was also distinguishable from the genetic variation that was seen at the level of an individual patient (ie, intrapatient variability). At the level of the individual patient, a swarm or quasi-species of highly related but distinguishable viral variants has been demonstrated throughout the course of HIV infection.[72-74] The genetic variation of HIV is hierarchical as depicted in the simplified schematic of subtype variation, interpatient variation, and intrapatient variation (Figure 1).

Remarkably, all the HIV-1 isolated from the United States and Western Europe through 1994 have been of a single subtype, B. Most of the diverse subtypes of HIV-1 have been found in sub-Saharan Africa. Subtypes A, C, and D in particular have been found more frequently than other subtypes in Africa. A high rate of spread of HIV-1 for Africa appeared during the 1980s, at about the same time the epidemic spread in the United States and Europe. The movement of populations and extensive international travel makes the likelihood of mixing subtypes inevitable, and non-B subtypes have already been identified in the United States and Europe.

In Asia, the introduction and spread of HIV-1 appeared about a decade later than in the West (see Chapter 9 for details). In Thailand, HIV-1 subtype B was detected in IDUs during the mid-1980s. During the late 1980s, subtype E was first detected. By the early to mid-1990s, HIV-1 subtype E had spread very rapidly among heterosexuals in Thailand, with the highest rates in the northern regions of the country.[78] Although apparently present earlier in the region, HIV-1 subtype B never spread enough to cause a major heterosexual epidemic, as did HIV-1 subtype E.

A similar situation occurred in India with HIV-1 subtypes B and C. While subtype B appeared to be introduced earlier among IDUs, this subtype did not spread as rapidly among heterosexuals as did subtype C. Previously associated with the massive heterosexual epidemic in southeastern Africa, subtype C also caused a rapid heterosexual epidemic in western India, initially spreading from the Bombay region.[78,79]

The results in Africa and Asia suggest that HIV-1 subtypes A, C, D, and E are well adapted for heterosexual transmission, while subtype B is less efficiently transmitted by this route. When HIV-1 subtypes move very rapidly through a new population, as has happened in Asia for HIV-1 subtypes E and C, the viruses isolated show relatively less diversity.[78]

An even more distant subtype, designated HIV-O, has been detected in Cameroon.[80] The viruses isolated from this subtype are even less related to HIV-1 subtypes A through H than either of the other subtypes are related to each other, yet HIV-O is more related to HIV-1 than to HIV-2.[81] To emphasize this distance, HIV-1 subtypes A through H are designated the major group (M), and HIV-O is designated the outgroup (O) (see Figure 1).[82] Despite extensive serosurveys, the distribution of HIV-O appears to be quite restricted.[83] While HIV-1 subtypes A through H probably had a common human progenitor ancestor, HIV-O no doubt entered independently from a chimpanzee host.[c] HIV-2 almost certainly entered independently from monkey species native to West Africa.[45,84]

The movement and distribution of HIV-1 subtypes throughout the world is often perplexing, particularly when subtypes such as E to H appear to be isolated more frequently in such places as Asia, South America, or Eastern Europe than in Africa, where they presumably originated.[90,91] However, the viruses that have been isolated and characterized were acquired for analysis from convenience samples and therefore may suffer from extensive regional selection bias and inadvertent clustering. In the future, it will be important to develop more consistent surveillance methods and full-length sequence analysis to generate a true global map of HIV subtypes. Table 1 presents a summary of HLTVs and HIVs with regard to their natural hosts and basic characteristics.

Emergence of HIV-1 Disease Phenotypes

Our understanding of the epidemiology and biology of different HIV-1 subtypes is critical to future intervention efforts, and further studies are clearly needed.[92] Studies have demonstrated differences in the ability of non-B and B subtype viruses to infect Langerhans cells, a critical cell in heterosexual transmission of HIV. This suggests that the viral properties of

TABLE 1. Overview of HTLVs and HIVs

Virus	Host	Characteristics
HTLV (I and II)	Human	• Low replication rate & degree of genetic diversity • Rarely causes lethal disease
HIV-1 Subtype A-H	Human Chimpanzee	• High replication rate & degree of genetic diversity • Genetic diversity occurs within & between geographic regions, populations, individual patients, and viral subtypes • Subtype A associated with longer AIDS-free survival than other subtypes
HIV-2	Human	• Low replication rate & degree of genetic diversity • Lower transmission rate compared with HIV-1 • Lower viral load compared with HIV-1 • Longer AIDS-free survival compared with HIV-1 • May offer protection against HIV-1 infection • Highly related to SIV
HIV-1 Subtype O	Human Chimpanzee	• More closely related to HIV-1 than HIV-2 but very distinct from Subtypes A-H

non-B subtype viruses would facilitate heterosexual transmission and may have contributed to the dramatic epidemic spread in Asia and Africa.[93] A cross-sectional study of heterosexual couples in Thailand suggests a higher risk of heterosexual transmission of subtype E compared with subtype B.[94] Studies in many African countries have described multiple HIV-1 subtypes, but it is not known if subtypes enter populations at different time points, or if the distribution of subtypes reflects the dynamics of different subtype-specific transmission potentials. Recent studies in South Africa and the Gambia demonstrate the association of certain subtypes with different modes of HIV transmission: subtype B viruses are associated with homosexual transmission, while non-B subtypes are associated with heterosexual transmission.[95,96] Future detailed studies of prospectively followed cohorts will be necessary to determine differences in pathogenicity and transmissibility of different subtypes.[92]

Host selection of HIV-1 subtypes for efficiency of heterosexual transmission may partially explain the high rates of heterosexual transmission seen with subtypes C and E.[97] HIV-1 subtype B, the major subtype in the developed world, appears to have undergone counterselection to lose the phenotypic property of efficient heterosexual transmission. If efficient heterosexual transmission requires a particular genotype for vaginal infection, such sequences may have been partially lost by these HIV-1 B "strains" that have been repeatedly passaged by blood exposure or rectal intercourse. Many of the non-B subtypes, on the other hand, could theoretically maintain vaginal phenotypic properties through regular heterosexual transmission in Africa and Asia.[98]

Based on prospective studies of female sex workers in Dakar, Senegal, we have recently reported on disease progression in non-B subtype infections with known time of infection. In evaluating AIDS-free survival curves of women with incident subtype A, C, D, and G infections, we have shown distinct differences in AIDS-free survival.[99] The comparison of non-A subtypes with subtype A demonstrated a significantly longer AIDS-free survival for women infected with subtype A. Due to the small sample size per subtype, our estimate of AIDS incidence should be considered imprecise, and further study is clearly warranted. Cross-sectional studies indicate a significant proportion of AIDS cases with subtype A infection in West and East Africa (PJK, unpublished data,1998). Further study of HIV-1 subtype natural history and progression from different geographic regions is clearly needed to better evaluate the role of viral subtype differences and AIDS pathogenesis.

HIV-Related Retroviruses of Monkeys

Soon after the recognition of clinical AIDS in people, several clinical reports described outbreaks of severe infections, wasting disease, and death in several colonies of Asian macaques housed at primate centers in the United States.[100,101] Due to their similarity to the human syndrome, these diseases were designated simian AIDS or SAIDS. As in the case of human AIDS, many possible causes were considered.[d] Following the recognition that SAIDS appeared to be of infectious origin, cytomegalovirus of monkeys was also considered as a possible etiologic agent.

However, seroepidemiologic screening revealed that a proportion of the SAIDS monkeys had antibodies that cross-reacted with HIV,[105] while healthy monkeys had no such antibodies. Although the antibodies cross-reacted with core antigens of HIV-1, they showed only very weak cross-reactivity with the envelope antigens. Further characterization of the cultures revealed the presence of HIV-like particles and antigens detectable with antibodies from either SAIDS monkeys or people with AIDS. The sizes of the protein antigens detected by radioimmunoprecipitation were similar to those of HIV-1. When these antigens were tested with sera from people with AIDS or healthy carriers, virtually all sera had antibodies cross-reactive to core antigens. This primate virus was named STLV-III due to its relationship to HIV-1 (which was then called HTLV-III and/or LAV), and later simian immunodeficiency virus or SIV.[107]

The pathogenic effects of SIV appeared to be species-specific. Unlike captive rhesus monkeys, whose SIV infection was associated with SAIDS, African monkeys infected with SIV appeared to remain healthy. Similarly, captive African mangabey monkeys infected with SIV revealed no disease symptoms. At least half of the healthy wild-caught African green monkeys showed evidence of exposure to SIV on the basis of antibodies.[e] Although it was possible that SIV caused some type of disease that had not been recognized, it was clear that the disease did not resemble the lethal immunosuppressive syndrome found in Asian macaque monkeys.

The possibility that SIV might be a rare cause of disease in African monkeys in advanced age could not be ruled out. The high prevalence of infection in wild-caught monkeys supported the notion that these African species of primates had evolved to a more benign coexistence with the virus in which infection did not affect survival. This was clearly different from the case of SIV in Asian primates or HIV-1 in people. Because wild macaques do not appear to be infected with SIV, and because the virus is limited to a small set of African primates, it appears likely that the virus accidentally infected captive rhesus monkeys in recent times. It may seem surprising that a virus that had coexisted for such a long period of time in African monkey species was not more widely distributed in different species of Old World primates, such as baboons. However, new SIVs are still being described,[f] and it is also possible that species specificity may play a role in the level of host-virus adaptation and, therefore, levels of population infection.[110] Limited studies to detect active immune responses in African monkeys have been disappointing, though soluble SIV-inhibitory factors have been found.[118,119]

HIV-2

Because a relative of HIV-1—SIV—had been found in wild African monkeys and was only about 50% related to HIV-1 at the genomic level, it seemed logical that viruses more highly related to SIV might also be present in human populations. Serum samples from West African prostitutes were examined to determine if they had antibodies that were more highly cross-reactive with SIV than with HIV-1.[47] Through Western blot and radioimmunoprecipitation methods, it became clear that a significant proportion of Senegalese prostitutes had antibodies that were highly reactive with all the major antigens of SIV detected by this technique.[g] When the same SIV antigens were reacted with sera from HIV-1–infected individuals of either European or Central African origin with classic disease manifestations of AIDS, little or no reaction was seen with the envelope antigens.[h] The class of reactivity seen with serum samples from West African prostitutes was in fact virtually indistinguishable from that seen with serum samples from African monkeys or captive rhesus macaques.[84,111,120]

With evidence that a virus more closely related to SIV than to HIV-1 was present in Senegalese prostitutes, more extensive studies were undertaken to determine if the SIV-related virus was more widely distributed in Africa in general, particularly in West Africa. The screening of more than 2,000 high-risk individuals from Central Africa, including many individuals with AIDS and other STDs, revealed no evidence that HIV-2 was present in the same regions in which HIV-1 was so common.[121] However, pockets of infection with HIV-2 were detected in Mozambique and Angola, which, though distant from West Africa, are often on the same Portuguese trade routes as Guinea Bissau and Cape Verde, both West African countries with some of the highest rates of infection.[122] Even within Senegal, prevalence rates for HIV-2 are substantially higher in the southern region of Casamance, which borders Guinea Bissau, than in the northern region.[123]

The transmission of HIV-2 appears to be significantly slower than that of HIV-1 by heterosexual sex.[105,124] Similarly, rates of perinatal transmission of HIV-2 appear to be low to negligible compared with HIV-1.[125-127,128]

While end stage HIV-2 disease appears to be similar to HIV-1–induced AIDS, the rate of disease progression is much slower than that of HIV-1.[62,129]

Although several cross-sectional studies of HIV-2 infection were conducted in the late 1980s, they were intrinsically limited in their ability to describe the natural history of HIV-2 infection, which required prospective studies.[130] Studies concerning the natural history of chronic infections such as HIV are difficult to achieve, particularly with minimal loss to follow-up; not surprisingly, such studies have been rare in developing countries, where viruses such as HIV-2 can be studied.

Our prospective studies conducted in a registered female sex worker cohort in Dakar, Senegal, have provided the unique opportunity of measuring the infection and progression rates of both HIV-1 and HIV-2 infections.[131-133] Kaplan-Meier analysis comparing HIV-2 (n=50) and HIV-1 (n=81) seroincident women were significantly different, with HIV-2 infected women demonstrating a slower progression to AIDS (Wilcoxon-Gehan test; P=.006). HIV-1 infected women with known time of infection had a 5-year AIDS-free survival of 66.9%, whereas in HIV-2 infected women, the 5-year AIDS-free survival was 94.7% (Figure 2). These differences in survival probabilities between HIV-2 and HIV-1 were also seen for CD4+ lymphocyte counts below 400 cells/mm^3 and below 200 cells/mm^3 as outcomes.[132,133]

In our prospective study of HIV-2 infected individuals, we also identified individuals who fit a definition of long-term nonprogression and can determine a rate of this phenotype in the study population. The Kaplan-Meier analysis of HIV-2 incident infected individuals indicate that 85% (95% CI = 50%-96%) remain AIDS-free after 8 years of HIV-2 infection. Using a definition of long-term nonprogression of >8 years infection in the absence of AIDS or related symptoms and stable CD4+ lymphocytes > 500 cells/mm^3, we found 39 of 41 (95%) of our women would be classified as long-term nonprogressors. This dramatic difference in pathogenicity provides a unique opportunity to identify viral and host immune mechanisms involved in a closely related and relevant virus system that is predicted to have a significantly slower course of progression.

Differences in Viral Load

Plasma viremia has become the standard surrogate marker of HIV progression.[134] Studies of long-term nonprogressors compared with rapid progressors during the early phases of their infection have consistently demonstrated lower plasma viral RNA and proviral burdens in the nonprogressors.[135-137] Nonprogressors have demonstrated lower seeding of virus in lymphoreticular tissues as well.[138] A quantitative assay has also demonstrated utility in SIV, where plasma viremia at 6 weeks post infection was predictive of disease outcome.[139]

We determined plasma viral load in individuals from the cohort of registered commercial sex workers in Dakar, Senegal.[i,50] HIV-2 viral RNA was detectable in 56% of all samples tested; the median load was 141 copies/ml. Levels of viral RNA in the plasma were inversely related to CD4+ cell counts. In a comparison of HIV-2 and HIV-1 viral loads, we found that the median viral load was 30 times lower in the HIV-2 infected women (P<.001, Wilcoxon rank-sum), irrespective of the length of time infected. This suggests plasma viremia is linked to the differences in the pathogenicity of the two viruses.[j]

The observations that HIV-2 infected carriers have lower loads of virus and slower rates of sexual transmission are compatible with observations that HIV-2 subtypes appear to evolve and deviate less rapidly than do HIV-1 subtypes.[51,52,145] This does not appear to be due to any reduction in the error rate of the HIV-2 reverse transcriptase.[146] However, the slower rates of HIV-2 replication and spread also help explain why the HIV-2 epidemic is largely restricted to West Africa. Furthermore, even within West Africa, some HIV-2 subtypes are essentially indistinguishable from the SIVs that occur naturally in monkey species living in the same area.[147,148]

The lower rates of replication for HIV-2 may also help explain why this virus appears less virulent than HIV-1 within individual hosts. Case reports and cross-sectional studies clearly reveal that some HIV-2 infected people develop clinical AIDS.[149,150] However, disease rates for HIV-2 are much lower than expected, based on HIV-1 associated disease with proportional prevalence rates.[151] One possible explanation for this dichotomy might have been that HIV-2 had entered the human population more recently than HIV-1. This was largely dismissed when it was recognized that HIV-2 rates had stabilized in West Africa. In some regions of West Africa it seems clear that HIV-2 had stabilized before HIV-1 had moved in.[152] In addition, West African sera stored from earlier time periods revealed that HIV-1 had been present in the region for an extended period.[153]

Demonstrated differences in the infectivity and disease potential of

HIV-2 compared with HIV-1 support the notion that HIV-2 might behave as an attenuated virus vaccine upon interaction with the more virulent HIV-1 infection. Studies from the Dakar, Senegal, cohort have shown that HIV-2 positive women were at lower risk of HIV-1 infection than were HIV negative women. The original report of 70% protection was based on 9 years of observation.[154] A recent update based on 11 years of observation indicates that HIV-2 protection ranges from 64% to74%, depending on the method of analysis.[155] Further studies of viral interaction are critical to confirming and defining the protective mechanism involved. In vitro studies of HIV-2 and HIV-1 suggest that viral determinants may be responsible for the inhibition of HIV-1.[156]

AIDS Denial

The recognition that AIDS is caused by HIV-1 was not easy for some to accept. A small group of scientists have persisted in denial of the overwhelming evidence for causation. Additionally, various conspiracy theories have emerged suggesting that HIV-1 was deliberately created by germ warfare scientists. While such proclamations seem silly or irrational to informed medical scientists, they interfere with constructive attempts to educate appropriate population groups.

One reason why some have been reluctant to accept that AIDS is an infectious disease caused by HIV-1 is the very prolonged induction period combined with a very high mortality rate. Most infectious diseases occur after a short induction period. Even for the small number of infectious diseases with a very long induction period caused by viruses, such as tropical spastic paraparesis, adult T cell leukemia, or shingles, only a small fraction of infected people experience that clinical outcome. The definition of AIDS as an amalgamation of clinical outcomes ranging from tuberculosis to chronic diarrhea to cancer (eg, lymphoma and Kaposi's sarcoma) also may cause confusion for those trying to accept HIV-1 as the single etiologic cause. This only becomes logical when it is recognized that AIDS disease is fundamentally an irreversible destruction of the immune system. All other outcomes are secondary to the immune destruction.

Another problem in understanding AIDS etiology may be a lack of appreciation of the discipline of epidemiology and dissension about the proper definition of cause. For epidemiologists, a very high-risk association, such as for tobacco and lung cancer, is sufficient to ascribe cause.

Using analogous logic, the causal association between HIV-1 infection and subsequent destruction of the immune system is overwhelming. In prospective cohort studies, almost all HIV-1 infected people eventually develop immune depletion. This association is much higher than for such viral infections as polio or flu. Concerning time and spatial geographic associations, clinical AIDS rates have exactly paralleled HIV infection rates, whether in Bombay, San Francisco, or Nairobi, allowing for the 5- to 15-year induction period.

Until recently, a lack of understanding about how HIV-1 caused immune depletion helped those who reject epidemiology to deny causation. This situation has changed dramatically, however, with the recognition that HIV-1 subtypes can be highly lytic for T4 lymphocytes,[157] and that very large numbers of T4 cells are killed by the virus in vivo.[158,159] Further, while the very low rate of infected circulating lymphocytes was interpreted by some as incompatible with the destruction of large numbers of cells, recent studies reveal that most HIV-1 is in lymph nodes rather than blood, and up to 25% to 50% of lymph node T cells may be infected.[160] HIV-1 is also highly unusual as a virus that targets T4 lymphocytes and macrophages, both essential components of the immune system (Chapter 2 provides an excellent overview of the virus' effect on the immune system). Finally, HIV-1 is transmitted in exactly the same way as clinical AIDS: by blood, by sex, and from mother to infant. When taken together, these various correlations provide inescapable evidence that HIV-1 must be the cause of AIDS.

Conclusions

Over the past two decades, we have learned a great deal about the virology of HIV and its close relatives. A large family of HIV-related retroviruses is present in humans and monkeys in sub-Saharan Africa. All members of this family have the same complex genomic structure, share at least 40% to 50% homology, and share cellular receptors. Although both HIV-1 and HIV-2 appear to have entered the human population several decades ago, HIV-1 is more virulent than HIV-2. The recognition of the different HIV-1 subtypes has led many to question whether properties of HIV-1 infection and its consequences as a whole can be generalized among different subtypes. The evolution of HIV-1 subtypes in human populations may have favored or even selected for diverse biological properties. Such diversity could potentially impact the overall efficacy of HIV therapy or intervention strategies. Thus, the study of the natural biological variation of the virus itself may provide important insights into the rational design of interventions to alter or interrupt disease progression.

At the same time, numerous SIV-type viruses are present at high rates in African monkeys, in which they appear to cause little or no disease. Although SIV in African monkeys is more closely related to HIV-2 than to HIV-1, the viruses in mangabeys and macaques are essentially the same virus as HIV-2. The macaque virus also appears to have originated from either a human or an African monkey source, as Asian primates show no evidence of natural infection. A chimpanzee virus, which is a logical progenitor of HIV-1, was also identified in Africa. It seems likely that additional HIV progenitor viruses will be identified in African primates. Understanding how subhuman primates naturally resist disease from HIV-related viruses should facilitate the development of new ways to treat and prevent HIV disease in people.

As research results have accumulated, we have grown to appreciate the tremendous biological diversity the HIV viruses possess at the level of genetic variability, epidemiologic patterns, and host pathogenesis. To better understand the virologic properties of these viruses, we must now attempt to link our observations from in vitro and genetic analysis studies to studies in infected populations. New and innovative technologies will be required to more readily diagnose subtypes and recombinants and to quantify the viral burden. Our understanding of HIV-1 subtype epidemiology is evolving, and future studies are likely to provide better data on the subtype distribution and their epidemiology. These studies will be critical to future predictions of the epidemic, and they may also indicate differences in transmission and disease potential that will affect the design of future global HIV interventions.

Summary Points

• The unique epidemiology of a new disease (AIDS) and the realization that the etiologic agent infected T lymphocytes guided efforts to identify and isolate the causative virus (HIV).

• Although human and simian T cell leukemia viruses rarely cause lethal disease, the HIV-1 causes AIDS, while the pathogenicity of SIVs appears to depend more heavily on the host species (ie, nonvirulent in natural hosts but induce a fatal immunosuppression in abnormal monkey hosts); the lower replication rate and degree of genetic variability of HIV-2 compared with HIV-1 may explain its reduced pathogenicity.

• A virus that could be a progenitor of HIV-1 was isolated from a chimpanzee in central Africa, and all HIV-1 viruses tested appear to be avirulent when inoculated into chimpanzees, strongly suggesting a subhuman primate origin for HIV-1.

• While HIV-1 subtypes A through H probably had a common human progenitor ancestor, HIV subtype O (restricted to Cameroon) no doubt entered independently from a chimpanzee host, and HIVs-2 almost certainly entered independently from monkey species native to West Africa.

• Viral subtypes have unique phenotypes and distribution: Subtype B appears to be transmitted primarily through nonheterosexual intercourse, subtype A is associated with longer AIDS-free survival than other subtypes, and subtype C is responsible for the newest and most frightening epidemics worldwide (especially South Africa, India, and China).

• HIV-2, which is more closely related to certain SIVs than to HIV-1, has low rates of heterosexual and perinatal transmission compared with HIV-1 and is also associated with a much slower rate of disease progression. In addition, HIV-2 may offer protection against infection with HIV-1.

Figure 1. Schematic representation of the phylogenetic relationship of SIV/HIVs and their genetic variability

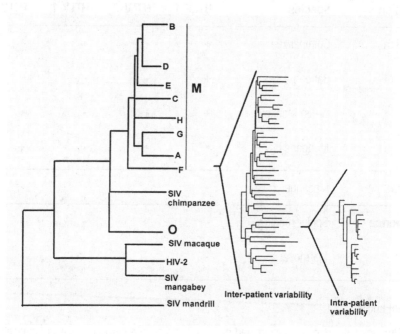

Figure 2. Kaplan-Meier AIDS-free survival probability comparing incident HIV-1 and HIV-2 infected individuals. Wilcoxon-Gehan, p value <0.01.

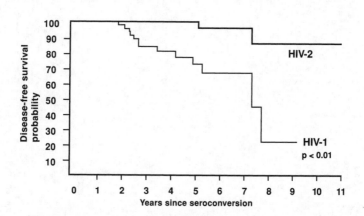

TABLE 2. Retroviruses Related to HTLV and HIV in Subhuman Primates

Region	Species	HTLV-1	HTLV-2	HTLV-1	HTLV-2
Africa	Chimpanzee	+	-	+	-
	Baboon	+	-	-	-
	Green Monkey	+	-	-	+
	Mangabey	●*	●*	-	+
Asia	Macaque	+	-	-	-‡
America	Spider monkey	-	+	-	-
	Marmoset	-	-	-	-

* Not known

‡ Although wild macaques examined have all been seronegative, monkeys in captivity have been infected with the virus that is essentially the same as the mangabey SIV and HIV-2.

CHAPTER 2

The Virus Versus the Immune System

Jeffrey Laurence

I n 1981, when AIDS was first recognized, the average person with active disease lived just over 6 months. Thirteen years later, survival reached a mean of 4 to 5 years, primarily due to better diagnosis and treatment of the opportunistic infections that characterize this syndrome. By the end of 1995, however, with the introduction of a new class of anti-HIV medications—protease inhibitors—the picture began to change dramatically. Protease inhibitors were combined with older and, by themselves, much less potent medications, the HIV reverse transcriptase inhibitors AZT, d4T, and 3TC. This combination therapy significantly reduced the amount of HIV in the blood, raised measures of immune function (ie, CD4+ T cell count), and lengthened the survival of many who otherwise would have died.

This shift, a Lazarus syndrome for some and a source of hope to many, led to the erroneous assumption that HIV may have been eradicated in some patients or at least blocked from doing any further harm. Until recently, this seemed a plausible outcome. Headlines in the popular press and in scientific journals heralded annual declines in AIDS deaths of 40% to 70% between 1996 and early 1998. However, viral factors, immune system damage, viral drug resistance, and social factors ensured that these salutary changes were not to last for long.

Data for 1998 indicate that the rate of decline in AIDS-related deaths has reached a plateau.[1] In New York City, this was true for all demographic groups except Hispanic males and those between 35 and 44 years of age. The number of people living with AIDS grew 22% during the observation period of 1995 to 1998.[1] Clearly not all HIV-infected individuals are receiving adequate treatment, or many are not benefitting from it.

Also disquieting and of relevance to a discussion of how HIV disrupts immune function is the change in diagnostic patterns. AIDS diagnoses are being made at higher CD4+ T cell counts since introduction of the new combination anti-HIV regimens, such as Highly Active Antiretroviral

Therapy or HAART. For example, in Australia in 1992, the median CD4 count at AIDS diagnosis was 50/mm^3 (normal values range from 500-1200/mm^3), but this measure doubled to 100/mm^3 in 1996 and almost trebled to 130/mm^3 by 1997.[2] The reasons for this are unclear.

Some of these earlier AIDS diagnoses may, paradoxically, reflect a good thing. New anti-HIV drugs suppressing HIV should improve at least some immune functions, perhaps stimulating immune cells to proliferate and concomitantly reactivating chronic bacterial and other viral infections. This is known as an HIV reactivation syndrome. However, other AIDS diagnoses may reflect a disconnect between HAART-induced increases in T cell numbers and how well, or how poorly, those T cells function.

The overall strategies by which HIV has been able to evade our immune defenses are shared by many microbial pathogens. The generation time of HIV—it can produce new daughter progeny within 12 hours of entering a permissive cell—is far shorter than that of its host cells. An entire pathogen population can thus respond quickly to selective pressures mounted by a single individual, be they through anti-HIV antibodies, natural killer cells, CD8+ T cells, or drugs.[3,4] The host can only hope to survive by having multiple means with which to defend itself.

The ability of viral and bacterial pathogens to interfere with both acute immune response and immunologic memory in chronic infection has been recognized for more than a century. For example, 19th century medical texts reported that measles predisposes to flare-ups of tuberculosis. Indeed, an ordinary measles virus infection temporarily weakens host immunity, an effect noted in 1908 by Clemens von Pirquet.[3] In people who have been exposed to tuberculosis and have acquired resistance to the disease, the injection of a small amount of tuberculin under the skin produces an observable immune reaction known as delayed type hypersensitivity. Von Pirquet observed that such sensitive individuals frequently lost their skin test reactivity during a bout of measles, although the reactivity returned later. A similar loss of delayed type hypersensitivity to tuberculin antigens and to proteins from other opportunistic infections common in AIDS occurs in people with HIV infection. But these losses, absent effective anti-HIV therapy, are permanent.

Similarly, chronic infections of a normal host by herpes viruses such as Epstein-Barr virus or cytomegalovirus remain for the most part subclinical and undetected. They create a problem only in the immune suppressed, whether due to a genetic disorder, cancer, cancer therapy, or a concomitant infection such as AIDS. Other chronic infections may lead to serious tissue injury and malignancy or death, even in normal hosts. This is exemplified by *Mycobacterium tuberculosis*; hepatitis B and C viruses; certain sexually transmitted diseases (STDs), such as chlamydia, papillomavirus, and herpes simplex; and, of course, HIV.

Dr. Frances Brodsky recently provided an excellent summary of the way pathogens in general subvert the immune system (condensed in Table 1).[4] HIV is a particularly formidable pathogen, as it utilizes virtually every one of these methods to survive. This is unusual, since viruses with genomes as small as that of HIV typically ensure their survival by exploiting gaps in their host's immune repertoire and replicating very rapidly. Much larger viruses produce a range of viral proteins aimed at disabling the host's immune response. HIV does both. Given these strategies and the formidable challenges they invoke to development of a completely effective anti-HIV vaccine, the world will likely confront HIV for many lifetimes.

At the beginning of an HIV infection, little sequence variation occurs in the viral swarms or "quasispecies" present in infected individuals. These viruses tend to use the cell membrane receptor CCR5, one of a family of signaling molecules that enable HIV to readily infect two key cells of the immune system (ie, the CD4+ T cell and the cell-eating, antigen-presenting macrophage). These "R5" viruses tend to replicate relatively slowly, with a low degree of damage to host cells. But with time, HIV evolves to show a much stronger attraction for T cells. Growth rates of these later viral swarms increase, they become more pathogenic, and they expand or switch their coreceptor usage to both CCR5 and CXCR4, or even CXCR4 alone. CXCR4 use limits HIV infections predominantly to the T cell.

T cells and macrophages infected with HIV lose a critical immune recognition molecule, MHC-I, which renders them invisible to anti-HIV killer T cells. The anti-HIV T cells must recognize viral proteins in the context of MHC-I molecules to ensure effective target killing. A similar effect renders many CD4+ T helper cell responses effete, as two "minor" HIV genes (These are the *nef* and *upu* genes, along with the HIV envelope gene *env*.)—not required for HIV growth, but very helpful to its immune suppressive capacity—decrease expression of the CD4 molecule itself. Helper CD4+ T cells, through secretion of immune hormones such as interleukin-2, recruit and multiply anti-HIV CD8+ killer T cells. As the loss of these helper cells accelerates with advancing HIV disease, so does the loss of the immune system's ability to defend itself via CD8+ killer cells.

**TABLE 1. Strategies Used by Microbial Pathogens to Avoid
         Immune System Recognition**

Evasive Strategy	Application in HIV Infection
Stealth	• Latency, characterized by infection in the absence of viral protein production, removing the antigenic signals to which immune receptors could respond.[5,6]
	• Epitope mutation, or changing key viral structures, via random mutations, to which the immune system's antibodies and killer T cells have been programmed to respond.[7]
	• Infection of privileged sites, including the brain, eye, and testicles, which normally exclude immune reactive cells.
	• Infection via immune receptors, so that the very molecules that identify an immune cell and are critical to its ability to recognize and respond to an invader serve as the door through which the invader enters.
Sabotage	• Inhibition of apoptosis or cell death (which would otherwise destroy the invading pathogen along with the host cell).
	• Inhibition of macrophage activation, so that the virus cannot be readily phagocytosed (ie, scavenged or consumed).
	• Down-modulation of immune receptors, interfering with the immune system's recognition of infected cells.[8,9,10]
	• Production of virus-encoded proteins that mimic host receptors and block extracellular immune signals (not used by HIV itself but employed by common viral opportunistic infections).[11]
Exploitation	• Lymphocyte activation, by which stimulation of a T cell or macrophage in the course of an immune response simultaneously activates growth of latent virus within those cells.[12]
	• Induction of immune cell attack on T cells by which CD4+ T cells are not destroyed by the virus itself but rather by the "good intentions" of killer CD8+ T cells.[11]
	• Adherence of HIV to lymph node cells, infecting lymphocytes passing through lymphoid tissue.[3]

An understanding of the changes in immune function seen after initiation of HAART is best approached by exploring how HIV kills T cells and suppresses their growth. Only a few years ago, we had the virus-immune cell dynamics all wrong.

First proposed in 1995, the "tap and drain" model of T cell loss hypothesized that great numbers of CD4+ T cells are infected with HIV and rapidly destroyed each day. An equal number of these T cells must then be produced to compensate for this loss, eventually "exhausting" the immune system. HAART, by suppressing HIV-mediated T cell killing, and prolonging the half-life of circulating T cells, should lead to a rapid and sustained increase in T cell count. The latter was, indeed, seen.

However, this conceptually pleasing scenario of viral invaders and valiant immune system defenders, fighting to the point of exhaustion, only to be rescued by an armamentarium of new drugs is incorrect.

First, the rapid movement or redistribution of T cells from lymphoid tissues such as the lymph nodes and spleen to the peripheral blood accounts for the dramatic rise in T cells characteristic of initial HAART treatment.[13] Although the mechanism for this abrupt change remains unknown, the shift can occur in HIV-negative as well as HIV-positive individuals. For example, health care workers accidentally stuck with a needle contaminated with HIV-infected fluids are typically given AZT or HAART as a preventive measure. This postexposure prophylaxis itself leads to dramatic rises in T cells, as the drugs redistribute lymphocytes among body compartments.

In the HIV-positive patient, this initial rise in T cells correlates with reduced production of immune system hormones, specifically proinflammatory cytokines. (The affected proinflammatory cytokines include interferon-γ, interleukin-1, and interleukin-6.) The early rise in T cells is also accompanied by decreased expression of proteins on the cell surface known as homing receptors (VCAM-1 and ICAM-1 are two prominent ones), which normally permit cells to locate and attach to appropriate tissues.

Second, T cell production does not increase in HIV infection, certainly not to the point of exhausting anything.[14] In fact, daily production of both CD4+ and CD8+ T cells is little altered until late stage disease, despite the fact that the half-life of T cells is decreased by at last two thirds in the setting of HIV.

Third, no correlation exists between levels of HIV in the blood (the plasma viral load or vRNA, typically counted as numbers of viral genome equivalents per milliliter of plasma and ranging from undetectable to several million) and T cell half-life or absolute rate of T cell production rate.[14,15] Why this is true remains unclear. It suggests that CD4+ T cell loss cannot be a consequence solely of direct virus-mediated cell killing. Other probable factors include:

- immune-mediated damage, by which killer T cells primed to destroy HIV also destroy healthy cells;

- bystander effects related to shed HIV envelope proteins; and

- blocks in T cell renewal in bone marrow and the thymus gland.[16]

An apparent paradox also exists. After HAART, the half-life of circulating T cells decreases more than in an untreated HIV-infected patient, even though the production rate of new T cells may double with drug use.[14] The increase in T cell production could reflect suppression of HIV growth, removal of blocks to such growth at the stem cell level, and renewed activation of mature memory T cells. These changes provide excellent motivation for using HAART. But what about the depressed T cell survival times?

T cells may be subdivided according to their function. CD4 (helper) and CD8 (killer and suppressor) T cells represent one such division based on function. HIV, of course, does a superb job in distinguishing between these two classes, as one of its receptors is the CD4 molecule. Another T cell subset subdivision contrasts naïve versus memory cells. Naïve T cells, commonly if incompletely defined by an antibody marker known as CD45RA, are produced by the thymus gland. They have the capacity to be educated: ie, to learn about new invaders and to distinguish its own body's cells from foreign material. These cells can mature into CD45RO memory cells, but the latter cannot functionally go backwards.

Naïve T cells are suppressed in favor of memory cells in HIV disease and are the last to return with HAART.[16] Indeed, virtually all of the new CD4+ and CD8+ T cells appearing in the blood after HAART are proliferating memory cells. Such cells, when activated, are programmed to die rapidly by a process of programmed cell death known as apoptosis.

Turning for a moment from T cell to virus, what is happening to HIV in the face of prolonged HAART? Virus production is suppressed but not eliminated. HIV transcription persists in peripheral blood cells, even in patients who have maintained undetectable levels of plasma viral RNA for three or more years. This suggests that HIV infection cannot be eradicated with current drugs.

Viral latency is another confounding issue. The reservoir of T cells harboring dormant, nonreplicating HIV capable of being activated to infect virgin T cells is minute. In a body with more than 100 billion T cells, fewer than one million are likely to contain dormant HIV. However, the mean half-life of these latently infected cells, 44 months, is identical in untreated patients. With prolonged use of effective HAART, estimates suggest that a century or more will be needed to eradicate even such an insignificant population of dormant virus from a given individual.

Strategies for augmenting immune function, particularly HIV-specific CD4+ T cells and the cytolytic killer T cells they help support, may be critical to making headway.[17] For example, significant frequencies of T helper memory cells capable of recognizing internal (*gag* or viral core) HIV proteins are detectable in most people with active HIV (see Table 2). The median frequency of these cells is more than three-fold higher in so-called HIV-positive nonprogressors, those people who may live for one to two decades or more taking no anti-HIV medications with little evidence of immune damage. HAART, in depleting circulating and tissue viral antigen, leads to a progressive decrease in *gag*-specific T cells after two years or more of continuous anti-retroviral treatment. Attempts to reverse this trend include early and repeated vaccination with HIV recombinant proteins and interleukin-2 treatment. It is hoped that one highly speculative strategy of "drug holidays" or "strategic treatment interruptions," which involve stopping anti-HIV medications for a few weeks every few months, will promote a transient return of HIV replication and perhaps a boost to the HIV immune repertoire.

TABLE 2. T Helper Memory Cell Frequency in Infected, Nonprogressing, and HAART-Treated Patients with HIV

Status	Median Frequency in Entire CD4 + T Cell Population
Active HIV Infection	0.12%
Nonprogressing HIV Infection	0.40%
HAART-Treated HIV Infection	0.03%

In closing, our view of viruses such as HIV solely as plague-carriers has shifted to recognize them as tools for investigating normal immune function and for enabling protection of those functions. Viruses that have coevolved with both bacteria and animal hosts for hundreds of millions of years have much to teach us. They also have great potential in immune therapeutics. One approach could be to leave the protein coat of HIV intact, allowing it to attack infected or infectable CD4+ T cells, but to remove its destructive genes. "Anti-sense" genetic material could be inserted into its genome, causing it to act as a Trojan horse, immunizing individual cells against intact HIV infection.[18] This method, now being tested clinically, represents the future of gene therapy for HIV and one means by which HIV, by virtue of its capacity to infect nondividing cells, may be exploited to carry useful genes into cells, in an attempt to cure disease rather than cause it.

Summary Points

• HIV replicates very rapidly (new daughter progeny within 12 hours) and uses stealth, sabotage, and exploitation to evade the host immune repertoire. While HAART has led to dramatic improvements in survival, the evasive strategies used by HIV prevent existing therapies from producing true cures.

• T cell production does not increase in HIV infection, and no correlation exists between levels of HIV in the blood and T cell half-life or absolute rate of T cell production rate. After HAART, the half-life of circulating T cells decreases, although the production rate of new T cells can double with drug use.

• Naïve T cells (capable of learning about new invaders) are suppressed in favor of memory cells in HIV disease and are the last to return with HAART.

• Virus production is suppressed but not eliminated during HAART; with viral latency, a century or more of HAART would be needed to eradicate dormant virus from a given individual. One highly speculative strategy of "drug holidays," which involve stopping anti-HIV medications for a few weeks, are hoped to promote a transient return of HIV replication and perhaps a boost to the HIV immune repertoire.

• One novel approach being tested involves leaving the protein coat of HIV intact and allowing it to attack infected or infectable CD4+ T cells, but replacing its destructive genes with "anti-sense" genetic material or even useful genes, causing it to act as a Trojan horse, immunizing individual cells against intact HIV infection.

CHAPTER 3

How Infectious Is Infectious?

Kenneth H. Mayer

n the mid-1970s, research in virology and immunology accelerated rapidly, yet many lines of investigation did not seem to be immediately relevant for patient care. Some well-characterized infections, such as influenza, measles, mumps, and rubella, could be prevented by effective vaccines, while the pathogenesis and control of other increasingly common viral infections, such as hepatitis A and B,[1,2] and *Herpes simplex*[3,4,] remained elusive. At that time, investigations had begun into the relationship between viral infections and the development of tumors.[5,6] Although many researchers throughout the 20th century examined the relationship of chronic viral infections, cancer, and immunosuppression, a great gulf existed between the lab and clinical practice prior to the advent of the AIDS epidemic.[7]

Researchers tended to approach the problem with perspectives limited by their specialties, which seemed to be a classic case of the blind men interpreting parts of an elephant in different ways. Based on the patterns of transmission that were initially described and the failure to find a readily culturable new pathogen, virologists believed the AIDS epidemic was most likely due to a virus, and they focused on trying to characterize the infectious particle. Epidemiologists tried to refine understanding of the specific behaviors associated with acquiring the syndrome, targeting each new population affected. Immunologists characterized the changes in the immune system that occurred in symptomatic and at-risk individuals as the syndrome unfolded. In the early AIDS era, researchers who collaborated with multidisciplinary teams were the exception rather than rule.[8]

However, due to the unique unfolding of the AIDS epidemic, major strides have been made in understanding viral-mediated immunopathogenesis, virulence, and patterns of disease dissemination. Moreover, the techniques needed to quantify HIV replication and how it affects the immune system have led to a radical transformation in the entire field of infectious disease. Changes have benefited how chronic viral infections are measured, how the risks of specific exposures to infectious disease are interpreted, and how hospital and health care workers avoid contact with infectious materials. In addition, infectious disease has developed into a clinical specialty that provides primary care for people living with HIV and AIDS.

How Viral Infections Are Measured

By the time the initial cases of AIDS were being identified, virology had made several major advances.[9] Researchers had observed that viruses are obligate intracellular parasites consisting of either RNA or DNA and that different viral strains could be isolated and grown in cell culture. The development of these very important techniques allowed for better characterization of specific viral strains and enabled researchers to better understand how to intervene against viruses.

The science of immunology developed in parallel, with the realization that many infections could be controlled naturally or through immunization by the development of antibodies that could neutralize viral infections.[10] Cell-associated immune responses also played a role in controlling infections by generating cytotoxic T lymphocytes, natural killer cells, and antibody-dependent cellular cytotoxicity. When the AIDS epidemic first appeared, we understood how the immune system controlled some viral infections, and some very successful vaccines had been developed (eg, polio, measles, mumps, rubella, influenza).[11] However, understanding of the immunology and the control of many other common viral diseases (eg, herpes simplex, Epstein-Barr virus) remained elusive.[12]

Prior research demonstrated that some viral infections could be chronic and latent, particularly those of the herpesvirus family.[12] These viruses had a propensity to enter cells, integrate into the host genome, and remain quiescent for many years postinfection. *Herpes zoster* infection commonly reactivated as shingles in the sixth, seventh, or eighth decade of life.[13] However, the same infection reactivating in persons in their 20s raised suspicions about an occult immunological problem. Thus, the concept of a chronic latent virus that could reactivate after patients became immunocompromised was accepted, but the linkage between a senescent immune system and a young person with leukemia, for example, was not manifestly clear in the early 1980s.

Another initially controversial concept was the fact that in some species, chronic viral infections were associated with the development of cancer.[14] Just prior to the discovery of AIDS, retroviruses were shown to cause feline leukemia and other nonhuman lymphoid tissue malignancies.[15,16] Human T cell lymphotropic virus (HTLV) was found to exist in at least two forms, causing hematologic malignancy in a minority of the people.[17] This virus could be present in infected hosts for many decades and not cause disease but still be transmissible to others. At the start of the AIDS epidemic, the epidemiology and immunopathogenesis of HTLV-1 and its minor variant HTLV-2 were just being described and greatly assisted researchers searching for the etiologic agent of AIDS. (Chapter 1 reviews in depth this search for the cause of AIDS.)

When AIDS was recognized as a distinct syndrome, infectious disease specialists, epidemiologists, public health researchers, and lab scientists had little information available with which to identify the likely cause of new outbreaks of immunosuppression in gay and bisexual men and in IDUs and their sexual partners. Some researchers postulated an immuno- logical "burn-out" hypothesis (ie, their immune systems were sorely taxed because of recurrent drug and sexual exposure that required them to respond to many different antigens). However, the discovery of disease in lower risk sexual partners with all the typical manifestations laid this theory to rest. Similarly, people with no risk factors who received blood transfusions were also reported to develop classic features of the syndrome. One of the early questions was whether an existing infectious agent (eg, cytomegalovirus) might have developed a virulent strain and be responsible for the transmissible immunosuppression. However, not all patients with manifestations of AIDS had evidence of prior cytomegalovirus infection, so researchers began to focus on the fact that this might be a novel agent.

In this early phase, many researchers used the hepatitis B model[18] and thought several outcomes could occur after becoming infected with the agent that caused AIDS. Some individuals, particularly those with low-grade fevers and chronic lymphadenopathy, were postulated to have mild disease, and researchers hoped they might be able to clear their infection and subsequently develop protective immunity. Investigators likewise thought another subset of individuals might be carriers of infection but remain asymptomatic indefinitely. AIDS researchers believed that a comparably effective vaccine could be developed based on the genera- tion of neutralizing antibodies. Subsequent studies showed that AIDS was caused by an agent that would be more difficult to neutralize since it was able to maintain latency in host cells that were intimately involved with the overall regulation of most human immune responses. New knowledge was clearly needed to determine how to understand and confront this unique human infection.

The recognition of a human retrovirus, HIV, as the etiological agent of AIDS[19] led to many subsequent advances in the field of infectious diseases. Although Pasteur, Metchnikoff, and other classical microbiologists appreciated the importance of leukocytes in controlling infections,[20] HTLV and HIV presented researchers with the first known human pathogens that selectively targeted the host immune system. (See Chapter 2 for an excellent discussion of the strategies used by HIV to attack the human immune system.) The systematic loss of specific immune functions due to progressive HIV infection allowed researchers to track the relationship of specific immune cells with the control of endogenous and exogenous microbial challenges.[21]

The development of immunologically specific histochemical staining techniques in the 1970s and early 1980s enabled researchers to characterize lymphocyte subpopulations by staining for different cell surface markers.[22] Specific groups of lymphocytes with different immunological functions could thus be classified. Some lymphocyte subpopulations were associated with priming host responses to produce antibodies and were known as B lymphocytes (because their site of origin in a chicken was the Bursa of Fabricus). Antibodies are proteins that specifically recognize markers (antigens) that the body perceives as foreign (nonself) and can coat these antigens to neutralize them or otherwise facilitate their removal. Another group of lymphocytes, the T cells, are derived from thymic tissue and are more frequently associated with producing the hormones (cytokines) responsible for cell-cell interactions and direct cell-mediated interactions with foreign antigens.[23]

Further elucidation of T lymphocyte subpopulations led to the characterization of helper/inducer lymphocytes, which are known as CD4 (or T4) lymphocytes, based on a classification system that was developed just before the emergence of the AIDS epidemic.[21] Another important T lymphocyte subpopulation is the cytotoxic/suppressor T cell group, known as CD8 or T8. The more closely immunologists looked, the more refined the subset divisions became, so that both the CD4 and CD8 subsets actually represent a heterogeneous array of cells primed for specific immunological functions. The different markers found on the surfaces of each group of lymphocytes were associated with the ability to either recognize different antigenic signals or perform different immuno-logical functions. Prior to the AIDS epidemic, we did not appreciate the importance of the cell surface markers in orchestrating the appropriate functioning of the immune system.

The finding of depressed CD4 counts (and frequently increased CD8 counts and inverted CD4/CD8 ratios) among a wide range of affected subpopulations (eg, gay men in California, IDUs in New York, monoga-mous women in Africa) helped epidemiologists postulate that the illness was possibly triggered by the same immunosuppressive agent. Prior to the identification of HIV as the cause of AIDS, the use of CD4/CD8 ratios and absolute and relative CD4 counts allowed investigators to track the spread of the virus into new communities and understand better the natural history of what is now known as HIV disease.

Immunologists have used an increasingly sophisticated system of immune cell profiling based on cell surface markers to describe the immunopathogenesis of a wide array of clinical diseases, to understand how immune cells regulate host response to antigenic challenges, and to develop new types of immunotherapy.[24] The CD4 cell, which is infected and depleted by HIV, has been shown to be the "orchestrator" of host immune responses. Several of the cytokines, such interleukin-1 and inter-leukin-2, have been used in clinical trials as adjunctive immunotherapy for several diseases, including non-AIDS cancers, as well as for HIV disease.[25]

Although serological tests for HIV antibodies were commercially avail-able by 1985, these tests were not helpful in monitoring the course of the disease. The presence of anti-HIV antibodies was diagnostic of infection. The analysis of specific antibody patterns, while of interest to lab scien-tists seeking to learn how the immune system recognized the virus, did not have clinically useful prognostic significance. The early clinical para-digm held that HIV was held in check after the initial bout of replication following the initial infection, and that the deep lymphoid tissues (eg, nodes, bone marrow, liver, spleen) served as the latent reservoir of the infection.[26,27] The virus later escaped immune surveillance, leading to immunocompromised status, opportunistic infections, and neoplasms.

To better understand the dynamics of HIV replication in host tissues, newer molecular genetic techniques were developed to be able to probe specific sites for HIV in its different forms. These techniques involved the tagging of lab-generated genetic sequences complementary to most HIV strains and amplifying the product of whatever bound to these probes.[28]

Three different methods have been developed: polymerase chain reaction (PCR), branched DNA (bDNA) testing, and nucleic acid sequence-based analysis (NASBA). These are known generically as viral load tests. Each can quantify the amount of HIV circulating in the blood or can be adapted to measure the extent of HIV infection in different tissues and body fluids.

Thus, the development of new nucleic acid probe techniques in response to the epidemic led to a fundamentally different understanding of the pathogenesis of HIV disease.[29-31] Moreover, the development of these techniques has had broad-based applicability to other poorly understood chronic viral infections, such as hepatitis C and cytomegalovirus. Because of the high rate of HIV turnover, the plasma viral load can rapidly decrease after a patient has been taking effective combination antiretroviral therapy for several days, so the tests are used to monitor therapeutic efficacy. This monitoring strategy has been extended to the clinical management of other chronic viral infections, which had not been the case prior to the advent of new molecular diagnostic monitoring techniques for the clinical care of HIV-infected persons.

Concepts of Per Contact Risk

Prior to the determination that AIDS was caused by HIV, no similar model existed for an inefficiently transmitted human virus that could cause serious clinical consequences following latency of more than a decade. The germ theory of infectious disease, in which specific pathogens were associated with specific clinical disease, was about 100 years old when the AIDS epidemic was first described.[20] Most prior, well-characterized epidemics had been associated with bacterial pathogens that tended to have incubation periods of weeks to months and could readily be identified using relatively simple histologic staining, bacterial culture techniques, and light microscopy. The use of cell and tissue culture to grow obligate intracellular pathogens, such as viruses, was well established by the time AIDS appeared. Thus, many agents associated with new diseases could be readily identified soon after their emergence.

Some of the major variables that determine whether an infection is transmitted from one infected person to another susceptible but uninfected person were well understood. Almost 150 years ago, John Snow, the father of modern epidemiology, demonstrated that, by removing the handle of the Broad Street pump in London, he could arrest a devastating cholera epidemic.[20] Later, Koch's Postulate stipulated the steps for proving that a disease was caused by a specific microbe. The potential pathogen had to be isolated from people who were sick with the disease, had to be capable of infecting an appropriate animal model and producing a comparable symptom complex, and had to be isolated once again from the sick animal. This hypothesis worked well to identify the infectious causes of a variety of syndromes, providing that the organism could be readily isolated and cultured and that an appropriate animal model could be found.

Several other parameters associated with the infectiousness of and susceptibility to specific pathogens were further clarified over the past century. For an infection to occur, the right amount of a specific organism had to be at the relevant site with the appropriate virulence characteristics in a susceptible host. Thus, in the example of cholera, because the organism does not have the capacity to readily bind to human respiratory tissue cells, cholera pneumonia is almost nonexistent, while cholera-associated diarrhea still ravages many parts of the developing world.

Pathogens need not bind to specific tissues to cause disease, since they can secrete toxins that subsequently cause cellular and systemic damage. However, for these toxins to be released, the pathogen must be in a permissive environment in the host's body. Some sites are more hospitable for a specific microorganism than others. For example, gonococci have the ability to bind to specific cells in the genital tract because of unique attachment proteins on their cell surface; thus, they are highly adapted to be a STD pathogen. The likelihood of becoming infected with a bacterial pathogen after an initial exposure could be relatively high, such as the more than one-in-four risk of becoming infected with gonorrhea after a high-risk sexual exposure with somebody who was already infected.[32]

However, the interaction between microorganisms and the human host is dynamic. Most tissues in the human body that interface with the outside would (eg, skin, oropharynx, alimentary canal, and urogenital system) are colonized with myriad microorganisms, most of which offer the host essential benefits.[33] Indeed, each gram of stool contains billions of commensal microbes. When the balance between good and bad microorganisms remains constant, health can be maintained.

As noted earlier, certain pathogens have highly adapted affinities for specific tissues. Other organisms become infective only in large numbers. For example, 100 to 1000 organisms of cholera would be insufficient to cause diarrhea, but the same number of *Shigella bacilli* would be capable of causing disease. In outbreaks of cholera, the excretion of human waste and poorly maintained water supplies allows for the microbe to grow in sufficient numbers to potentiate an epidemic focus. On the other hand, basic hygienic practices, such as boiling water, can decrease numbers and mitigate such an epidemic. In the case of *Shigella*, the organism is so virulent that it can be transmitted by food handlers and sexual contact as well as via infected food and water supplies.

Susceptibility to infection may vary as well, both in specific situations and from host to host. Most people have chronic, low-level colonization of skin and mucous membranes with *Candida* and other fungi but rarely experience clinically significant recurrent infections. However, giving an immunocompetent woman a broad spectrum antibiotic to treat a urinary tract infection will also kill off the "good" microflora that suppress the growth of *Candida*, allowing them to flourish and cause vaginitis or thrush. These factors may also play a role in whether an individual is transiently colonized and develops symptoms or remains relatively immune despite exposure to an infectious pathogen.

The relative immunity of the host varies according to the specific microorganism. For example, women who have diabetes may be more susceptible to recurrent yeast infections because of a subtle abnormality in polymorphonuclear cell function associated with hyperglycemia, but they rarely develop systemic fungal infections. On the other hand, people who have hematologic cancer and receive chemotherapy that suppresses white blood cell count may be at a particular risk for systemic candidemia (ie, fungal invasion of the blood stream). People who have foreign bodies that may track organisms from their skin to deeper tissues, such as in-dwelling intravenous catheters, are also at risk for systemic *Candida* infection, since the lines may serve as a nidus for deep tissue colonization and subsequent propagation of the organism in the blood stream.

The advent of the AIDS epidemic dramatically altered the way in which epidemiologists, microbiologists, and infectious disease specialists came to understand infectiousness and susceptibility.[34,35] In the early 1980s, the only human model for a chronic viral infection that resulted in a variety of clinical outcomes was hepatitis B infection.[36] Careful epidemiologic studies had indicated that hepatitis B was transmitted by blood-borne contact, initially identified as a cause of transfusion-related hepatitis[37] and subsequently found to be increasingly common among

IDUs who shared their paraphernalia. Occupational transmission from infected patients to health care workers also helped underscore submission of the agent through parenteral blood contact. Other investigators found that men who have sex with men, particularly those who had multiple partners, and the offspring of women with chronic hepatitis had a higher rate of hepatitis B than did the general population. The isolation of the infecting particle permitted the devising of a test that could identify a marker of the infectious agent as well as the development of antibodies against the virus surface, which was found to be protective. This discovery allowed researchers to identify clinical syndromes specific to hepatitis B and to separate out those that were associated with other viruses capable of invading the liver.[38]

How Viruses, Cancer, and Transmissable Immunosuppression Interact

In 1903, Rous found a virus that could reliably cause sarcomas (deep tissue tumors) when injected into chickens.[20] Since then, the question of the extent to which viruses were responsible for the development of cancer in humans has remained controversial. The development of tissue culture systems allowed scientists to study the effects of infections with different chronic viruses in specific cell lines and to establish correlations between these viruses and the development of unregulated cell growth. The discovery of animal viruses that attacked the immune system and caused malignancy helped refine the understanding that viruses could enter cells and be immunosuppressive or oncogenic (or both).[14-16] Likewise, the recognition that some viruses remain latent, including integration into cellular host chromosome, led to the realization that chronic viral infections in humans could reactivate when the host became immunosuppressed.[12] Researchers were concerned that latent integrated viral reactivation could lead to serious clinical consequences, including cancer or infection that opportunistically developed due to inadequate host defenses.

Just prior to the AIDS epidemic, Temen and colleagues identified an enzyme called reverse transcriptase, which inverted the genetic code and enabled RNA viruses to replicate as DNA forms, which could in turn be integrated as proviruses within the host cellular genome.[15] These proviruses could remain latent in inactivated cells for years and later replicate when the cell was activated by exogenous stimuli. HTLV was identified as an RNA retrovirus that increased the risk of developing rare forms of leukemia and other hematologic cancer in chronically infected persons (see Chapter 1).[17] Some HTLV-infected individuals tended to develop other atypical problems (eg, lymphoid infiltration of the skin), but no pattern of severe, life-threatening opportunistic infections arose similar to that seen in individuals who developed AIDS. Moreover, patients with leukemia or lymphoma tended to have increased numbers of lymphocytes, whereas individuals who developed AIDS showed a marked depletion of specific types of white blood cells.

HTLV provided an oncogenic retrovirus model, and its discovery expedited the search for the etiologic agent of AIDS.[39] As noted earlier in this chapter, the identification of different subsets of white blood cells with discrete functions in regulating host immune responses was very helpful in identifying specific markers for the diverse array of syndromes associated with AIDS. During the earliest days of the epidemic, a common feature of AIDS was the depletion of T helper lymphocytes and the increase in the helper-to-suppressor/cytotoxic T cell ratio.

The realization that the AIDS virus could be chronic, produce a variety of syndromes (including cancer), and be immunosuppressive facilitated the development of an integrative hypothesis. The common element associated with men who had sex with men (MSM) developing Kaposi's sarcoma, women dying of disseminated tuberculosis, and IDUs developing cytomegalovirus retinitis was a progressive depletion of the T helper cells, mediated by an agent that was transmitted by sex and blood contact. Once three independent labs isolated a unique human retrovirus and developed antibody tests that reflected the epidemiologic patterns of the AIDS epidemic, the pieces of the integrative hypothesis fell rapidly into place.

The ability to track this array of chronic immunosuppressive clinical sequelae, rendered by a progressive depletion of CD4 lymphocytes, has established specific connections between the control of the immune system with specific host cellular functions and the development of specific infectious diseases. The search has progressed rapidly to delineate the specific mediators known as cytokines, which enable T-helper cells to mediate host responses, to better understand how and when opportunistic infections develop.

By pinpointing the cause of AIDS and developing a readily available antibody test, initial epidemiologic insights regarding the infectious etiology of AIDS was greatly expedited. Once a marker for HIV infection was obtained, researchers were able to correlate specific behavioral practices of well-defined cohorts with the rates of transmission of infection. From these cohort studies, we learned that HIV transmission is most readily accomplished through anal intercourse but is also efficiently transmitted vaginally.[35] Oral transmission was documented to occur in a few carefully followed cases but was found to be much less efficient than the other modes. These epidemiologic findings preceded the development of the field of cell-surface biology and enabled researchers to better understand why some individuals are more likely to become infected with HIV than are others.

Impact of the HIV Epidemic on Infection Control Policy

The initial cohort studies increased understanding of the natural history of HIV transmission and quickly indicated that the hepatitis B model was not appropriate. Although HIV and hepatitis B shared transmission routes, HIV was transmitted with much lower efficiency. For example, per-contact risk was more than 100 times greater among health care workers exposed to a hepatitis-infected patient (30% risk)[40] than to an HIV-infected patient (0.3% risk).[38] On the other hand, while the majority of hepatitis infections are eventually cleared, almost no one infected with HIV becomes free of the virus; patients are presumed to be infectious for life. In addition, only 5% to 10% of HIV-infected patients are nonprogressors (ie, live for more than a decade without any evidence of immunologic decline), compared to the majority of those infected with other chronic, latent viruses.

The availability of definitive diagnostic tests removed some of the hysteria that initially characterized the epidemic. Being a member of a "risk group" did not automatically mean having a subclinical form of AIDS. Careful studies suggested that arthropod-born transmission did not occur, nor was HIV transmitted through casual contact. Attention now focuses on the rationale for public health policies and practices that are predicated on the actual transmission dynamics, including the relatively low per-contact risk of specific types of exposures.

Since ancient times, we have recognized that those who care for the sick might be at risk for acquiring illness themselves. This was particularly true in epidemics that devastated large populations, such as the bubonic plague in the 14th century and influenza outbreaks after major wars.[20] Even before the development of germ theory, careful observers noted patterns of transmission in specific epidemics, such as the role of blood, bodily fluids, skin contact, or airborne expulsion (eg, sneezing or coughing). These astute individuals could also assess the lag time between contact with an infected person or material and the development of disease. However, rational infection control policies did not develop until researchers and public health officials understood the structure and life cycles of bacteria, viruses, and other infectious agents and were capable of accurate diagnoses and quarantine measures.[41]

The potential for iatrogenic transmission of disease was noted in the mid-19th century by Semmelweis when he demonstrated that puerperal fever (ie, streptococci) could be transmitted by physicians and other clinical staff who did not wash their hands between obstetrical cases.[20] His careful demonstration of the importance of handwashing, and the subsequent popularization of antisepsis in the United States by Oliver Wendell Holmes Sr., created the framework for the modern science of infection control.

However, it was not until the demonstration that inadvertent needle sticks and other sharp exposures could effectively spread hepatitis B that health care providers fully realized their risk of becoming infected with serious blood-borne pathogens. Nonetheless, this awareness of the potential occupational risk to health care workers did not lead to immediate changes in the disposal of sharp objects nor to the universal administration of the protective hepatitis B vaccine.

During the early years of the HIV epidemic, tremendous concern arose among heath care workers because of the lethality of this untreatable disease that was ravaging stigmatized groups. Initially, many patients with HIV were placed in strict isolation. Concerns regarding the possibility of a silent carrier state often led to the presumptive isolation of individuals deemed at increased risk for HIV acquisition, such as gay men and IDUs, even when their presenting complaints were clearly unrelated to the emerging immunodeficiency epidemic. The subsequent elucidation of the etiologic agent of AIDS provided a scientific framework for understanding the mechanisms of HIV transmission, but many of the original fears persisted. Moreover, early case reports of health care workers acquiring HIV infection, without other risk factors for its acquisition, led to further anxiety and presumptive protective measures in clinical settings. In the global literature over the two decades of the HIV epidemic, occupationally acquired HIV fortunately remains a rare event (ie, less than 1000 reports after millions of needle-sticks and other occupational exposures), but its impact on the management of occupational health has been enormous.

In response to many reports of inappropriate professional behavior and denial of care for at-risk individuals, public health authorities, particularly the CDC, began educating clinical workers and the general public about what was then known about HIV transmission. Careful studies documented ways in which health care workers became infected with HIV, pointing to high-risk behaviors associated with HIV acquisition as well as preventable infection (ie, negligent disposal of sharp, blood-contaminated objects).

The recognition that the misplacement of sharp objects that came in contact with blood often led to inadvertent needle-stick injuries resulted in the development of several infection control practices (eg, never recap needles but instead place impermeable sharp instrument disposal units wherever these objects might be used). Following several highly publicized lawsuits over HIV transmission to health care workers, the importance of infection control policies became more widely appreciated by clinical professionals, their employers, and the general public. Hospital administrators recognized the importance of training and maintaining special personnel to oversee the implementation of infection control policies. Hospitals also began to provide adequate in-service education to health care workers on protecting themselves against inadvertent exposures and to carefully document the adequacy of protection available.

Although it was known prior to the AIDS epidemic that the administration of purified serum proteins, particularly γ-globulin, could protect against the development of hepatitis A or B after an initial exposure, no federal programs routinely mandated occupational protective services directed against these pathogens. With the heightened sensitivity to the risks that health care workers may encounter after exposure to bloodborne pathogens, comprehensive exposure reduction programs have evolved that address how worker risk from all transmissible agents may be minimized. Health care facilities are now required to provide postexposure prophylaxis for health care workers after potential contact with sharp objects or mucosal splashes from specimens that could transmit HIV. Thanks to enhanced scrutiny regarding HIV protection, health care facilities are mandated to protect health care workers against all potentially transmissible agents: eg, vaccination programs to protect against hepatitis A and B and skin testing, chest x-rays, and prophylaxis for employees exposed to tuberculosis.

Evaluation of health care facilities by accrediting agencies, whose approval is necessary for licensure, now includes an assessment of the adequacy of each institution's provision of exposure-specific education, protective vaccination, and other services to limit workers' risks of becoming infected with transmissible agents. In several states, physicians and other health care professionals are obliged as part of their licensure renewal to complete continuing medical education courses that review the current status of protective measures to avoid and manage exposure to blood and other bodily fluids.

On the other side of the patient-provider equation, the AIDS epidemic has highlighted several underlying tensions. Some health care workers argued that it would be desirable to screen every patient for HIV infection. The practicality of this was quickly challenged, since the prevalence of HIV in the general population is less than 1 in 10 000. Others believed that routine screening of all at-risk patients for HIV was essential to protect them against inadvertent HIV transmission. However, many indeterminate and false positive results would require the use of more sophisticated and expensive confirmatory examinations with the likelihood of detecting few new cases. At the time, such screening tests could not be processed quickly enough to provide health care workers with HIV status information in a timely manner. Newer rapid assays are available but are considerably more expensive and still cannot provide results for emergency medical situations.

Some health care workers and politicians then suggested testing only high-risk patients and segregating all HIV-infected patients.[41] This simplistic solution did not take into account the stigma that many HIV-infected persons experienced in the early days of the epidemic, which would result in many individuals wanting to misrepresent their HIV risk status. Several public health leaders suggested that false confidence might ensue from health care workers using different levels of caution in patient care based on perceived risk status. Patients who were declared HIV-negative might have other infectious agents in their blood, which could be transmitted to careless health care workers. In addition, as the HIV epidemic spread and atypical populations were infected, the neat categories of "risk group" were blurred. For example, in Rhode Island by the mid-1980s, almost one of three HIV-infected persons was a woman, and more than half of them never injected drugs.

Thus, mandatory testing of patients for HIV has not been generally adopted as a useful protocol in most settings. Instead, protocols of "universal precautions" were developed that instructed health care workers to treat all bodily fluid contacts "as if" they were capable of transmitting HIV or other serious pathogens.

However, advances in the clinical management of HIV disease have led to a new emphasis on earlier identification of HIV infection among exposed individuals (see Chapter 11). Early diagnosis of infection improves the likelihood that AIDS antiretroviral therapy (HAART) and prophylaxis against opportunistic infections will reduce morbidity and mortality. Several studies have shown that patients who start these medications prior to reaching an advanced stage of immunocompromise tend to have more favorable clinical outcomes and fewer side effects. In addition, pregnant women who take short courses of antiretroviral therapy (even a single dose) prior to delivery significantly reduce their infant's risk of becoming HIV infected. Where resources are limited, knowledge of HIV status during pregnancy may still reduce likelihood of transmission by forgoing breast-feeding. Finally, women in the United States and developing countries suffer gender inequities that place them at great risk yet keep them ignorant of their partners' status. Routine testing and subsequent triage to primary care may be the only way that these disenfranchised women might learn of their HIV status. (For a thorough discussion of this issue, see Chapter 6.)

Recent attention to the possible use of antiretroviral drugs by occupationally exposed health care workers has also sharpened the debate about the right to know the HIV status of the patient to whose blood or other fluids they were exposed. Several lines of evidence support the use of postexposure antiretroviral medication. These include animal experiments, clinical trials on the prevention of maternal transmission with antiretroviral regimens, and a retrospective case-control study of occupationally exposed health care workers.[40] The efficacy of postexposure prophylaxis appears to be greatest if a 4-week course is started as soon after a relevant exposure as possible (generally with 24 to 72 hours; but the sooner, the better). The side effects of these medications in exposed health care workers resulted in discontinuation rates of 50% to 65%, underscoring the desirability of using these expensive medications only after a high-risk exposure to a known infected source. This had led some health care workers to suggest that testing and identifying as many HIV-infected individuals as possible would lead to a more judicious use of prophylaxis in occupational settings; however, such an approach still does not solve the emergency room scenario that commonly arises.

Tension also exists between the patient's right to autonomy in deciding whether to undergo screening and the providers' desires to minimize their risk of becoming infected from an occupational exposure. The complex issue of how the final decision is made when there is a disagreement about the willingness to be screened has not been fully resolved. In settings where the state (eg, correctional facilities) or treatment programs (eg, methadone maintenance centers) can establish mandatory protocols, routine HIV screening and flagging of results is standard protocol, but breaches in confidentiality have been documented in these settings. On the other hand, most states still maintain anonymous HIV testing facilities to entice at-risk individuals to undergo screening in settings where they need not fear discrimination or the loss of confidentiality. (These issues are considered at length in Chapter 11.)

On the other side of the equation is the concern that HIV-infected health care workers could transmit HIV to their patients. Once again, hepatitis B provides a timely model. The transmission of hepatitis B from surgeons to patients had been a known, albeit rare event. Subsequent guidelines recommended that if health care workers performing invasive procedures were known to have a more infectious variant of hepatitis B (as measured by the presence of the "e antigen" in the blood), they were enjoined from using sharp objects without first informing their patients. In many health care settings, professionals may be routinely screened for hepatitis B, and if found to have chronic infection, they may be told to change their career to one that does not involve the use of sharp objects. Fortunately, hepatitis B is now a vaccine-preventable disease, so the number of newly diagnosed infectious chronic carriers in the United States is decreasing.[11]

Awareness of provider-patient transmission of hepatitis B greatly heightened concerns raised by the AIDS epidemic. Even though HIV is up to 100-fold less infectious than hepatitis, calls were raised in many quarters that all HIV-infected health care workers should be promptly identified and removed from clinical practice. These calls became especially urgent after five people in Florida not otherwise at risk for HIV were infected by their dentist.[42] However, public health officials argued that the cost of creating and enforcing such a system did not justify the ends, given the low likelihood of transmission and the ability of HIV-infected clinicians to provide exemplary care. Other problems included the frequency of retesting and the employer obligation to workers who test positive and must be removed from the position for which they were hired. Currently, the onus is on individual providers and their institutions to decide how to best protect the health of their patients, and it is acknowledged that one blanket policy will not be sufficient.

Provision of Care to Chronically Infected Persons

The emergence of the AIDS epidemic has radically transformed the delivery of health care to chronically infected individuals. Prior to the onset of AIDS, infectious disease specialists did not generally provide primary care for patients, since many infections (eg, most bacterial infections) resolved, following appropriate treatment, whereas chronic infections might be associated with an underlying disease (eg, cancer). The primary care providers for persons who were predisposed to develop serious chronic infections tended to be hematologists, oncologists, rheumatologists, and general internists. The role of the infectious disease specialist was to consult with the primary provider and assist in the diagnosis and therapy but not to become involved in actual patient care.

This arrangement continued at the outset of the AIDS epidemic. The major diagnostic and therapeutic challenges were related to the patients' opportunistic infections, so the infectious disease consultation was important. Early on, health care providers caring for HIV-infected persons needed well-honed pastoral skills, given the high mortality. In addition, at-risk patients often engaged in behaviors not sanctioned by society and therefore sought practitioners with clinics open to gay men and IDUs. Thus, the initial providers of care in the epidemic were a diverse group of caregivers (see Chapter 11).

Since there was no cure and no fixed paradigm of optimal care for HIV, no discussion was possible regarding the credentialing of providers of HIV care. Moreover, due to the stigma associated with the risk behaviors that exposed one to HIV, many medical providers emphasized the need to "mainstream" the education of those who would provide care for HIV-infected persons (ie, training all health professionals in the rudiments of HIV disease management). In this manner, new cases could be readily identified, and infection with HIV could be recognized as something other than a marker of stigmatized behavior.

Over the past two decades of the epidemic, advances in the ability to diagnose, monitor, and treat HIV infection have decreased morbidity and mortality but have increased the need for intensive education and hands-on training of health care providers. Several studies indicate that patients fare better if they receive care from experienced providers who are interested in acquiring new knowledge. In other words, HIV has evolved from an often rapidly fatal disease requiring primary and supportive care with episodic expertise from a specialist to a chronic, manageable, but complex infectious disease.

The shift in professional opportunities and obligations for infectious disease specialists is the major reason why the Infectious Disease Society of America (the professional association of these specialists) quintupled its membership between 1980 and 1999. Infectious disease outpatient practice was almost nonexistent in the pre-AIDS era, since simple bacterial infections were usually treated by primary providers, such as pediatricians or internists, and serious infections generally required hospitalization. Now discussions by several national groups are underway as to whether providers of HIV care should have specific training and undergo subspecialty licensing exams.

The future of HIV care is in flux at the beginning of the third decade of the epidemic, but the emergence of the epidemic itself has had multiple unanticipated consequences. Optimal care for persons living with HIV necessitates a broad-based team of care providers, including medical, mental health, and supportive services ranging from access to complementary/alternative medicine therapies to social service case management (see Chapter 11 for details). The integration of clinical research with primary care has been another key feature of HIV care. The advent of AIDS has resulted in the unique recognition of how viruses interact on molecular, clinical, and community levels, and the mobilization to confront the epidemic has profoundly altered how care is being delivered. The incursion of the virus has truly been a catalytic event.

Summary Points

- Advances in immunology and virology assisted efforts to identify the infectious agent that causes AIDS. Conversely, research into HIV and AIDS has greatly advanced knowledge in both immunology and virology, particularly the functions of lymphocyte subgroups and their cytokines through cell surface markers and molecular genetics techniques.

- The span of time spent on the identification of HIV was prolonged because of its many unique features: extended latency prior to symptom onset, ability to cause cancer and immunosuppression (among other clinical syndromes), choice of host cell (lymphocytes integral to immune response), and the disparate and stigmatized groups initially found to have the syndrome).

• The AIDS epidemic had a profound impact on infection control policies, particularly the management of sharp objects that may have been in contact with blood or other body fluids.

The Response of Quantitative Scientists to Challenges Posed by the AIDS Epidemic

Victor DeGruttola

The potential for HIV to spread rapidly throughout communities across the world was not the only reason for its destructive impact. Crucial to its spread was lack of adequate warning about the true level of risk those communities faced. This lack of warning resulted in large part from the complexity of the statistical problems posed by the epidemic. Sophisticated statistical counsel was neither provided to nor sought by health authorities making public statements about risk until years after the first cases of AIDS were identified. The large amount of statistical and epidemiological research conducted in response to the epidemic demonstrates how understanding the AIDS epidemic depends on high-level expertise in quantitative science. As a result of this research activity, public health scientists and policy makers now have new research tools to aid in characterizing the epidemic.

Early mistaken beliefs about the risks associated with HIV resulted as much from statistical naïveté as from a lack of relevant information. In fact, within a short time after the first described case, the Centers for Disease Control and Prevention (CDC) had developed surveillance procedures that produced a wealth of data about the spread of AIDS and some important information about its natural history as well. However, misinterpretation of these data contributed to the complacency and inaction of the early 1980s, as described by Shilts.[1] Recognition of the estimation problems described below might have spared the public from such misinformed ideas as:

- the latency period of the infection and the onset of symptoms is one to two years

- only "promiscuous homosexuals" and IDUs are at risk of AIDS

- only 5% of those infected with the virus become ill

- the supply of blood and blood products was essentially safe prior to the development of widespread tests

Beliefs about the epidemic eventually changed, thanks largely to the combined efforts of statisticians and epidemiologists. Impressive bibliographies compiled by Jewell[2] and by Brookmeyer and Gail[3] reflect extensive research activity in the late 1980s and 1990s. With few exceptions, however, adequate statistical treatment of the crucial issues did not begin to appear until 1986. One important paper from that year by Brookmeyer and Gail dealt with epidemic projection. Thereafter, an increasingly sophisticated body of work addressing the AIDS epidemic appeared in scientific journals and contributed to an accurate though bleak assessment of the menace of AIDS.

The areas of statistical and epidemiological innovation resulting from the AIDS epidemic might comprise, by themselves, a course in public health methods:

- natural history of HIV (including distribution of time between infection and onset of AIDS as well as decline in measures of immune function)

- studies of HIV transmission

- design of surveys to establish HIV prevalence

- screening and accuracy of testing

- projection of AIDS incidence

- epidemic transmission models

- design of therapeutic trials

Studies of natural history were among the first to make use of statistical methods in a serious way. AIDS patients infected through contaminated blood provided information about the delay between transfusion and onset of clinical symptoms. In fact, these observations led to the early estimates of average latency of one to two years. In 1986, Lui et al[4] correctly recognized that the observations on time between transfusion and onset of AIDS symptoms were truncated, and this realization led to estimation of the mean latency period of four to five years using a parametric approach (ie, assuming that the data followed a particular

mathematical shape). Although somewhat naïve—parametric assumptions
are influential and cannot be validated from such truncated data (With
truncated data, sample values exceeding or falling below a fixed constant
are not observed or recorded.)—this work at least alerted people that the
average latency was much longer than had been thought and helped
interest other statisticians in the problem. Since the paper by Liu, a
number of statisticians have considered this problem. A variety of
approaches have been published that differ in the way they condition on
times of transfusion and in the degree of parameterization. Building in
part on some earlier work by Jewell (1990), Brookmeyer and Gail
showed the relationships among the approaches that have been taken to
solve this problem.

The impact of recognizing statistical problems such as truncation and
using very simple approaches to accommodate data that arise in such a
setting can be demonstrated in a fairly straightforward way. The
approaches described by Brookmeyer and Gail could easily be used to
characterize latency and risk to the blood supply based only on transfusion-related data available in 1983. These analyses make clear that by
1983, one could have inferred that the hazard of AIDS increased rapidly
for at least four years after infection; in fact, students could make this
inference as part of a homework assignment. (Students attending a course
in methods for AIDS research at the University of Washington were asked
to use appropriate methods to characterize latency and risk to the blood
supply based only on transfusion-related data available in 1983. They had
no difficulty doing so.) Though estimation of risk beyond four years was
not possible at that time, there was no reason to believe that the hazard
would end abruptly. A longer average latency implied by such analyses
also permits the inference that, by late 1983, thousands of people had
already been infected through the blood supply (and, by analogy, other
blood products) and that an epidemic of what was then called HTLV III
had become widespread.

Studying the natural history of HIV infection also required development of new statistical methods, especially those for analyzing
interval-censored data, using both parametric and nonparametric
approaches. Such problems first arose in AIDS research in the study of
cohorts of hemophiliacs. In several cohorts, stored blood samples could
be used to determine the interval in which serological evidence of HIV
infection was observed. In some cases, these intervals could be fairly
wide, and estimates obtained from assuming that seroconversion occurred

at the midpoint of the interval could be biased. In addition, variance estimates developed from such assumptions would be overly optimistic. Development of appropriate methods allowed estimation of precise HIV incidence curves for hemophiliacs. Such curves show that hemophiliacs in France continued to be infected for about a year after such infection had ceased in the United States.[5] In addition, application of such methods to cohorts of people at risk of HIV infection, such as hemophiliacs and participants in hepatitis clinical trials, also permitted estimation of the risk of onset of symptoms of AIDS after seroconversion. Even by 1987, such work had shown that, unlike most other infectious diseases, the risk of clinical symptoms in untreated patients rises during the first five years after infection and then remains fairly constant for many years thereafter.

An important development in understanding the epidemiology of HIV infection was the development of a method sometimes referred to as backcalculation. Backcalculation is a method for estimating the HIV infection curve and using it to project AIDS incidence based on data from AIDS surveillance and from cohorts of HIV-infected people. In 1986, Brookmeyer and Gail first published a paper using these methods to demonstrate the extent of the epidemic. This early work helped to mobilize resources to combat AIDS. More recent efforts have characterized the uncertainty of these procedures. This work is important not only in using backcalculation to forecast AIDS case load but also in evaluating the degree to which surveillance data reflect the public health impact of treatment strategies. One important source of uncertainty arises from the assumption of independence in annual AIDS incidence. A more recent approach by Pagano[6] allows for plausible dependence in annual AIDS incidence. In all cases, these activities owe a great debt to CDC for collecting and making available extensive surveillance data related to the spread of AIDS.

Mathematical complexity also characterizes the field of epidemic transmission models. Almost in parallel to the work of epidemiologists, applied mathematicians have published extensively over several decades on modeling epidemic dynamics. The complexity of approaches that model the connection between different "compartments" or categories of people at risk of infection implies a need for an enormous amount of information. It may be this feature that causes such work to be more prominent in biomathematical journals than in the biostatistical literature. As Brookmeyer and Gail[3] have pointed out, so many parameters are required by such models that their usefulness in case projection is limited.

However, qualitative findings from such models might help characterize the conditions likely to be necessary for an epidemic to take place. These models are also useful in establishing the potential benefit of a treatment strategy such as needle exchange in settings where controlled studies may be difficult. The result adds to the arsenal that a quantitative scientist can summon in fighting for the interests of people vulnerable to the effects of AIDS.

In addition to epidemiologic methods, much work has been undertaken in the design and analysis of clinical trials. Perhaps most important is work investigating the role of viral load as a surrogate endpoint for the effect of treatment on clinical progression of disease. While it has been observed that patients with undetectable virus have low risk of clinical disease progression (provided that their immune systems were intact at the time treatment was initiated), it has not been demonstrated that those treatments with the best short-term effect on viral burden are the best overall. Analyses that investigate the role of a surrogate endpoint, such as viral burden, sometimes make use of a metric called the "proportion of treatment effect" that can be accounted by the surrogate. Lin et al[7] and De Gruttola[8] have demonstrated the inherent instability of such analyses as well as problems in interpretation. Work by Daniels and Hughes demonstrates how meta-analyses—pooling data across studies—can be used in investigating the value of a surrogate marker. Such work will become increasingly important as the number of new treatments increases, as does the pressure to rapidly evaluate them.

Although many antiretroviral drugs in several drug classes have recently become available and have had considerable impact on AIDS morbidity and mortality, the frequent onset of resistance to these drugs reduces their periods of usefulness. The advent of techniques for rapid sequencing of virus has made it possible to study the patterns of genetic mutations that are associated with drug resistance, but the large number of such mutations and of potential drug combinations complicates such investigation. To address this problem, a variety of statistical methods, including cluster analysis (the elements of a population are arranged in groups or clusters, and some clusters are selected at random for subanalysis), recursive partitioning, and linear discriminant analysis (each possible set of linear combinations of values for one or more cariables with a set of threshold values in a classification procedure), have been used to investigate the relationship between genetic sequences and response of plasma HIV-1 RNA to therapy.[9] Such efforts improve the ability of physicians to target therapy to the resistance profiles of viruses with which their patients are infected.

In the interval between the first description of AIDS (1981) and the first statistically accurate description of the epidemic of HIV infection (1986), hundreds of thousands of people were infected with HIV in the United States—perhaps 10 000 to 15 000 through blood transfusions alone.[10] Added to the cost in terms of destruction of lives and disruptions of families and careers is the financial cost of treating these patients— perhaps tens of billions of dollars. What might have been achieved, if people at risk had been correctly informed of the jeopardy they faced? In places where the epidemic hit later and more time was available for warning, considerable evidence exists to support the importance of wide- spread, protective changes in behavior. Even if such measures prevented only a tiny proportion of cases, earlier investment in applying sophisti- cated statistical ideas to the problem of AIDS would have reaped enormous returns. At least the recent work of statisticians and other quantitative scientists help assure that appropriate methods will be used in the future—not only in AIDS research but in related problems as well.

Summary Points

• Late involvement of epidemiologists and statisticians led to several misconceptions about the AIDS epidemic and delayed identification of key features that may have been useful in reducing disease spread.

• Epidemiological studies of the natural history of HIV and AIDS helped define the latency period between infection and onset of symptoms.

• New statistical methods were developed to characterize the HIV/AIDS epidemic such as backcalculation, with which HIV incidence is estimated based on known AIDS cases and in turn future AIDS cases are forecast.

• Complex mathematical theories have been used to model epidemic dynamics and to establish the potential benefits of prevention strategies such as needle exchange.

• As part of ongoing clinical trials, statistical methods are being used to identify the relationship between genetic sequences and response of plasma HIV-1 RNA to therapy.

• Issues surrounding the testing of health care workers and patients remain controversial, pitting privacy concerns against occupational safety priorities and clinical advances capable of preventing the establishment of HIV infection (following high-risk exposure) and of slowing disease progression.

• As the AIDS epidemic progressed and HIV treatment became more widely available, infectious disease specialists moved from a consulting to a primary care role. However, questions regarding the need to certify specialists who provide HIV care remain unanswered.

Section II: Social Concerns

The three chapters in this section address broad social themes that have relevance far beyond HIV: gender inequity, racism, homophobia, poverty, access to health care, drug use, and much more. Addressing the concerns raised will improve the health and well-being of American society as a whole. If the prescribed efforts to reduce HIV transmission are implemented, other conditions associated with economic and social deprivation (eg, premature births, infant mortality, drug and alcohol use, violence, hypertension, asthma, etc.) will benefit as well. Conversely, if interventions focus too narrowly on HIV prevention alone without addressing underlying behaviors and socioeconomic conditions at the heart of the problem, other epidemics may arise with equal lethality. The upcoming lessons to be learned are essential for overcoming HIV/AIDS ... and much more.

CHAPTER 5

Sex and Drugs and the Virus

David G. Ostrow

I n the early 1980s, the idea that drugs alone, apart from needle sharing, played a role in the transmission of HIV was not popularly accepted. Drug users and gay men were viewed as separate populations.[1] This situation has since reversed itself to the extent that nonintravenous "recreational" drug use is well recognized as a significant factor in the homosexual transmission of HIV and other STDs. This chapter reviews the history of sex-drug research during the US AIDS/HIV epidemic and addresses questions such as the extent to which researchers studying gay/bisexual men have succeeded in addressing the important issue of nonparenteral drug use and HIV risk.

That researchers and policy makers are still grappling with this issue is illustrated by the most recent Research Synthesis Symposium on HIV Prevention in Drug Abusers. Among 39 formal research presentations and discussions, none focused on substance abuse issues in gay or bisexual men.[2] Moreover, the popular and scientific literature barely mention that more than one half of all new AIDS diagnoses in the United States, and at least one third of incident HIV seroconversions, still occur among and drug-using men who have sex with men (MSM).[3] A central thesis of this chapter is that researchers working to prevent the spread of HIV among drug-using MSM must address two of the most stigmatized behaviors in our society—homosexuality and drug use.

Early Years of Denial

In 1984, data from the Multicenter AIDS Cohort Study (MACS) and the San Francisco Men's Health Study confirmed that men who reported using "recreational drugs" (then mainly marijuana, "downers," and volatile nitrites or "poppers") were at higher behavioral risk and were less likely than abstainers to report reductions in risky sexual behaviors between their first and second semiannual assessments.[4] As soon as the HIV antibody test was available in 1985, we confirmed that the drug-using men were not only more likely to already be seropositive upon entry into the study, but had seroconversion rates 2 to 3 times that of the abstinent men between visits 1 and 5.[5] When these data were presented at the First International AIDS Conference in Atlanta in 1985, symposium chair James Curran, then Director of HIV Prevention for the CDC, asked rhetorically what could be done if unlimited funds were available to intervene with gay men around their sex-drug usage.[6]

Dr. Curran's question is just as difficult—if not more so—to answer now as it was then. In the early phase of research on the epidemiology of HIV among drug users, efforts focused on drug users only as injectors and sharers of needles. This led to intervention programs that did not adequately address the sexual risk behaviors of drug-using gay/bisexual men, IDUs, or women. Some of those interventions, such as the provision of sterile needles and syringes, have been so successful that new IDUs are more likely to get HIV infected from unprotected sex than from using contaminated "works."[7] Yet politicians and community leaders who feel that needle exchange programs send a message condoning drug use still vigorously fight them. Meanwhile, gay/bisexual men appear to be abandoning safer sex messages in increasing numbers as a result of "safer sex burn-out" or thinking that HIV is not the serious threat that it once was.[8]

In the mid-1980s, the nonparenteral sex-drug connection seemed more like an epiphenomenon than a serious and worthwhile research endeavor.[9] Public attitudes about AIDS and persons living with HIV infection were so negative that proposals to isolate people with AIDS were frequently being discussed.[10] To say any consensus existed on how to most effectively prevent the spread of HIV infection among any at-risk group (except blood product recipients) would deny the vigorous debates that often pitted public health against privacy concerns.[11] As research data accumulated showing how fast and widespread the epidemic was growing among homosexual men,[12] the early years were marked by public health policy that was mostly reactionary—that is, reacting to some of the worst human emotions—fear, disgust, guilt, shame, and stigma.[13]

Many gay community organizations and activists took a stance against the implication of recreational drug use in the spread of HIV, not to mention those who vigorously denied any role of HIV in the pathogenesis of AIDS.[14] No one wanted to indict pleasurable drug use as a cofactor, unless the epidemic could be blamed entirely on drug use and thereby restore safety to unprotected anal sex. However, data from the MACS and

San Francisco Men's Health Study cohorts showed that recreational drug use was associated with relapse to risky sexual behaviors and HIV seropositivity and that specific drugs were associated with higher rates of seroconversion. Indeed, HIV infection rates paralleled over time the rates of sex-drug usage (eg, volatile nitrites, cocaine, and downers) among seronegative members of the cohorts.

Issues in the 1990s

Despite increasing interest from the CDC and other agencies in funding interventions involving drug-related HIV infection, drug-using MSM were rarely included in such studies. If drug use were not enough of a disincentive, the fact that many of the men at highest risk met the DSM-IV criteria for both drug abuse and antisocial or borderline personality disorders[15] would certainly contribute to the barriers. The number of persons working in this area has stayed relatively constant, and we frequently gripe among ourselves about the difficulty to find research funding and to maintain community support for what is unpopular research.

However, the NIDA has committed a sizable amount of its AIDS research dollars toward funding studies with drug-using persons at risk of HIV who are not necessarily IDUs. Increasing numbers of community-based organizations have reoriented their HIV prevention programs to target MSM who use drugs as well as engage in risky sexual behaviors. Specific research initiatives at NIMH, NIAAA, and NIDA now fund studies of the basic mechanisms linking drug use to sexual HIV transmission.[16]

Some progress has been made since Dr. Curran asked his rhetorical question in 1985. For example, we have learned to avoid stigmatizing sex between men and recognized the urgent need to revise the entire outcome measurement side of our research to become current with trends in sexual behavior. As HIV-infected men plan their sex lives on the basis of feeling healthier from potent combination therapies and the hope that they are no longer infectious, prevention studies will have to take into account the new strategies of avoiding HIV transmission by choosing seroconcordant partners or using postexposure prophylaxis.[17] It is no longer adequate to measure the number of times anal sex occurs with or without condoms or the number of partners with whom it occurs and merely examine changes in these figures to determine intervention success. That most men consistently adhering to "negotiated safety" are also abstaining from the use of alcohol or drugs during sexual activity should be taken as a positive indication that at least some of our educational messages about the dangers of combining sex and drugs do reach their target audience.

Another trend during the past five to six years has been the adaptation of harm reduction techniques. First introduced into interventions for IDUs, these programs supplemented the goal of abstinence with interventions to reduce the risk of HIV infection through the sharing of nonsterile injection equipment. We have further adapted this technique in our Awareness Intervention for Men (AIM) model. AIM focuses on primarily on raising awareness of how participants are using drugs to satisfy their sexual and intimacy needs, then helping them plan for future sexual encounters that might include drugs, and finally motivating them to put these harm reduction plans into action.[18,19]

Barriers to Sex-Drug Research

Prior to the AIDS epidemic, research on the links between drug use and sexual behavior focused mainly on the effects of alcohol and alcohol expectancies on sexual and social behaviors.[20] Pioneering research in the 1960s showed subjects given either vodka or vodka-flavored water who were told that they would be "disinhibited" by the drinks would respond as suggested.[21] The only other sex-drug research ongoing in the pre-AIDS era was laboratory studies of the effects of drugs on male erectile function. Some of this research was beginning to move in the direction of studying drugs of abuse, such as marijuana and cocaine, rather than alcohol and prescribed medications, when political considerations, including Congressionally mandated bans on the funding of most human sexual behavior research, brought sex-drug research to a virtual halt.[22]

Not surprisingly, when the AIDS epidemic hit the United States in the early 1980s, we were totally unprepared; basic research on drugs and sexual behavior needed to understand the epidemic from the beginning was nonexistent. The only information published on pre-AIDS gay male sexual behavior came from comparisons of the gay male cohorts participating in the Hepatitis B vaccine studies of the late 1970s with the early AIDS natural history cohorts such as the MACS.[23]

Today, hundreds if not thousands of published reports address the correlation between drug use and risky sexual behavior in a wide range of populations. However, great hesitation remains on all sides to accept the importance of these findings and to move on from correlative and mechanistic studies to true intervention studies.

Not only are funders and policy makers hesitant. The gay community is understandably hesitant to admit that the problem of recreational drug use, which fueled the explosive growth of the AIDS epidemic, remains 20 years later.[24] Corporate sponsors of large gay community fund-raising parties ("circuit parties") threaten to cancel sponsorship if anyone admits that drugs are consumed at parties bearing their names, even when the sponsor is a vodka or volatile nitrite ("popper") manufacturer.[25] Bars and bathhouses are reluctant to admit researchers who might suggest to their patrons that the alcohol and drugs consumed on the premises might be bad for their health. The larger community, including many activists, seems reluctant to accept research that could be used to apply the same labels to gay men that form the basis of anti-gay discrimination.[26]

We have seen one notably egregious example of official denial of the sex-drug problem in the way the US government has regulated the sale of poppers.[27] When research showed that poppers were definitely associated with HIV infection and unprotected anal sex, Congress banned the sale of butyl nitrites in 1988 and alkyl nitrites in 1990; but, since they were actually marketed as room fresheners and not pharmaceuticals, Congress gave the enforcement of the ban to the Consumer Product Safety Commission, not the Food and Drug Administration. Once manufacturers and distributors of poppers saw that no effective enforcement of the ban was forthcoming, they returned to openly advertising and selling their versions of room deodorizers and tape head cleaners. Sales of poppers are now back to where they were before AIDS. Simultaneously, research on the popper-HIV connection has virtually dwindled to zero.[12,28,29]

The history of poppers reminds us that we should not forget the commercial interests that are at stake in the sex-and-drugs arena. Bars are still the social and financial underpinnings of most gay communities. Drugs are still the central focus of circuit parties and raves, and there is money to be made. When a gang in Brooklyn began selling phony ecstasy tablets to ravers, the counterfeit drugs (usually aspirins with "trademark" logos pressed into them) were so popular that they drove the legitimate drug dealers out of the clubs.[30]

In addition, while gay AIDS activists were very eager to trumpet data showing dramatic changes in mens' sexual behaviors in response to the epidemic, they were much less eager to embrace later findings showing that numbers of gay men were "relapsing" to unprotected anal intercourse despite the risk of HIV infection.[31] AIDS behavioral

researchers may have made a mistake by calling the phenomenon
"relapse" because of its clinical implications and suggestions that something was pathological about anal intercourse. This is an important
problem of semantic clarity that sexual behavior researchers in the AIDS
era face on a daily basis.[32] Since the goal is to prevent the spread of a
deadly disease, we have been forced to view the very sexual acts that
define homosexuality as "bad" and have been accused of disgracing
homosexual behaviors. It is very important then that we avoid the use
of words such as "relapse" without the important explanation that we
are not talking about a pathological behavior per se but rather about
basic human sexual needs and functions. Only when a virus such as
HIV is transmitted is the sexual act made pathological. With the advent
of protease inhibitors and more potent combination antiretroviral therapies that possibly reduce the risk of HIV transmission between infected
and uninfected partners during unprotected sex, as well as the continuing controversies over the safety of unprotected oral sex, "relapse" is
even more difficult to define.[33]

Relationship between Sex, Drugs, and HIV Infection among MSM

Because drug use per se cannot be proved to cause AIDS, it best serves
as a behavioral marker for high-risk sexual activity and a cofactor in HIV
transmission. The search for causal mechanisms responsible for these
associations take on significant importance for primary and secondary
AIDS prevention among gay men. As outlined in one of the earliest
papers on this topic,[4] the behavioral connections between substance use
and unprotected anal intercourse among gay men can be conceptualized
as belonging to several general categories, though other factors likely
contribute as well (Table 1).

Many of these mechanisms occur in combination, leading to
extremely high risk for HIV transmission (particularly among members of
a closed network). In fact, by combining high-risk behavior with a
concentration of HIV risk among partners, the ideal situation is created
for saturation of the network with HIV infection.[35] This is certainly the
case among persons who combine IDU with the sharing of unclean
needles within a "shooting" network in a high prevalence location.[36]

Different theoretical models of how drug use is related to sexual
transmission of HIV are of much more than academic interest when it
comes to testing and designing effective interventions. Each model implies

TABLE 1. Mechanisms by Which Sex-Drug Activity Serves as a Cofactor in HIV Transmission

Category	Causal Mechanism
Pharmacologic Actions	Increased sexual desire
	Increased intensity of sexual experience
Cognitive Inhibition	Decreased awareness of risks involved
	Ineffective use of safe sex measures
Underlying Vulnerability	High-sensation seeking behavior
	Sexual compulsivity
	Risk-taking personality traits
Escapist[18,19]	Use drugs to escape awareness of risk
Network Pathway	Sex-drug use within networks of members seeking risky sexual gratification
Biological Cofactor Actions[34]	Local drying or irritation of mucosal membranes
	Vasodilation
	Acute immunosuppressive effects

different routes and determinants of unsafe sex, different ways in which drug use impacts on sexual decision making, and different points in the sequence at which intervention to prevent risky behavior can occur.

The direct causal theories imply that if drug abuse is treated, a reduction in sexual risk will follow. Indeed, many recent publications, reviews, and studies assert that "drug abuse treatment is HIV prevention."[37] While this may be true for intravenous drug use, where the drug-use behavior is that through which HIV is being transmitted, it is more complex for nonparenteral use of "softer" drugs. If there is indeed a shared underlying vulnerability, such as extreme sensation seeking, stopping the use of a particular drug may be replaced by another drug or addiction to another high sensation-producing situation. If the sexual component of the "addiction" is not addressed, it is unlikely that recreational drug treatment will produce long-term reduction in sexual HIV transmission.

In contrast, common underlying vulnerability theories imply the need to affect both the drug use and high-risk sex or the common underlying vulnerability trait. Very few reports in the literature discuss attempts to change sensation-seeking traits or risk-taking personalities as related to sexual risk-taking, but there have been attempts to treat other compulsive behaviors, such as gambling, in this way.

The network aspect of this conundrum is one that might be amenable to relatively straightforward intervention. Many effective cocaine treatment programs require that participants sever their ties with drug-using friends and develop new social networks of abstainers. While an effective intervention for those who can uproot themselves and remake their social network, it does not require that the person fully overcome the underlying personality vulnerabilities or even their cravings for the drug. For those individuals unable or unwilling to leave their social drug-using network, network-based outreach interventions might be feasible and less socially disruptive than the therapeutic community approach. Either form of intervention is likely to be quite expensive, however, and will require the cooperation of the larger community as well as the social network.

The escape or AIM model implies that interventions targeted at the use of drugs to escape conflict between ones' desires and social prohibitions could ultimately be very effective. Again, very little published literature addresses this subject, although we are currently testing this model in the AIM Project among drug-using MSM in Chicago.

Finally, because a combination of 3 or 4 mechanisms may be acting to increase the sexual transmission of HIV and other STDs when drugs are used, a multifactorial intervention will likely be needed to stop sex-drug related transmission. Perhaps therapeutic communities must be brought back and applied to this problem, as they were designed to provide the type of behavioral/social/personality "modification" that could not be achieved through simple workshops or even intensive psychotherapy.

Sex-Drug Research Today

Causal theory interventions are often linked to shared vulnerability interventions in the following ways: "Addicts lead chaotic lives. This chaos results, at least in part, from the organization of their conscious lives around their drug taking and obtaining drugs. The result of that chaos and overriding preoccupation with drug finding is a release of the ego-driven inhibitions on conscious control of risky behaviors, perhaps through sublimation of sexual inhibitions to the overriding immediate needs of drug-seeking. Thus, if addicts can be weaned from their drug-seeking and -taking preoccupation, their lives will normalize, including reinhibition of sexual and other risky behaviors." Whether or not such links between causal and common underlying vulnerability theories are explicitly acknowledged, the links between normalization and reorganization of a recovering addict's life and reduction in risky sexual behavior is often explicitly acknowledged in the design and implementation of causal-based interventions for drug users.

Obviously, the literature is predominated by interventions for IDUs that have as a specific component reduction in heterosexual risk taking.[37,38] Two reports of interventions designed specifically for at-risk drug-using MSM based on causal attributions are those published by Stall and colleagues (polydrug-using alcoholic MSM in San Francisco)[39] and by Reback and Shoptak (amphetamine-using MSM in Los Angeles).[40] The two trials differ in obvious and important ways. The Stall intervention recruited alcoholics participating in a day treatment program located in a predominantly gay/bisexual section of San Francisco. In contrast, the Los Angeles intervention targeted amphetamine-abusing MSM not in treat-ment. Both interventions used control groups to separate the direct effects of the intervention from nonspecific impacts of being in treatment and from community-wide changes in risk behavior.

The results for both studies, however, were remarkably similar: men in treatment, regardless of whether the treatment was specific for drug-related sexual risk or was a nonspecific "control" intervention condition, improved in terms of sexual risk in a somewhat dose-response manner. These findings would on the surface be interpreted as favoring the direct causal model of drug-related sexual risk. However, several cautions need to be made. In both interventions, it was difficult to prevent contamina-tion of the "control" intervention by essential elements of the sex-drug specific intervention (ie, a Hawthorne effect or effect of observation, in which subjects' awareness of the study alters the observed outcome). It may be extremely difficult to prevent the host treatment center from adopting a drug-sex intervention on a center-wide basis during the active treatment phase of an investigation if they are favorably impressed by the reductions in HIV risk-taking seen among early study participants.[41] This highlights a concern among all investigators working in the midst of an epidemic. Limiting intervention activities and enforcing the control arm to satisfy statistical power requirements becomes difficult, time-consuming, and ethically questionable while simultaneously trying to prevent HIV transmission within a vulnerable target community. This serious moral consideration does not disappear as the urgency of the epidemic recedes and has no simple answers.

AIM Model

Efforts to develop an intervention flexible enough to accommodate mixed causal mechanisms among risk-taking, drug-using MSM resulted in the AIM model. As described in two recent review articles, the AIM model seeks to increase awareness of the tactical use of drugs prior to sexual encounters, whether these drugs are used to escape awareness of the risk involved (escape theory) or to increase sensations associated with risk taking (sensation-seeking theory). Regardless of the exact mechanism, the AIM model uses a three-step process to first increase awareness, next to make a plan to avoid taking sexual risk to obtain the gratification being sought, and finally to implement these plans in future encounters. Thus, AIM is an extension of standard cognitive-behavioral/skills development interventions[42] that incorporates "readiness to change" concepts and can be added to standard small group interventions targeted at drug-using MSM.

As was expected, limiting exposure to the experimental intervention among control subjects proved difficult with the AIM model. Since participants in both study groups are recruited on the basis of their drug use and drug-associated sexual risk taking, all those enrolled spontaneously bring up their drug use and its motivations during discussions of risk triggers and moderators. Although a significant Hawthorne effect will no doubt arise, questions added to the 12-month follow-up assessments will attempt to define and quantify these effects on the final outcome.

In addition, while AIM has encountered no problems identifying and enrolling appropriate subjects, tremendous difficulty arose when trying to motivate these same men to return for the actual small group interventions, which were held on two successive Saturdays for five to six hours each. Despite repeated attempts, less than half of the qualifying men completed the full intervention. This experience is quite similar to that of other investigators (C. Bartlett, personal communication, 1997) who have attempted to work with high-risk, drug-using populations. Moving the intervention directly to sites where subjects engage in risky sexual behaviors or obtain sex-drugs may overcome the low turnout seen for clinic-based interventions and expand recruitment to less motivated men.

Not surprisingly, it has been quite expensive to field the AIM model in a controlled clinical trial setting. Future studies must focus on more cost-effective ways to identify, recruit, and motivate men who combine drug use with high-risk sexual behaviors.

In addition, men at highest risk of STD infection are the very ones least likely to ask for or to receive preventive interventions.[43] This modern-day demonstration of Hart's Law of Inverse Care Access[44] has important implications for the future application of HIV and STD interventions targeted at lower socioeconomic high-risk persons. The use of any technological innovations, such as HIV vaccines and postexposure prophylaxis, will require that we reach the highest risk "core" populations. If we truly wish to see preventive interventions used by the persons at highest risk of becoming HIV infected, we must design studies that reflect the real world circumstances in which these strategies will be utilized, while also examining innovative means of delivering those interventions to those at greatest need.

This brings us full circle in this review of sex-drug research with gay or bisexual men during the first two decades of the HIV epidemic. As HIV increasingly becomes an STD concentrated in lower socioeconomic status, minority, and marginalized individuals in our society, the relevance of prevention intervention research conducted among predominantly with white, gay-identified, upper socioeconomic status men is increasingly questioned. Similarly, the experience of middle-aged, white, gay, male researchers is sometimes deemed irrelevant to the behavioral research needs of younger men and women of color and other vulnerable populations.[45]

Conclusions

Because HIV has affected the gay community disproportionately (and will continue to do so as long as the community is more widely defined as MSM), more information is needed about the impact of various HIV/STD prevention treatments on gay men and MSM specifically. Further, despite near universal awareness among gay/bisexual men about HIV and how it is transmitted, few data explain why seroconversions still occur and why they seem to occur disproportionately among younger and minority men. Obviously, our existing interventions are failing or not reaching these men.

Other factors operative in HIV seroconversion among drug-using MSM include both drug use and sexual sensation-seeking. What remains to be demonstrated is whether or not sexual risk reduction follows from alterations in the sex-drug using/seeking behaviors or vice versa, and whether sensation seeking and other contributing psychological traits can be changed. All intervention research studies should use theory-based interventions, and those interventions and their theoretical underpinnings should be thoroughly described. Too often, published studies do not adequately explain the intervention or the application of the underlying theory to the intervention design. This robs the scientific community of the information needed to interpret study findings and to refine and disseminate the intervention components in a cost-effective manner.[41] By successfully fielding innovative, theory-based interventions, we can learn a great deal about the underlying causal mechanisms linking sexual and drug risk behaviors.

We must also develop more realistic measures of behavioral intervention outcome. Especially in this "post-AIDS" and "post-condom" era,[25] insisting on total adherence to condom use every time with every partner cannot remain the expected outcome. Instead, researchers must focus on how changes in knowledge and attitude translate into fewer HIV-transmitting behaviors and eventually into reduced rates of HIV seroconversion over time.

Likewise, we must reconsider why so few studies have examined reducing HIV risk among drug-using MSM in the context of the barriers identified earlier in this chapter. For one, the target population of drug-using MSM is neither an identifiable homogeneous "community" nor a group of men who self-identify themselves as having a problem in need of research and intervention. This may be an issue of education regarding the continuing problem of HIV seroconversion related to sex-drug use, as has been attempted by the Substance Use Counseling and Education program at Gay Men's Health Crisis of NYC.[43] However, when actual field outreach has been attempted, the targeted population has shown little interest. Similarly, we have yet to develop an effective recruitment strategy for those individuals whom we feel are the most at-risk MSM, but who are also in denial about their substance abuse problems.

Finally, we must find more effective ways to join together the experience of older, established researchers with the talents and connections of a new generation of talented community-based prevention experts. Partnership with community-based organizations that are doing innovative prevention can benefit both parties while providing the setting necessary for the development and testing of real world interventions. Public policy advocates have previously used this partnership to test new models of health care delivery. Extension of this partnership model to include prevention intervention research and policy development can help to both focus our research efforts and ensure the dissemination of useful prevention programs.

If we can accomplish just some of the recommendations given here, we may achieve increased interest in and support of basic and applied behavioral research. Sustained over the long term, increased interest in sex-drug research has the potential to consolidate and further the progress that has been made in the last 20 years. Such advances will in turn continue to break down the barriers to recognizing and understanding the roles that drugs play in the sexual lives of men who have sex with men.

Summary Points

• The epidemic of HIV/AIDS among drug users and MSM are not separate, as considerable overlap exists in terms of risk behaviors among drug-using MSM.

• Even those who learn the mistakes of the past are still prone to repeat them in the future when it comes to the scientific study of stigmatized behaviors such as sexuality and recreational drug use.

• Recently discovered infectious agents, such as hepatitis C, could easily replace HIV/AIDS as STD epidemics if behavioral interventions focus only on HIV and not the sex and drug risk behaviors through which these agents are being transmitted.

• The use of "party drugs" in the context of sexual encounters presents enormous barriers to behavioral modification based on cognitive change/skills development interventions as the sex-drug party scene effectively operates to suppress cognitive inhibitions and the application of safer sexual skills.

- Just as has been observed in research with IDUs, the prevalence of HIV in the sexual and drug use networks of sex-drug using MSM is both an important determinant of HIV incident infections and a potent tool for effective interventions.

- Enhanced sexual sensation seeking appears to be a common characteristic of both men who engage in risky sexual behaviors and men who combine "party drug" use with sex. New and innovative interventions for high sensation seeking men need to be developed and effectively marketed to "party drug" users who do not recognize themselves as being in need of treatment.

CHAPTER 6

Social Inequality and HIV Infection in Women

Sally Zierler, Nancy Krieger

S ocial inequality plays a significant role in HIV infection among US women. To explain which women are at risk and why, we will review the epidemiology of HIV and AIDS among women in light of conceptual frameworks that link health with social justice. We will review data linking inequality of class, race/ethnicity, sex, and sexuality to the distribution of HIV among women. Although we primarily limit our analysis to research on US women, we believe our framework and its applications are relevant to women in other countries. Our major premise is that the work of public health is not only to reduce human suffering but also to envision and create dyanmics that promote human health.

In 1981, six women in the United States were noted to have an unexplained underlying cellular immune deficiency.[1] It was a description of the same phenomenon among five previously healthy young gay white men that prompted the 1981 *Morbidity and Mortality Weekly Report*, now viewed as the first official recognition of AIDS.[2] A retrospective study of underlying causes of death suggested that 48 women unknowingly had died of AIDS in the years 1980-1981.[3]

Although not described in that report, these women were probably young, between the ages of 15 and 44 years. They likely lived in poor neighborhoods, and if they could get work, they rarely earned sufficient wages to pay for food, child care, clothing, and shelter. Most of these women almost certainly depended on public assistance and men for economic survival. Most were also likely to have been women of color—African American, Hispanic, Haitian, American Indian—who were raising young children. Unlike white gay men diagnosed with AIDS, sickness among these women was not unexpected. It was part

With permission from the *Annual Review of Public Health,* Volume 18 (1997, by Annual Reviews, www.AnnualReviews.org)

of the ongoing, usual excess morbidity and mortality among the poor and racially oppressed.

Eighteen years later, as the proportion of women among AIDS cases continues to rise—from 6% in 1984 to 23% in 1999—the vast majority of women with AIDS in the United States are still poor women of color, of whom 80% are in black or Hispanic racial/ethnic categories.[4] By mid-1999, a total of 114 621 women with AIDS had been reported to the CDC. Among states reporting incident HIV infection from July 1998 through June 1999, 32% of adult cases were women; 77% of women were in black or Hispanic categories. Among the youngest adults (13 to 24 years), 49% of new infections were among women. HIV infection is the fourth leading cause of death for women age 25 to 44, following cancer, unintentional injuries, and heart disease.[5] As a cause of death among black and Hispanic women in this age group, HIV infection ranks second. How we understand and reduce HIV infection among women depends in part on the conceptual frameworks that guide data collection and interpretation as well as program design and implementation. To date, much of the literature on women and HIV has relied on biomedical,[a,6-8] lifestyle,[b,8-10] and psychological[c,11-15] explanations of disease causation. This review instead uses frameworks that make connections between disease and inequality and between health and social justice (Table 1).

Economic Inequality

Economic forms of gender inequality that increase HIV risk include factors that preclude women from earning comparable wages and having access to jobs, as well as from receiving compensation for responsibilities of child and other family care. Many studies have documented how such dependence translates into women being in the difficult position of having to risk loss of income, food, housing, and social nurturing requiring money (eg, theater, traveling, music, and recreation) to prevent HIV infection from men who may not be willing to use condoms.

Among the first public health articles to frame women's experience with HIV infection within the larger social and economic conditions in their lives was the powerful commentary published in the *Health/PAC Bulletin* by Anastos and Marte, which drew on both feminist and political economy analyses.[16] Noting the invisibility of women in the CDC surveillance definition, research agenda, and prevention programs, the authors highlighted the public health portrayal of women as vectors of transmission to babies and to their male sexual partners with little regard for women's rights. They urged that health professionals care about women not because they may be pregnant, mothers, prostitutes, caregivers, or sexual partners, but because women were deserving of good health and fair access to medical resources. The authors wrote not about drug use and sex, but rather about where women were situated geographically and socially. "... for many women," Anastos and Marte noted, "their address alone places them at risk ... poor black and Latina women are at unduly high risk for infection, whatever their life-style, because poverty and lack of resources and opportunity keep them in areas of high HIV seroprevalence."[16]

Few studies have linked regional economic conditions in the United States with prevalence of HIV. Among them is a set of studies by Drucker[17] and Wallace.[18,19] Building upon a political economy of health framework, they dissect relationships between urban crises in housing, depleted city budgets, poor schools, and unemployment, and how these economic conditions led to dislocation of residents, dissolution of family and other social networks, and spread of AIDS. One study, for example, employed analytic techniques of population and community ecology, quantitative geography, and epidemiology to link reduction in public services to poor neighborhoods in the Bronx to subsequent high concentrations of HIV prevalence:[18]

> Where communities once lived, hulks of burned and abandoned buildings and vacant lots remained ... Both the devastated zones and nearby communities experienced rising rates of homicide, suicide, drug and alcohol abuse, HIV infection and AIDS ... the fate of the South Bronx reflects the vulnerability to HIV infection created by processes of urban decay already widespread in many US cities.

Four additional US studies provide population-based evidence of strong relationships between incidence of AIDS in large urban areas and neighborhood level income.[20-22] Linking AIDS incidence data to 1990 census-based socioeconomic data from the zip code or census tract level, these studies analyzed socioeconomic inequalities in AIDS occurrence within three cities: Philadelphia,[6] Newark,[21] and Los Angeles.[22] They found that incidence of AIDS was between 2 and 13 times higher in

low-income areas compared with high-income areas. One study reported
an inverse relationship between AIDS incidence and income among four
racial/ethnic groups (white, black, Hispanic, and Asian/Pacific Islander
Americans).[22] The fourth study identified the cumulative incidence per
100 000 for low-income US census block-groups in Massachusetts: 442
cases among black nonHispanic women, 352 among Hispanic women,
and only 13 among white nonHispanic women. The risk for black
women was 34 times that of nonHispanic white women, while Hispanic
women had 27 times the risk of nonHispanic white women. All of these
women were living in poor neighborhoods where 40% or more of the
population lived below the federal poverty level.[23] Several studies have
noted more specific conditions of poverty and accompanying economic
challenges in the lives of women with or at risk of HIV infection. For
example, an ongoing 5-year NIDA study to reduce HIV occurrence
among women who have injected drugs and smoked crack described the
extent of social and material deprivation among 887 women from low-
income, inner-city neighborhoods in Los Angeles.[24] Most of the women
received their primary economic support from male sex partners or from
public assistance programs. Nearly all of the women reported a monthly
income of less than $1000.

Similar levels of economic poverty have been reported by two
ongoing national cohorts based on populations of HIV-infected women
from ten major US cities: the HIV Epidemiology Study (HERS) and the
Women's Interagency HIV Study (WIHS). Together enrolling nearly 3000
women with HIV infection and a comparison group of approximately
1000 seronegative women, these studies confirm that most women with
HIV in the United States are living and often also caring for children
amidst severe poverty.[25,26]

Data also suggest a bleak picture of women with or at risk of HIV
infection being economically more destitute than their male counterparts.
Data from the NIDA National AIDS Demonstration Research (NADR)
programs for 6609 female IDUs showed that women are much less likely
to earn a legal income than men. Nearly 30% of the women depended on
male partners for economic support, and 42% said they relied on illegal
means of income, mostly involving sex work. These women were also
two times more likely than men to have children living with them,[27]
implying that their already low incomes needed to be stretched that
much further.

Similarly, an interview-based study[28] of 428 women and 2470 men diagnosed with AIDS in 11 states examined education, recent household income, and current employment. Women fared worse than men for all three measures. Overall, half the women had not completed high school, most were unemployed, and 77% had an annual household income of less than $10 000. Nearly all black women interviewed (versus three quarters of the white women) had an annual family income under $10 000. Additionally, among women living with AIDS and reporting a history of injection drug use, black women were nearly two times more likely not to have completed high school than US black women (63% vs 32%); for white women, the corresponding proportions were less divergent (29% vs 20%). The authors noted that although employment and income data may have reflected consequences of AIDS rather than conditions at time of diagnosis, their report included data on persons infected with HIV but free of AIDS-defining symptoms. Among this subgroup, 84% of women and 58% of men were unemployed.

An analysis of social class and HIV in Brazil described conditions comparable to women in US cities.[29] This cross-sectional study of 600 women in 3 cities who depended on sex with men for money, drugs, or gifts at least once in the previous month found that lower social class position was associated with higher prevalence of HIV infection. In fact, women in the lowest social class stratum were more than four times more likely to have HIV infection relative to women in higher social class stratum (17% vs 4%), independent of HIV prevalence in the cities where women lived and worked.

Several anthropologic case studies and ethnographies likewise document the central role of economic resources in the prevention of HIV infection in women.[30-33] Farmer has tracked rising water from construction of a hydroelectric plant that dammed Haiti's largest river to the spread of AIDS among families forced to relocate from their original farmlands to higher, less fertile ground. In a context of deepening poverty, Farmer tells the story of women becoming sexually involved with men who might offer women alternatives to destitution in their lives. As said by Acephie Joseph, who later dies of AIDS, "... I looked around and saw how poor we all were, how the old people were finished ... It was a way out, that's how I saw it."[31]

Political economy of health analyses link the spread of HIV to development projects funded by the World Bank and International Monetary Fund.[30,33-36] Schoepf has described how women in Zaire have survived amidst conditions that underscore already pervasive gender inequality in the labor market and in childbearing decision-making. Strapped with responsibilities for childcare and wage-earning amidst extreme conditions of poverty, women "engage in ... activities in the informal sector," usually involving sex for material sustenance, sometimes at the request of their families for purchasing land or building materials or to repay debts. Men, less constrained by caring for children, have sought wages from jobs that involved traveling or living away from home for long periods of time. These labor migrations became a source of HIV infection among men as they sought sexual contact with women or men along their routes. Upon returning home, these men then introduced HIV into their families.[33] Analyses of women and AIDS in Zimbabwe[34] and South Africa[35] have identified similar patterns of disease spread.

Finally, use of race/ethnicity as a marker for social class has been inferred by a number of US studies.[5,37] The underlying assumption has been that higher rates of HIV infection among populations of color reflect the greater poverty among them than among white populations. However, without explicit data to separate economic from racial/ethnic factors, such studies cannot rule out racism as a dimension in the prevalence of HIV and AIDS in minority groups.

Racial Inequality

To the best of our knowledge, no published studies have measured racism in the lives of women at risk for or living with HIV infection. Instead, most investigators have interpreted their findings in one of four ways:

- racial/ethnic differences reflect underlying biologic differences[38,39]

- race/ethnicity is a marker for social class position

- racial/ethnic categories reflect culture

- racial/ethnic disparities result from social processes of racial domination, subordination, and resistance, reflected in US history of expropriation, conquest, slavery, and discrimination

Interpreting racial differences as markers for biological differences is problematic because race is a social rather than biologic or genetic construct.[40-42] As this scholarship has demonstrated, racial categories instead have been created by subjective systems of race relations that emphasize distinctions based on selective physical characteristics. The weak link between these characteristics and so called race-specific disease accounts for only a minute percentage of each racial group's overall morbidity and even less of their mortality.[43] Sickle cell anemia, for example, the one known potentially fatal black-linked disease, accounted for only 0.3% of the 37.0% higher age-adjusted death rate in 1977 for the US black compared with white population.[40]

Although disparities in socioeconomic conditions may partially explain inequalities in health, these racial/ethnic differences in AIDS incidence persist within class strata.[22,23] Persistence of these differences may reflect residual confounding due to inadequate measurement of socioeconomic position, noneconomic aspects of racial discrimination, or differences in cultural practices unrelated to inequality. We recognize that important dimensions of race/ethnicity derive from shared culture, ancestry, and also, histories of racial/ethnic domination and struggle.[40,44,45,d]

How might racism affect HIV risk in women? Several commentaries on racial/ethnic disparities in AIDS have called attention to economic inequalities rooted in racial discrimination as a cause of HIV infection.[45-52] Using a political economy of health framework (see Table 1), these commentaries emphasize that excess relative risk of AIDS among communities of color, notably African American and Hispanic people, reflect underlying forces of discrimination in employment, housing, earning power, and educational opportunity.[49,51,53] Living amidst such constraints, social and economic strategies for work, play, and love may involve more risk for drug use, partnerships with drug users, and income-earning strategies that include sex and drugs than among people living free of constraints imposed by racial subordination.

Noneconomic expressions of racism can also increase risk of HIV infection among women. In response to daily assaults of racial prejudice[54] and denial of dignity,[55] women may turn to readily available mind-altering substances for relief and for self-medication of depression.[56,57] Seeking sanctuary from racial hatred through sexual connection as a way to enhance self-esteem, gain social status, and feel emotional comfort may offer rewards so compelling that condom use becomes less of a priority.[58] Women are at particular risk if such drug and sexual activities occurred within communities affected by residential segregation. Such segregation, enforced by racial discrimination in housing and limited economic options, creates concentrated pockets of HIV and other STDs. These other STDs, left untreated due to inaccessible health care services or inhospitable treatment, have been implicated as cofactors for vaginal susceptibility to HIV infection.[59]

Additionally, racism construed as a psychosocial stressor could increase biological susceptibility to infection, since studies have found that social stressors may impair immune function.[58] Although studies have not yet measured how racism and resistance to racism may affect women's risk of infection, the effects of racism on health have been demonstrated, including elevated blood pressure[60,61] and impaired mental health.[57,62,63]

Although not specific to women, some research has documented how recent awareness of atrocities of scientific misconduct in the 40-year Tuskegee Syphilis Study has carried over into suspicion of the origins of AIDS and motives for public health and medical interventions.[46,49,51] A 1990 survey of 1054 African American church members conducted by the Southern Christian Leadership Conference reported that 35% of people believed that AIDS was a mechanism of racial genocide; 30% were unsure if this was true.[53] In addition, public health messages that women with HIV should use condoms and not become pregnant ignore a legacy of sterilization abuse and other forms of population control against women of color. As Levine and Dubler wrote:[64]

> One need not accept the concept of an active governmental policy of genocide to appreciate the power of the loss of a generation of men through societal neglect and the community's desire to replace them through the birth of a new generation.

On the other hand, racial injustice may be a basis for collective resistance and the generation of responses that protect communities from HIV infection. Some investigators have recognized the power of social networks in affecting social change among subordinated groups.[17,47,45] As Friedman has noted, this approach moves[47,65] beyond the common view of minorities as deprived and subordinated, and thus, as less able than whites to protect themselves against the epidemic, while recognizing that blacks and Hispanics are indeed subjected to relations of dominance and inequality that leave them with lower levels of material resources and of formal education than whites. ... In addition to deprivation, subordination, and pathology, however, minorities are constantly developing resources and dynamics of their own that aid their individual and collective struggles for survival, dignity, and happiness.

For example, in the AIDS Community Demonstration Project in New York, women sex workers organized with HIV investigators to bring effective race-conscious messages for rebuilding community at the same time as they teach women how to protect themselves from HIV transmission.

Gender Inequality

The proportion of AIDS cases in women attributed to sexual intercourse with men has steadily increased from 15% per cent in 1983 to 38% in 1995. In 1995, among women reported to have acquired AIDS from sex with men, 37% of cases were attributed to sex with men who injected drugs. The remainder of AIDS cases among women having sex with men were attributed to sex with a partner with HIV infection whose risk was unreported or unknown (54%), sex with a bisexual man (7%), sex with a transfusion recipient (1%), and sex with a man with hemophilia (1%).[4]

Although injection drug use remains the predominant mode of transmission among women with AIDS in the northeast, the number of women reported to have acquired HIV from sex with men exceeds the number infected through injection drug use in the south, the midwest, and the west. Nonintravenous drugs, in particular smokeable freebase cocaine ("crack"), have been linked to male sexual transmission of HIV to women (see Chapter 5 for thorough review of nonintravenous drug use and HIV risk).[66-68] Among crack users, the practice of exchanging drugs for sex with multiple partners has led to intersecting epidemics of syphilis and HIV, each enhancing transmission of the other.[66,67]

Women's sexual experiences with men may include unsafe sex with the possibility of HIV transmission within a consensual context. However, when expressions of sexuality preclude condom use due to fear of loss of material support, beliefs that women should not make sexual demands of men, or fear that partners will react violently to discussions of low-risk sex, gender-related sexual inequality drives a women's risk of HIV infection.

Studies document that economic dependence on men who are primary partners affects women's perception of or practice in influencing partners' use of condoms.[69-71] A study of African American women in Los Angeles found that women who depended on their male partners for financial assistance for housing were more likely to have sex without condoms than women who did not depend on men for economic reasons.[72] By contrast, among women who expressly have sex with male clients for economic purposes, condom use was more frequent in that setting than with their primary partners.[29]

Noneconomic disparities between women and men also affect risk. Amaro summarized interviews with[25-27] Latina women in the Northeast United States on reasons for engaging in sex with men who do not use condoms. Women "expressed feelings of powerlessness, low self-esteem, isolation, lack of voice, and inability to affect risk reduction decisions or behaviors with their partners."[69] Studies also found that condom use was less likely among women who reported needing men for social status[71] or physical protection,[73] and among teenage and young women engaged in sex with older men.[74,75]

Gender-Based Violence

Among women, past and present experiences with violence can affect risk of HIV infection in several ways. Childhood sexual abuse, noted to have occurred in an alarmingly proportion of women currently infected as well as women living amidst conditions of increasing risk for infection, has profound, long-term effects on psychological and physical health. Most relevant to HIV risk are sequelae that include high-risk sex, prostitution, crack use, injection drug use, recurrent sexual assault, homelessness, and incarceration.[76-81] Studies of incarcerated women,[82,83] homeless women,[73] women in drug treatment programs,[79] and drug-dependent women[78,80,81,84] report prevalence of early sexual abuse ranging from 30% to 80%. Among women living with HIV infection, nearly half report forced sexual experiences in childhood or teenage years.[81,85-87] The preponderance of evidence that childhood and adolescent sexual abuse predisposes young women to drug using and sexual experiences links this trauma to HIV risk.

Teenage girls and women most at risk for HIV infection are likely to have witnessed or been affected by violence in their neighborhoods. Among 246 inner-city, mostly African American youth (ages 18 to 23) from Detroit, 42% had seen someone shot or stabbed, 22% had seen someone killed, and 9% had seen more than one person killed.[88] Studies from other cities[89-91] find similar estimates of exposure, even among very young children. One in ten children (average age 2.7 years) treated at Boston City Hospital had witnessed a shooting or stabbing before the age of six, half in the home and half in the street.[91] In a recent study of young adult women prisoners' experiences with violence, over 85%

reported at least one victim experience, nearly 70% reported abuse by male sexual partners, and 75% reported being robbed or physically or sexually assaulted by strangers.[92]

The between violence and HIV infection in women can be drawn from the effect of violence or fear of violence on women's ability to protect themselves sexually.[87,93] A study of more than 2000 women in drug treatment programs or sexual partners of male injection drug users found that 42% of women were sexually active with men who physically hurt them, 45% with men who had threatened women with violence, and 21% with men out of fear of physical harm if they refused.[84] A recent Baltimore study among women during their most recent childbearing year revealed that those living in the poorest neighborhoods with high unemployment and high HIV prevalence were found to be most at risk for partner violence.[94] A study of Brazilian sex workers further found that 23% of women reported fear of violence if they insisted that clients wear condoms, and the prevalence of this concern tripled when requesting condom use with men whom they regarded as "non-clients."[29]

The relationship between HIV risk and violence likewise emerges in a context of homelessness among women. Among homeless women, 22% to 86% cite domestic abuse as their reason for being homeless.[73,95,96] Without a safe place to live, women face dangers of street life that include exposure to HIV from rape, sex for economic survival, and drugs. A study of women who had been homeless for at least 3 months reported that 15% had been raped while homeless in the last year.[73] Interestingly, the authors noted that homeless women with the least risk for HIV infection were those who asserted they did not have male "protectors" in the streets.

If women at risk for HIV infection are living within relationships that include violence, women already infected may be living in similar conditions. In the WIHS multisite cohort study of HIV-infected women, 67% reported sexual or physical violence by a current or past partner, and in nearly one third of women, this occurred in the past year. Prevalence of partner violence in this cohort jumped to 83% among women who were current injection drug users and 81% among women who depended on sex for money, drugs, or shelter.[85] Limited empirical data indicate that a woman's disclosure of HIV infection itself may be a trigger for partner violence.[97,98] Based on these findings, Rothenberg and others[97,99] have suggested that state-level policies of partner notification may be dangerous to women (see Chapter 10 for a review of partner notification and privacy issues). This danger stems from a premise that disclosure obligations may risk harm to women if they are required to inform violent sexual partners of possible exposure to HIV infection.[98,99] Indeed, the risk of violence women face by disclosing their HIV status may exceed the risk their male partners face from female-to-male sexual transmission of HIV.[100]

A political economy of health framework (see Table 1) underscores that men inflicting this violence are also likely to be living amidst conditions of economic and social hardship. Men carry distinct gender authority and social roles that, in a context of poverty, have limited room for healthy expression. As people who may use violence against women, these men also may have experienced assaults against themselves through racial discrimination, economic impoverishment, and the social alienation that accompanies it. Thus, the brutally logical concurrence of violence and HIV happens within a larger structural control of social and economic resources and their distribution.

Gender Inequality and Drug Use

Gender inequality may affect the social pattern of illicit drug use and in turn women's risk of HIV infection. This social patterning spans from onset to dependency and extends to drug treatment. Many studies report that heterosexual teenage girls and women are more likely to begin and to continue drug use with boyfriends and male partners. Men, on the other hand, are more likely to begin and then continue to share drugs with male friends and associates.[27,101-104]

The effect of these patterns on HIV risk vary according to the social networks and HIV prevalence in the region where the networks form.[105] Friedman and colleagues[106] reported that among IDUs living in a high HIV seroprevalence area who had been injecting drugs for fewer than 10 years, women were more likely than men to become infected. This observation was most apparent among women using drugs in "high risk networks," which included older and therefore more likely HIV-infected injectors, or injectors only recently known to women, suggesting more rapid turnover and thus exposure to a greater number of high-risk injectors over time. One study reported that women injectors with at least 3 different male sex partners in the past 6 months were 5.1 times more likely to seroconvert than women injectors with fewer than 3 partners over that same period.[104]

Preliminary findings from ethnographic research note that once a pattern of regular drug use has begun, women's networks are more likely to depend on men for locating, purchasing, and bringing home drugs (P. Case, personal communication, 1995). Women's autonomy in engaging in harm reduction (eg, needle exchange programs) or drug treatment may be met with resistance by male partners. Studies have documented that, compared with men, women were less likely to receive support from primary partners and from family members for seeking treatment of drug addiction.[101,108]

In fact, recent reports from needle exchange projects suggest that women's positions in social networks of drug use reflect larger social roles and expectations.[65] Women tend to present at needle exchange sites at lower proportions than men, with various sites reporting that 25% to 32% are women.[109] This may reflect a lower proportion of female IDUs, but women may not use needle exchange sites for several reasons related to gender.

In a heterosexual construct, social norms dictate that men handle tasks of obtaining drugs and syringes for their women sexual partners (P. Case, personal communication, 1995). Data supporting this dynamic come from a Boston study in which, among adults who shared syringes, 70% of women reported sharing only with their male sexual partner, in contrast to 16% of men who reported sharing syringes only with their female sexual partners (P. Case, unpublished data, 1996). In other words, the men share needles with a wider range of people than do women, who tend to stick with their partners.

In addition, male partners may not allow women to participate in needle exchange programs, as suggested by observations at a San Francisco needle exchange program. One woman stated, "He told me either he goes [to the needle exchange site] or nobody goes" (S. Murphy, personal communication, 1996). Women at this site also reported being intimidated by male drug and sexual partners who threatened to withhold drugs and sterile equipment if women tried to get them for themselves (S. Murphy, personal communication, 1996).[110]

Women may also avoid scoring drugs or visiting needle exchange sites because the neighborhoods to which they must travel are too dangerous. At the San Francisco program, women felt harassed as they waited in line to exchange their needles by men wanting to give them drugs or to have sex with them. Women may also avoid traveling to these programs because public identity as a drug user carries more stigma for women than for men,[93,103] thereby reducing women's willingness to be seen in programs exclusively designated as needle exchange sites.

Finally, mothers risk criminalization for their drug use and subsequent loss of their children. At the same time, treatment programs for pregnant and parenting women are relatively few and often full. A New York City survey of 78 drug treatment centers[70] found that 54% of them excluded pregnant women, and 87% denied services to pregnant crack users, even if they had Medicaid insurance to pay for them. Thus, criminalization of both drug use and pregnancy in a context of drug dependence forces women to hide their drug use,[111] which in turn limits their access to programs available to them and their children, prolonging use and increasing risk of HIV infection.[64,112]

Sexual Identity as a Source of Inequality

Five instances of female-to-female sexual transmission of HIV have been documented in the literature.[113-117] In a review of AIDS cases in women who reported sexual contact only with other women, 152 women (93%) injected drugs, and 12 (7%) had a history of a blood transfusion before March 1985; no cases were attributed to female-to-female sexual transmission of HIV.[118] In a serosurvey of 498 women who have sex with women recruited through public venues, 1.2% were HIV infected; all infected women reported either a history of injection drug use or sexual contact with men.[119] Data from the National AIDS Demonstration Project reported 2.1% HIV seropositivity among female IDUs who had sex with women.[105] The authors attributed this level of infection to social networks of women drug users who were likely to have shared drug injection equipment and to have had sexual activities with women and men who were sexual with men. In 1997, the CDC reported that of 333 women reporting sex exclusively with women, only 9 (3%) reported no other risk factor.[120]

Inequality resulting from sexual identity may also affect women's HIV risk. Legal rights of lesbians and gay men are not protected under federal law, although some states and municipalities have passed laws that prohibit discrimination in the areas of housing, employment, and public accommodation. State sodomy laws are often selectively enforced against gay people, and their existence underscores a social message that sexual intimacy and love between women is unacceptable and perhaps even dangerous to society. In such a climate, women who identify themselves as lesbian and who also live in conditions of poverty, drug dependence, and reliance on sex work for economic support face considerable challenges in avoiding HIV infection.

To our knowledge, no studies have examined how sexual identity as lesbian may influence risk of HIV infection. The sparse data published or presented on lesbians and HIV infection suggest that apart from sexual identity and frequency of sex with men, lesbians share similar conditions of poverty and gender and racial/ethnic subordination as women who are heterosexual or bisexual.[121] Because data on sexual identity were not included for most published studies on HIV infection in women, distinctions between identity (as lesbian, bisexual, or heterosexual) and practice (sex with women, with men, or both) have been blurred. These distinctions may matter, since women who identify as lesbian may have experiences of social isolation and discrimination beyond those resulting from class, gender, and racial/ethnic position.[121,122]

The 2 largest ongoing cohorts of women living with HIV infection reported that 18%[121] and 25%[25] have had sex with other women, but across both studies, less than one fifth actually identified themselves as lesbian. Moreover, between 10% and 20% of these lesbian-identified women reported recent sexual activity with men. Among women in the WIHS, 11% of HIV positive and 9% of uninfected lesbians, and among women in the HERS, 19% of seropositive and 14% of seronegative women reported sex with men in the previous 6 months.

Community-based agencies may be unaware that their messages to women for HIV prevention typically assume heterosexual identity. By excluding those who identify as lesbian, these agencies may erroneously signal that lesbians are not at risk. Furthermore, safer sex messages directed to lesbians have emphasized prevention of woman-to-woman transmission despite the fact that the overwhelming experience of lesbians with AIDS is in a context of injection drug use and sex with men.[25,119,121,123,124]

Conclusions

Returning to our initial question—what accounts for the distribution of HIV among women in the United States—the data we have reviewed offer an explanation for causes of HIV incidence among women. Fundamental determinants of HIV risk among women include social inequality related to class, race/ethnicity, gender, and sexuality. This inequality and women's responses to it explain why the women most afflicted by AIDS in the United States are predominantly African American and Hispanic women living in conditions of economic hardship. Research explicitly investigating how social inequality affects women's risk of HIV is in its infancy and must be expanded.[125,126]

Surveying the first decade of public health efforts to understand and prevent the AIDS epidemic, Freudenberg concluded that "The future direction of this epidemic depends as much on what happens in the political arena as it does on new discoveries in the laboratories or on hospital wards. ... AIDS prevention effort has to be connected with a vision of a better world."[127] Research primarily concerned with measuring and promoting use of condoms and clean needles, sustaining energy of AIDS workers, and even "mobilizing communities to protect themselves," Freudenberg notes, will not be enough. Rather than promoting mostly defensive approaches that focus on "the negative image of protecting oneself from a deadly disease," he calls on us to imagine what it would mean to live in a world without AIDS, and to connect our daily lives to making it happen. The vision he invokes is one where everyone is entitled to comprehensive education about sexuality, drugs, and health; a world where those who need treatment for drug addiction can get it on demand; a world where basic health care is a right, not a privilege; a world where gay men and lesbians, women and people of color, are not discriminated against; a world where alternatives to drug use exist for the young people this country; a world where no one has to die on the streets because there is no home for them.[127]

What would it mean for epidemiologists and other public health researchers to integrate this vision into the daily work of HIV surveillance, research, and prevention efforts? We call on these investigators to draw upon social justice frameworks described earlier and in Table 1 to develop measurable surveillance tools.

To begin, surveillance data on HIV and AIDS among women can be linked to existing databases that routinely document social, economic, and political conditions at local, state, and national levels. A conceptually valid and cost-effective approach to adding socioeconomic data to HIV/AIDS surveillance records would be linking street addresses of cases to census data, using the technique of geocoding.[128] Census-based socioeconomic data at the level of census block-groups, which on average contain 1000 people, provide more valid descriptions than census tracts, which on average contain 4000 people. Block-groups tend to be more homogeneous with respect to social and economic composition.

Geocoding HIV/AIDS surveillance data to incorporate census-based socioeconomic information would permit characterizing socioeconomic conditions of neighborhoods (at the block-group level) and also of state economic areas and regional economies in relation to trends in HIV incidence and AIDS diagnoses. The same could be done with other routinely monitored health outcomes related to the AIDS epidemic, such as tuberculosis and selected STDs. Census data offer several markers of poverty, including population density, class composition, household income, percentage of female heads of household, adults with less than high school education, persons with income at a certain percentage of the poverty line, home ownership, and more.

Other links to surveillance data on the incidence of HIV and AIDS among women at the level of census block-groups include police data on frequency of domestic violence calls within block-groups boundaries; court records documenting frequency of restraining orders for streets within those block-groups; and arrests for drug-related activities, prostitution, and more explicit economic crimes, such as check forgery. Availability of civil services such as fire, police, public libraries, community centers, parks, playgrounds, and functional street lighting are examples of resources in neighborhoods that provide protection from as well as alternatives to drug-related crime. At the county, state, and regional level, it would also be possible to analyze data on occurrence of HIV among women in relation to public assistance programs, tax policies, and levels of industrialization. One application would be to develop what Friedman has named "AIDS impact statements," similar to the environmental impact statements that are now required to anticipate effects of diverse economic policies upon the environment.[129]

Research driven in part driven by descriptions emerging from expanded surveillance data would require development of valid measures of discrimination and subordination as well as resistance to inequality. Such data would provide documentation to advance legislative and regulatory action toward reducing HIV transmission and other conditions associated with economic and social deprivation, such as premature births and infant mortality, other effects of drug and alcohol use, violence, hypertension, and asthma, among many others. Examples of measurable social determinants of HIV infection among women are listed in Table 2. We recommend measuring these factors at the individual, household, neighborhood, and regional level and over women's lifetime.

It is likely that the moment of HIV transmission into women's bodies is a very private moment, whether in the embrace of a lover or shared injection of a drug. Yet the chosen or imposed isolation of this moment hardly measures the enormous public force that culminates in this irrevocable transference of viral particles. Social, economic, and political frameworks for HIV infection among women call for epidemiologists and other public health researchers to name and measure the impact of these public forces. We believe these factors are not immutable or inevitable but instead offer many opportunities for advancement in the development and implementation of public health policy and practice.

Summary Points

• The vast majority of women with AIDS in the United States are poor women of color, many of whom rely on male partners for economic support, housing, drugs, and protection. These women are likely to be unemployed, lack a high school education, and have a family annual income of less than $10 000.

• Racial discrimination, both on an economic and a noneconomic level, may increase risk of infection (greater exposure) and may impair immune function (greater transmission).

• Gender inequity with regard to sexual intercourse often precludes a woman from insisting on condom use (eg, fear of losing housing, material support, drug access, etc.).

• Women may face hostility from male partners if they participate in needle exchange or drug treatment programs, and they fear greater stigma and potential removal of children if they attend these interventions.

• Overall, the fundamental determinants of HIV risk among women include social inequality related to class, race/ethnicity, gender, and sexuality.

TABLE 1. Frameworks for Studying the Cause and Prevention of HIV Infection in Women

Framework	Assumptions	Possible Applications
Feminist	• Gender inequality affects health	• Gender disparity in power & risk of HIV
		• Gender differences in socially sanctioned sexual expression
		• Sexual & physical violence against women as determinants of HIV risk
		• Reproductive autonomy & HIV testing among pregnant women
Sociopolitical	• Economic & social relationships affect health	• Socioeconomic status & HIV infection
		• Social welfare policy, economic dependence on men, & risk of sexual HIV transmission to women
		• Racism & onset of drug use in women at risk of HIV infection
		• Reduction in municipal fire protection, destruction of housing, & HIV incidence
Ecosocial	• Biology interacts with social, economic, & political conditions to affect health	• Thinness of peripubescent vaginal mucosal lining & vaginal susceptibility to HIV infection among girls dependent on older men
		• Age-specific vaginal tract inflammation & HIV among women
Human Rights	• Violations of human rights affect patterns of disease	• Legal barriers to educating women & HIV incidence
		• HIV incidence among drug-using pregnant women in states that criminalize drug use during pregnancy
		• Enforcement of domestic violence & marital rape laws in relation to HIV incidence among women

TABLE 2. Measures of Social Inequality Related to HIV Incidence

Category	Markers
Economic	• Income (source, fluctuations, earnings, # supported, % federal poverty level) • Health insurance (including access to care) • Proportion of income for food, housing, medications, illegal drugs • Housing (status, crowding, quality, safety) • Transportation (public, private, shared) • Education (literacy, language, skills) • Recreation (access, affordability)
Political/legal	• Voter registration/participation & awareness of elected officials • Awareness of legal rights • Neighborhood activism & social advocacy • Workplace rights/organization • Awareness of eligibility for economic resources & how to access them • Police interactions (protection, arrest/incarceration, threats)
Racial/ethnic	• Racial/ethnic composition of neighborhood • Participation in cultural/ethnic events & resources • Experience with racially motivated discrimination • Participation in civil rights activities • Awareness of family history & ancestry
Gender	• Social & economic use of sex • Sexual identity • Sexual & reproductive autonomy • Awareness & use of women's health services

- Participation in women's groups (political, church, social, medical)
- Parenting & other caregiving responsibilities
- Marital/partner status
- Experience with discrimination (gender, sexual identity, martial/parent status)

Violence	• Experience of violence (related to race/ethnic group, gender, sexual identity)
	• Exposure to street, workplace, or home violence (victim, witness, participant)
	• Ownership or use of weapon (gun, knife, mace, other)
	• Response to violence (observed, experienced, inflicted)
	• Gang membership (self, partner, friend, family)
Networks	• Family, friends, sexual partners
	• Spiritual
	• Workplace
	• Drug-related (use, prevention, treatment, needle exchange)
	• Network membership turnover

CHAPTER 7

Gender Equity in HIV/AIDS Clinical Trials

Carola Marte, Terry McGovern

G ender equity in HIV clinical research raises several distinct issues for a clinician or lawyer working with HIV-infected women. First, most HIV-infected women come from impoverished communities that are underserved, "hard to reach" and historically underrepresented in clinical trials. Second, sex-specific data and studies have been neglected for all women, especially low-income women, and even more so low-income, HIV-infected women. Third, reproductive risk (ie, endangerment of fetuses or children) represents a commonly cited obstacle to the participation of women in clinical trials.

Since the 1980s, HIV/AIDS clinical trials have depended heavily on enrollment of gay white male subjects: those individuals who had knowledgeable personal physicians, or who attended HIV clinics at academic centers and were often eager to explore new therapies for their life-threatening illness. By comparison, women, persons of color, and drug users, who increasingly bear the burden of the epidemic from a demographic standpoint, remain under-enrolled and are slow to benefit from the newest antiviral medications.

However, for more than a decade, women have had the steepest annual increases in rates of reported AIDS cases. A 63% increase in female AIDS cases from 1991 to 1995 was the greatest rate of increase for any subpopulation defined by sex, race/ethnicity, or mode of transmission.[1] Rates among men but not women began to decline in 1996.[2] In 1992, heterosexual transmission overtook intravenous drug use as the primary risk factor for HIV infection in US women,[3] and sexual exposure is the only risk factor for most younger and adolescent women, who will appear in Centers for Disease Control and Prevention (CDC) statistics as persons with AIDS when they reach their 20s.[4,5]

Neglect of Women in the HIV/AIDS Epidemic

Historically, women's health has been overlooked by clinical investigators.

Female symptoms, illness, and treatments rarely serve as the focus of major research efforts.[6-8] Until recently, women were excluded from most large studies on hypertension[9] and coronary disease,[10] usually on the grounds that they dilute the homogeneity of an all-male population and are subject to cyclical hormonal changes that could influence drug pharmacodynamics.

This neglect has been especially discriminatory among HIV-infected women.[11-14] The HIV epidemic was characterized early on as one of gay men and Intravenous Drug Users (IDUs). A common misconception is that women became infected much later than men and in insignificant numbers. The epidemic in women was ignored for nearly a decade, and research in HIV-infected women was delayed even longer.

Indeed, in 1981, after receiving early reports of *Pneumocystis carinii* pneumonia (PCP), Kaposi sarcoma, and other opportunistic infections in young gay men in San Francisco, New York, and Los Angeles, the CDC began monitoring a newly recognized constellation of diseases called AIDS.[15] The surveillance focused on disease progression in primarily white gay male populations. The case definition of AIDS was expanded in 1985 and again in 1987.[16] In 1987, the addition of extrapulmonary tuberculosis, wasting syndrome, and encephalopathy resulted in a 25% increase in reported AIDS cases.[17] While these cases occurred primarily among heterosexual African American and Hispanic individuals and included high numbers of IDUs, the definition still omitted important disabling conditions common to women and poor communities.[18]

The CDC's narrow surveillance excluded illness already in existence prior to the advent of HIV but exacerbated in a person infected with HIV. In other words, when defining AIDS, the CDC did not allow for the possibility of converging epidemics.[19] By October 1990, several studies linked HIV infection with higher mortality and morbidity rates in persons with pulmonary tuberculosis[20] and bacterial pneumonia.[21] Studies also indicated that HIV-infected women were at greater risk for a more aggressive form of cervical disease[22] and a spectrum of gynecologic and sexually transmitted diseases, including pelvic inflammatory disease.[23]

Many HIV-infected women had severe undiagnosed and untreated gynecologic problems, and most were not receiving routine care. The rate of abnormal Pap tests among HIV-infected women was many times higher than that usually seen in populations with high rates of sexually tranmitted diseases (STDs). Yet no published studies or data addressed either abnormal Pap tests or other common gynecologic conditions in HIV-infected women at that time.[24]

As the HIV epidemic moved into its second decade, a few clinicians, alarmed at the neglect of the gynecologic disease they were observing, began to collect data. One early study was a review of abnormal Pap test rates by a small group of women professionals. The decision to pool the results of their clinic experiences for presentation at the Sixth International AIDS conference was a calculated response to the disturbing disregard of a major and potentially precancerous gynecological condition, cervical dysplasia, that was neither being researched nor appropriately diagnosed and treated in HIV-infected women.[25] That the study provided data on a larger number of women than previously described resulted directly from the clinicians' longstanding experience in women's health. Each had gone against the grain of prevailing infectious disease practices by establishing on-site gynecologic services for their patients.

Around the same time, HIV-infected women and their advocates began to challenge the very definition of AIDS. On October 1, 1990, a class-action lawsuit filed against Louis W. Sullivan, MD, Secretary of the US Department of Health and Human Services (DHHS),[26] alleged that the Social Security Administration was denying disability benefits to many claimants who were physically disabled by HIV disease. The plaintiffs were severely disabled with HIV-related illnesses, yet adjudged "able to work" because they did not have "AIDS." In December 1991, more individuals intervened in the lawsuit.[27] The plaintiffs claimed that the CDC surveillance definition was unduly restrictive and excluded the illnesses experienced by women and low-income individuals.

Pressure created by the litigation and research, along with the evolution of a strong grassroots movement, forced the federal government to expand its definition of disabling HIV disease and AIDS. On July 2, 1993, in the context of the emerging litigation, the Social Security Administration established a new and final listing for the evaluation of HIV infection.[28] This listing includes conditions common to women and other low-income populations.[29] In November 1993, the CDC announced that it was expanding the surveillance definition, effective January 1, 1994, to include the three conditions that the community had proposed: recurrent pulmonary tuberculosis, bacterial pneumonia, and advanced cervical disease, as well as any HIV-positive individual with CD4? counts of 200 or less.[30]

The first major prospective study of a gynecological condition, the

New York Cervical Dysplasia Study, began enrolling in 1991, 12 years after the initial reports of AIDS in women. The Women's Interagency HIV Study (WIHS), the major women's natural history study, began enrolling only in late 1994. Thus, the natural history of HIV in the absence of anti-retroviral interventions can no longer be elucidated for women as it has been for men in industrialized nations.

Government Policy on Women as Research Subjects

The dominant issue of gender equity in clinical research, at least in public health and governmental policy, has been the exclusion of women from clinical trials on behalf of their future offspring. Concern over unknown mutagenic and teratologic effects has provided a rationale for excluding all women of "child bearing potential," that is, any premenopausal woman who is not surgically sterilized. Since HIV is contracted most often by younger women, this practice excludes nearly all HIV-infected women from clinical trials. As with hazardous occupational exposures, the risks arising to offspring from paternal exposure in clinical trials have been disregarded.[31-33]

In addition, virtually all sex-specific HIV research until the past few years examined women as vectors (ie, sex workers or pregnant women). In a 1993 review of HIV publications referring to women, the subject of nearly one half was vertical transmission, and less than 1% were concerned with gynecologic disease or female-specific conditions.[34] The predominant research objective has been to prevent transmission to men and infants rather than to learn how HIV manifests in women themselves or how physicians can best manage HIV in their female patients.

In fact, since the mid-1970s, the exclusion of pregnant women from clinical trials was codified in a regulation entitled "Additional Protections Pertaining to Research, Development, and Related Activities Involving Fetuses, Pregnant Women, and Human in Vitro Fertilization."[35] The purpose of this regulation—evidenced in the title by placement of the fetus first—is to put unborn children at minimal risk. The regulation further requires that the "father of the fetus" give his consent to the pregnant women's participation in research. In this case, the fetus, not the women, is treated as the trial participant.

For many years, the Food and Drug Administration (FDA) directly encouraged the exclusion of women from clinical trials. A 1977 FDA guideline barred women of childbearing potential from early phases of clinical trials or until certain segments of animal reproduction studies were completed.[36] Although women with life-threatening disease (eg, HIV/AIDS) were an exception, drug companies routinely excluded women with AIDS from the early phases of clinical drug trials.

Medically, the 1977 guideline denied treatment for women, ignored the potential reproductive effects a given drug may have on men, and ignored the importance of sex differences in drug research. Although the analysis of sex-related drug response differences is necessary if the FDA is to fulfill its mandate, one major consequence of the 1977 guideline was the marketing of drugs that were not tested in women. Thus, the adverse effects of a given drug might be discovered only after the drug had been marketed for the general public (including women of child-bearing potential), rendering the labeling for women inadequate.[37] Not surprisingly, physicians complain of a general lack of understanding as to how a drug will affect women and an unawareness of a drug's side effects in women.[38]

A 1988 FDA guideline suggested a by-sex analysis, but the analysis outlined would detect only relatively large sex-related differences not likely to be clinically important. In addition, the trial sponsors were not mandated to undertake the suggested analyses. They were only required to report the total numbers of men and women enrolled. If the sponsor did comply and pharmacodynamic differences were indicated, a sponsor could, but was not required to, conduct additional studies.

Beginning in 1990, the HIV Law Project represented many women who were excluded from Phase I trials due to their reproductive potential or who were forced to use surgical or detectable birth control. Clearly the FDA's policies were obstructing the access of HIV-infected women to clinical trials.[39] On December 15, 1992, the HIV Law Project, the NOW Legal Defense and Education Fund, and the American Civil Liberties Union AIDS Project submitted a citizen petition requesting the Commissioner of the FDA to amend the 1977 FDA guideline as discriminatory.[40]

On July 22, 1993, the FDA published a "Guideline for the Study and Evaluation of Gender Differences in the Clinical Evaluation of Drugs" as a revision of the 1977 FDA guideline.[41] The 1993 guideline states that "in some cases, there may be a basis for requiring participation of women in early studies." The disease must be "serious and affect women" and "especially when a promising drug for the disease is being developed and made available rapidly under the FDA's accelerated approval or early access procedures." In these instances, the guideline states that a case can be made for requiring the participation of women in clinical trials at early stages.[42]

However, the 1993 guideline still allows trial sponsors to exclude women of childbearing potential, whether or not evidence of fetal toxicity exists, and it does not define the criteria used in determining whether a significant risk to the fetus exists.[43] Specifically:[44]

> Except in the case of trials intended for the study of drug effects during pregnancy, clinical protocols should include measures that will minimize the possibility of fetal exposure to the investigational drug. These would ordinarily include providing for the use of a reliable method of contraception (or abstinence) for the duration of drug exposure (which may exceed the length of the study), use of pregnancy testing (beta HCG) to detect unsuspected pregnancy prior to initiation of study treatment, and timing of studies (easier with studies of short duration) to coincide with, or immediately follow, menstruation.

While recommending mandatory birth control and pregnancy testing for all women of childbearing potential, the FDA simply suggests a risk-benefit analysis for men of child-producing capacity.[45] The risk-benefit analysis need only be performed if reproductive studies have shown abnormalities of reproductive organs or their functions (ie, if abnormal sperm production has been observed in experimental animals).

It is important to note that, at least in some cases, teratogenicity can be traced to alterations in the male gamete.[46] Mutagenic effects of a drug are likely to be more intensified in men because male germ cells, due to their rapid multiplication, are more susceptible to the effects of mutagens than are female germ cells.[47] These findings have been interpreted to mean that males of reproductive potential who participate in clinical trials might also cause harm to their potential offspring.[48] Significant evidence indicates that generational male-mediated effects do occur.[49]

The 1993 guideline emphasizes that women, not men and women, should be fully informed of the status of the animal reproduction studies and of any other information about the teratogenic potential of the drug. If the animal reproduction studies are not complete, the 1993 guideline states that other pertinent information should be provided, such as a general assessment of fetal toxicity in drugs with related properties. The 1993 guideline goes on to state that "if no relevant information is available, the informed consent should specifically note the potential for fetal risk."[50] However, such informed consent often excludes pregnant women with life-threatening illnesses.[51] Thus, the FDA is in effect shirking its duty to investigate the risk of adverse reproductive effects and shifting the responsibility for avoiding fetal toxicity or generational effects exclusively to women.[52]

In contrast, the National Institutes of Health (NIH) has worked to a certain degree to overcome gender inequity in clinical trials. In 1986, the NIH published a statement urging applicants to include women in clinical studies.[53] A 1987 inventory of all research activities found that only 13.5% of the NIH budget was spent on women's health issues.[54] Subsequent investigations by the General Accounting Office (GAO) found that the NIH's stated policy had not been implemented throughout the agency.[55] NIH officials had not required or even requested that researchers analyze study results by sex.[55] Later GAO investigations confirmed earlier findings that women were generally underrepresented in the trials surveyed, and although there were enough women enrolled in some trials to detect sex-related differences in response, the data were not so analyzed.[55]

In March 1994, the NIH established guidelines on the inclusion of women and minorities and their subpopulations in research involving human subjects, including clinical trials. The NIH's 1994 guideline added three major conditions to previous policy. Women, minorities, and subpopulations must be included in all human subject research and specifically in Phase III clinical trials so valid analyses of differences in intervention effect can be established. In addition, cost was no longer an acceptable reason for excluding these groups, and outreach efforts were to be initiated to recruit these groups into clinical studies.

However, several exceptions render the recommendations quite weak.[56] Women and minorities can be excluded if the clinical research is inappropriate with respect to the health of the participants or to the purpose of the research. For clinical trials, the participation of these population groups is not required if scientific data demonstrate no significant difference exists in the effects of the variables studied on women or members of a minority group compared with the general population. Women and minorities can also be excluded if their inclusion is deemed inappropriate under such other circumstances as the director of the NIH may designate. Moreover, these guidelines have no enforcement mechanism.

Liability Concerns

Many pharmaceutical trial sponsors assert that the risk of future liability for the teratogenic effects of drugs tested on fertile women is sufficient to justify a blanket exclusion of women of childbearing potential from the early phases of clinical trials. Any question of the adequacy of the informed consent could conceivably come before a jury; even though a plaintiff might never prevail, defending such a lawsuit would be expensive. Federal policy makers assert that a mandate to include women in industry-sponsored clinical research would be a disincentive for drug development.

Currently, regardless of whether a drug is toxic to fetuses or has reproductive effects, a woman will be asked to use hormonal contraception or surgical and detectable barriers and pregnancy testing. Historically, pharmaceutical companies have been overzealous in their application of this proviso to require "detectable" birth control. For women fighting severe HIV-related gynecological infections, the requirement of "detectable" birth control has prevented their enrollment in trials.

In reality, the unjustified exclusion of women may result in greater and more immediate liability for trial sponsors than would careful, informed inclusion. Under the equal protection clause's standard for review of government action that discriminates against women, such a policy can only be sustained if the party seeking to uphold it shows by "exceedingly persuasive justification" that the classification serves "important governmental objectives and that the discriminatory means employed are substantially related to the achievement of those objectives."[57] Wholesale exclusion of women from the early phases of drug trials cannot be used as a proxy for an analysis of reproductive effects; the Supreme Court has held time and again that "administrative convenience" cannot serve as a rationale to justify sex discrimination.[58] FDA policies regulating experimental drug trials must therefore meet constitutional equal protection requirements. This is particularly true where, as in the HIV and AIDS context, access to the experiment may itself be of significant benefit.

In addition to the equal protection clause, the 1977 FDA guideline also violated women's constitutional right to privacy, which has been interpreted by the Supreme Court to guarantee autonomy in the exercise of reproductive choice. For women who are not pregnant and women in the early stages of pregnancy, the constitutional right to privacy and autonomy outweighs any nonspecific governmental interest in avoiding fetal toxicity.[59] By supporting the exclusion of women of childbearing potential from drug trials—an exclusion that, in practice, extends to women with life-threatening diseases seeking treatment—the 1977 guideline placed an undue burden on these women's exercise of reproductive choice.[60]

The FDA has allowed the pharmaceutical industry's assumption that the exclusion of women minimizes the potential liability of drug manufacturers to drive federal policy.[61] However, this fear of liability does not justify differential treatment based on sex, particularly in an experimental setting.[62] Since the drugs tested in clinical trials are by definition experimental and are not being marketed to the general public, strict liability does not apply. Manufacturers can guard against potential liability in negligence by scrupulous use of adequate warnings and informed consent. Nonetheless, the pharmaceutical industry has been reluctant to change their exclusionary practices despite recent changes in FDA policy that encourage sex-specific analysis of data and inclusion of fertile women in earlier phase trials and the inclusion of pregnant women in the case of an incurable illness such as AIDS.[63] On average, women are enrolled in clinical trials for unlicensed HIV/AIDS drugs 9 to 12 months before completion of animal studies.[64,65]

In June 2000, the FDA published a regulation that would permit it to place a clinical hold on investigational studies of drugs for life-threatening illness if reproductive potential is a criterion for excluding otherwise eligible subjects. The FDA's expressed concern is over the ongoing exclusion of women from some clinical trials on these grounds despite its previous guidelines affirming the potential for therapeutic benefit from inclusion and the lack of a convincing rationale for exclusion.[66] This regulation had been drafted in 1995 by the HIV Law Project and was proposed and approved by the National Task Force on AIDS Drug Development that same year. However, four and one-half years elapsed before the FDA published it as a regulation.

Consequences of Excluding Women

The importance of publishing sex analysis of clinical trials data was underscored in the influential 1992 GAO report[67] and subsequently by the FDA.[68,69] Sex effects are acknowledged to be of significance and have been clearly demonstrated, including those relating to drug pharmacokinetics, efficacy, and toxicity.[70-72] A recent study reported that blood levels of delavridine, an antiretroviral drug, were higher in women than men in a study of combination therapy.[73] Several recent studies have noted differences between women and men in their experience of adverse effects to protease inhibitors, which has implications for adherence to and therefore efficacy of these regimens.[74,75]

Women have been excluded particularly on the grounds that female hormonal variations complicate data interpretation and require larger and more costly enrollments for studies. But a more compelling argument would be that hormonal changes require enrollment of women to understand potential hormonal influences on pharmacologic agents.[76] Clinicians have little information about whether menstrual cycles or endogenous hormonal changes from HIV infection itself should be taken into account in selection or dosing of antiretroviral agents. Exogenous hormonal therapies such as contraceptives are known to have metabolic interactions with many of the antiretroviral agents. The changes in blood levels of contraceptive hormonal agents varies with different HIV medications, causing either increases or decreases in an unpredictable pattern depending on which antiviral is involved. Many medications now carry explicit warnings about potentially lower effectiveness of oral contraceptives in women on certain antiretrovirals, but the clinical significance of these interactions has not been studied and is not known.

Lack of data on the safety and efficacy of medications during pregnancy presents the same difficulties. The current standard of care requires clinicians to recommend combination therapy with multiple antiretroviral agents. When prescribing these agents for pregnant women, information on the safety or dosing of combination therapies for the woman or her fetus are severely limited. Azidothmidine (AZT) monotherapy prevents at least two thirds of neonatal infections and has an acceptable safety profile in the short run for infants. Long-term risks, including for the more than two thirds of children who will not be infected, are unknown. Some preliminary evidence suggests the possibility of carcinogenic[77] and neurotoxic complications.[78] What level of risk is acceptable for neonates, most of whom will be uninfected, should be an issue of active debate.

The lack of longitudinal and natural history of HIV in women also affects clinical trials. Quantification of HIV "viral load" in blood specimens and of the immune system's CD4? cells are commonly used as surrogate markers to guide when to initiate antiretroviral therapy or prophylaxis against opportunistic infections. Although applied to the care of women as well as men, this surrogate marker information has been derived from male subjects, primarily from those in the MACS observational cohort, which enrolled exclusively gay male subjects, mostly Caucasian.

In reviewing applications for new drugs against HIV, the FDA accepts use of these surrogate markers as endpoints in clinical trials as a way to speed up approval and marketing of effective agents because these data can be collected much more rapidly than data on clinical outcome. In the third decade of the HIV epidemic, data suggest that women may have lower viral loads than men at the same stage of disease.[79,80] If this proves to be true, clinical guidelines may need to be modified for women.

Due to the late start for research on gynecologic problems of HIV-infected women, adequate data do allow for use of female-specific clinical benchmarks for HIV progression (eg, recurrent vaginal yeast or bacterial vaginosis) in clinical trials.[81,82] In addition, clinical trials of treatments for gynecologic conditions have not been adequately addressed. For example, the increased risk of cervical dysplasia in women who are HIV infected has been well established, but clinical trials on treatments for dysplasia are still ongoing, and no data are available to guide treatment decisions.

Data from clinical trials that enroll selected cohorts may not be applicable to clinical care of patients at large.[83-85] Patients face substantial hurdles in dealing with multiple medications, unpleasant side effects, and difficult dosing regimens. Protease inhibitors, the backbone of highly active antiviral therapy (HAART) regimens, are particularly demanding, and trying to match medication requirements of up to a dozen pills two or three times daily with normal family routines is unlikely to be successful. Many patients who cannot adhere to the required schedules may decide (especially if they understand that strict adherence is required to avoid resistance and failure of the therapy) to defer use of antiretroviral medications, even when this is inadvisable given their stage of disease.

Given its importance on measuring clinical effectiveness and pharmacologic efficacy, improving such adherence should be a research priority.[86,87] However, behavioral issues have barely been addressed in HIV research, despite the impact of depression, unstable housing, domestic violence, and active substance use on adherence and retention in clinical trials as well as in clinical care. If ease of adherence and minimization of side effects were considered a priority, clinical trial regimens and measures of treatment outcome would be designed differently from the outset.

Trends in Recent HIV Clinical Trials

The issue of diversity in clinical trials has been taken seriously by the HIV professional community. Discussion has paralleled, or even preceded, the revised policies of federal agencies.[88] By 1990, a consensus was building that HIV clinical trials should enroll representatives of those populations for whom the medications were intended, both to capture differences arising from sex or ethnic/racial differences and to ensure equal access to the perceived benefits of research care and medications. These concepts were formally discussed during conferences on HIV/AIDS clinical trials at Tufts in 1992[89] and at the Institute of Medicine in 1993.[90]

In trials funded by federal agencies or nonprofit organizations such as American Foundation for AIDS Research (AMFAR) and Community Research Initiative on AIDS (CRIA), efforts were made to increase enrollment of women, minorities, and past or present substance users through intensified recruitment, less stringent exclusion criteria, and allocation of increased resources to improve retention. Investigators recognized that subjects from populations who feared misuse or had experienced stigma could not readily be recruited into traditional academic research settings.[91] In part to improve accrual and in part to increase diversity, the National Institute of Allergy and Infectious Disease (NIAD) established a Community Program for Clinical Research on AIDS (CPCRA) as a kind of affiliate and complementary agency to the AIDS Clinical Trial Group (ACTG). Establishing the CPCRA clinical trial track made it possible to locate some of these research centers in health care institutions where impoverished populations receive their medical care.

Federally funded NIAID programs, especially the ACTG and CPCRA, record demographics for individual protocols. Industry trials include demographics when the results are published in professional journals, but no composite trade source exists for this information. In 1991 the Pharmaceutical Manufacturers Association (PMA) issued a report stating that most major industry trials collect data on gender differences.[92] However, these data are not available through PMA. Most industry trials of HIV medications still do not include sex-specific analysis of their results, and enrollment remains heavily weighted toward gay white males.

In a report on ACTG accrual of women from 1987 to 1990, 6.7% of ACTG participants were female at a time when 9.8% of reported AIDS cases nationally were in women. Just over half of the enrolled women were nonwhite, compared with 73% of AIDS cases in women nationally. Among female ACTG participants, 23% were past or present intravenous drug users (nearly all were past users), compared with 51% nationally.[93]

Between 1990 and 1993, female ACTG enrollment increased from 6.7% to 11.4%. For comparison, 19.3 % of CPCRA accrual during this period was female.[94] Most of the increase was attributable to two protocols, both beginning accrual in 1991: ACTG 076, the AZT perinatal transmission study (26% of all women who were newly enrolled in any ACTG trial in 1992 were in this study) and ACTG 175, for which recruitment of women was a specific goal.[95]

Overall, a significantly greater proportion of women enrolled was involved in treatment studies of asymptomatic individuals (eg, those with less advanced HIV disease).[96] Such trials investigate whether drugs already tested in advanced AIDS patients may work as an early intervention. By contrast, women were less well represented in Phase III trials designed for individuals with advanced disease. They were also less well represented in Phase I and II trials, where benefits and toxicity of new experimental regimens are first defined. Phase I and II trials generally have relatively small enrollment compared with Phase III trials, but exclusion of women from early trials has important ramifications, as discussed earlier in this chapter.

ACTG protocol 175 compared AZT monotherapy with combination therapy for individuals in early stages of HIV infection. A specific enrollment goal of at least 15% women was set, and gynecologic and adherence substudies were included. The protocol succeeded in enrolling 18% women, the highest proportion for any ACTG clinical trial open to both sexes. One factor in the final study design was the establishment of an ACTG Women's Health Committee in 1991.[97] With its conscious and successful effort to enroll a representative number of women, ACTG 175 had a noticeable impact on ACTG accruals. The 444 women who participated in this particular protocol represent 7.5% of cumulative female accruals from 1987 through 1996.

By May 1997, the cumulative proportion of women enrolled in ACTG protocols (since 1987) reached 15%.[98] At this time, women represented 20% of AIDS cases reported to CDC.[99] However, the ACTG figures include persons with HIV infection who do not yet have AIDS as well as those with AIDS. Since the annual rate of increase of HIV is greater in women than in men, the proportion of women with HIV is higher than that of women with AIDS. CDC has estimated that 30% of HIV infection reported in 1996 was in women[100]—twice the percentage of adult women enrolled in ACTG trials.

Comparisons with national statistics are necessarily imprecise for several reasons. ACTG demographics are published as cumulative totals, not annualized figures. Although annual totals are available for the number of subjects enrolled in active studies (a subject is counted in each calendar year he or she participates in a given protocol), demographic ACTG data are published only as cumulative totals. In addition, ACTG enrollment figures represent accruals, not participants (eg, one individual enrolled in two trials is counted twice). Data are not available on whether multiple ACTG enrollments show sex or ethnic/racial differences. Overall, demographic analyses that would provide the foundation for a policy ensuring equitable access to ACTG clinical trials are not available.

Table 1 shows the proportion of female and male ACTG accrual. Combining adult and pediatric accrual distorts the apparent proportion of women involved because younger subjects are recruited equally. In fact, perinatal trials, together with two small gynecological trials (112 enrollees), represent nearly a quarter (24%) of total adult female accrual. Subtracting such accruals in women-only trials shows that women represent 11% of total adult accrual in ACTG clinical trial protocols for HIV therapies tested in both sexes.

Although calculations based on cumulative ACTG data seem less impressive when broken down, women clearly made significant gains in the 1990s. The overall participation of women in clinical trials increased; there was one large and important antiretroviral trial that successfully enrolled close to the national proportion of women with AIDS and that also included gynecologic endpoints; and some gynecological treatment protocols have entered trial. In contrast to cumulative data, the ACTG data on the proportion of women enrolled in active studies in a given year show a gain from 12% in 1991 to 25% in 1996 (including studies addressing perinatal transmission of HIV from pregnant women to their infants).

Unfortunately, some of these gains may be lost. In 1996, NIAID held a competitive renewal for ACTG sites. Seven sites were discontinued, including one minority site (institutions with over 50% minority patients) and six from the urban Northeast. Of seven sites nationally that had succeeded in enrolling 20% or more women, four were not renewed in 1996 (three in New York City and one in New Haven).[101] More than one half of the women enrolled in New York City had been enrolled by the sites that were discontinued. SUNY-Brooklyn alone had accrued up to one third of women and minority participants involved in trials nationally, including the only significant ACTG gynecologic clinical trial (cervical dysplasia treatments).[102] Middle West and West/Northwest sites, whose relative representation in the ACTG was increased in 1996, enroll a proportion more representative of the background seroprevalence rates in their geographic areas.[103] They enroll fewer total women than do Northeastern sites, where the absolute number of infected women is enormous, approaching half of the national total.[104] One quarter of national female AIDS cases are reported from New York City alone.[105]

Only perinatal transmission trials are likely to escape this trend, but their success in reducing rates of vertical transmission will be compromised if the absolute number of infected women continues to escalate. Improving HIV prevention strategies and access to prenatal care, especially for marginalized women, will be essential for reducing the number of neonatal infections and, especially, orphaned children. If infection rates among women are not reduced, the number of uninfected as well as infected children who become orphaned during childhood by the death of their HIV-infected mothers will continue to climb.[106-108] Indeed, the number of orphans is estimated to be as high as 125 000 to 150 000 children by the year 2000.

Increasingly in HIV medicine, access to clinical trials not only represents better care;[109-111] it often serves as the only access to care. This is in part because HIV is a life-threatening disease without a cure, and experimental therapies provide a last resort. Largely through the efforts of gay advocacy groups, promising treatment options are available in clinical trials well before they achieve FDA approval, even allowing for the remarkably accelerated approval that is now accorded to many new anti-retrovirals. In an increasing number of states, clinical trials provide the only access for most patients to expensive therapies. Many states now ration HIV medications, especially protease inhibitors, available through Medicaid or federal drug assistance programs because of their unwillingness or inability to provide additional funds to ensure access to these "standard" recommended therapies for all HIV-infected persons.

Little evidence suggests that women should be excluded from HIV/AIDS clinical trials on the grounds that they are noncompliant or difficult to recruit.[77-113] Women have been successfully recruited in clinical trials, including many of the ACTG and CPCRA sites.[114] Significantly, the best accrual rates tend to be at sites with female principal investigators.[115]

The same influence of provider gender has been observed in clinical care generally.[116]

Recruitment and retention of women for research protocols do not present different problems than ensuring access to effective health care. A large number of HIV-infected women wish to participate in research, often motivated by a desire to increase knowledge about HIV in women[117] apart from their personal need for potentially life-saving therapy. The under-enrollment of women in research has arisen in part because many career researchers are not actively engaged in clinical care and therefore are inexperienced with the necessary remedies for barriers to access. Participation by low-income women in clinical trials requires material support (eg, child care and transportation) and access to essential health-related services. Treatment for psychiatric illness and chemical dependency are of particular importance due to the severe shortage of these services exactly in those communities with the highest prevalence and greatest need.

Successful enrollment of women with HIV/AIDS as research subjects means recognizing and correcting the traditional problems for women in our health care system as a whole, especially fragmentation of services for women and their children and inadequate support services. It has been argued that providing these services to ensure participation of women in research is an unjustified expense, and that access to clinical trials is not an entitlement. However, excluding women from research because adequate health care services are not available in the first place is compounding one inequity with another.

Conclusions

An analysis of the history of efforts to achieve gender equity in HIV/AIDS clinical trials highlights the importance of advocacy efforts integrating the expertise of physicians, legal advocates, and a patient/client-based grassroots coalition. Were it not for the combined efforts of these forces, the FDA might never have lifted the 1977 restriction on the inclusion of women of childbearing potential in early phases of clinical trials. If physicians had not identified the woefully inadequate understanding of gynecological manifestations of HIV disease in women, and if activists had not been persistent in their efforts to protest the unfairness of resulting policies, litigation concerning the inadequacy of the AIDS definition could not have succeeded, and the federal government would not have initiated relevant research in women.

Significantly more advocacy is needed before we will achieve gender equity in clinical trials. In 1999, no regulation or guideline requires that women be included in statistically significant numbers in clinical trials or that sex-specific analysis be conducted. This remains true despite mounting evidence that additional sex analyses would yield more a ccurate dosing and side effect data for women. Bias and misconceptions continue to hinder recruitment efforts as well. The same coalition of legal, medical, and client/patients must continue to push the federal government to end the historical discrimination against women in drug development, particularly in the HIV/AIDS epidemic.

Summary Points

• Early surveillance of HIV focused on white gay male communities, and the definition of AIDS omitted conditions common to women. Mounting pressure forced the federal government in 1993 to include conditions found among women and low-income populations in its definition of HIV and AIDS.

• The first major prospective study of an HIV-related gynecological condition (cervical dysplasia) did not launch enrollment until 12 years after the initial reports of AIDS in women, and the only major study of the natural history of HIV in women began 15 years after these initial reports.

• The FDA actively encouraged the exclusion of women from drug trials for many years and recommended mandatory birth control and pregnancy testing of all women of childbearing potential. A June 2000 regulation now allows the FDA to suspend clinical trials of drugs for life-threatening illness if reproductive potential is a criterion for excluding otherwise eligible subjects.

• The NIH urged clinical investigators to include women in their studies but did not establish guidelines defining the level of participation required until 1994, and these guidelines allow exceptions that render the recommendations weak (and unenforceable).

• Pharmaceutical companies claim risk of future liability as justification for the exclusion of women rather than employ appropriate warnings and informed consent.

• Longitudinal and sex-specific data for women are lacking for all aspects of HIV and AIDS diagnosis, treatment, and monitoring despite known sex effects related to drug pharmacokinetics, efficacy, and toxicity.

• Women remain underrepresented in HIV and AIDS trials due to the early absence of recruitment goals, larger issues related to access to health care, and the loss of ACTG trial sites where HIV-infected women live.

TABLE 1. Cumulative ACTG Accrual by Sex (through May 1997)

	Female		Male	
	N	%	N	%
Children	4701	50%	4659	50%
Adolescents	386	48%	417	52%
Adult	6266	15%	35 705	85%
Total	11 353	22%	40 781	78%

Section III: Policy Implications

As this final section so clearly demonstrates, public health professionals have been at the forefront of the AIDS epidemic. Ongoing requirements for surveillance, screening, prevention, counseling, education, and clinical and social service referrals have stretched your efforts to the limit, and you have met each challenge in a timely and respectful manner. You have been forced to walk a fine line between meeting the broad needs of the whole population while not infringing on the personal rights of individual patients. You must continually consider the legal implications of planned strategies to control and monitor disease transmission. You have been pushed to adapt your traditional STD paradigm to this new and sometimes overwhelming infectious phenomenon. You have been obliged to make sense of different disease patterns throughout the world in populations stressed by a wide range of economic, social, and medical factors. Although many issues remain unresolved, you have been forced to work miracles ... and you have done so ... and the world is grateful.

CHAPTER 8

HIV as an STD

Sten H. Vermund, Sibylle Kristensen, Madhav P. Bhatta

H IV can be spread via infected blood or blood products, and from mother to child, either peripartum or via breast-feeding. These routes of transmission can be controlled.[1,2] However, the dominant route of HIV spread throughout the world is sexual. The straightforward statement that HIV is a sexually transmitted infection has proven controversial when traditional sexually transmitted disease (STD) control measures are proposed. This chapter places the HIV epidemic in a historical content, reviews the biological interaction of HIV with other STDs, and discusses the use of efficient STD-related public health measures to limit HIV spread.

Historical Perspectives on STD Control and HIV

Eighteenth and nineteenth century efforts to control STDs focused on female prostitution, considered the principal nidus of infection by the male-dominated political leadership.[3] European cities such as Paris and Berlin enacted laws requiring regular medical inspection and registration of female prostitutes and the reporting of all cases of syphilis and gonorrhea.[4] STDs were especially common among men in the armed forces.[5] The threat to military efficiency posed by the high incidence of syphilis and gonorrhea was apparent to political leaders, which led the English Parliament to require the registration and examination of prostitutes when STDs were found.[6] In St. Louis and Cincinnati, mandatory physical examination and segregation of infected prostitutes[4] proved more successful than similar measures in California, New York, Pennsylvania, and the District of Columbia.[7-9] Despite substantial legislation regulating prostitution on both sides of the Atlantic, these approaches had no measurable impact on the incidence of STDs.[10-12]

Notable advances were made in the field of venereology in the first decade of the 20th century. In 1905, German scientists Fritz Schaudinn and Erich Hoffmann identified *Treponema pallidum* as the causative agent of syphilis.[13] In 1909, immunologist Paul Ehrlich discovered salvarsan, an arsenical compound capable of killing the treponeme, and August Wassermann and his colleagues Neisser and Bruck developed the first good serologic test for syphilis.[14]

Scientific progress was accompanied by social and public health reform.[9] The Social Hygiene Movement (also known as the Purity Crusade) was a US coalition of physicians, public health and welfare workers, "purity" crusaders, and women's rights advocates who recognized that STDs were prevalent in the general population.[5] Their approach included improved medical and public health care, legislative changes, and a massive social hygiene educational campaign focused on increasing the public's fear of STD infection.[5] The social hygienists argued that unless people had basic knowledge about STDs, their modes of transmission, and their prevention, it would not be possible to reduce STD incidence. While the educational campaigns may have raised fear of infection, the stigma associated with STDs may likewise have been exacerbated, discouraging many persons from seeking care.[9]

By World War I (WWI), STDs were a major public health problem.[10] Deaths due to congenital syphilis in 1917 were 1 in 500 live births.[13] STDs were the leading cause of rejection from active duty in the military; one million men were rejected by the draft in 1918 for having syphilis.[6] Incapacitation of troops by STD symptoms was more common than war-related injury. The entry of the United States in WWI resulted in a major shift in the public and government attitude towards STDs and their control. Public concern about military readiness was strong enough to override opposition towards STD control efforts.[9] In 1917, the United States Public Health Service (USPHS) initiated a cooperative venereal disease (VD) control program in partnership with state and local health departments and with the private sector, including medical practitioners, hospitals, and voluntary agencies.[15] Since STDs in the military could not be controlled unless they were reduced in the general population as well, Congress created the Venereal Disease Control Division within the USPHS, appropriating funds for research and for administration of state treatment programs.[5] Its essential elements included case reporting, widespread availability of testing, the provision of arsphenamine, promotion of condom prophylaxis, establishment of treatment facilities, and public education programs conducted at the level of state and local health departments.[5]

After WWI, public and political interest in STD control diminished in the United States, and the US Congress cut funding in half.[6] In 1922, Congress discontinued altogether the appropriation for diagnosis and treatment clinics, and VD control programs were neglected for more than a decade.[5]

Rising STD rates were recognized as a health menace by leaders in the public health and medical communities.[13] In 1936, the Surgeon General of USPHS, Dr. Thomas Parran, revitalized the VD control programs, including such measures as:[9]

- a trained public health staff

- case finding through serological testing or Gram stain for gonorrhea

- premarital and prenatal serodiagnostic testing

- establishment of diagnostic services

- availability of treatment services

- distribution of drugs for treatment

- routine serodiagnostic testing

- a scientific information program including public education

Enough political support was obtained by Parran to permit launching key elements of the control effort. The high rejection rates among World War II (WW II) draftees due to syphilis and the increased absenteeism resulting among military personnel from syphilis and gonorrhea led to intensified STD control efforts.[13] Once again, STDs incapacitated many more troops than did war-related injuries.

The military STD control program combined massive education programs, condom advocacy and distribution, and prompt diagnosis and treatment without punitive measures.[13] The USPHS working with the Conference of State and Territorial Health Officers planned and implemented a nationwide civilian VD program. As in WW I, cooperative agreements were set up between the USPHS and the US military.[15] The control measures taken during WW II contributed to a decrease in the prevalence of syphilis from 271/100 000 in 1946, to 197/100 000 in 1949.[9]

Paradoxically, the discovery of the one-shot penicillin treatment for syphilis and the success of WW II control programs in both military and civilian sectors minimized the significance of STDs as a public health priority in the minds of the public and politicians.[14] While syphilis reached a nadir of 76 cases per 100 000 persons in 1955, the decline in STD rates was short-lived.[16] Between 1965 and 1975, cases of gonorrhea increased three-fold, rising to over 1 million per year.[16] Similarly, from the mid 1950s to the mid 1970s, cases of syphilis more than quadrupled.[17] Although some observers attribute this rise to the three Ps of the 1960s— permissiveness, promiscuity, and the Pill—little evidence suggests that any of these factors affected STD incidence.[9] However, when government spending on VD control programs peaked in the early 1950s, the rate of infections dropped to their lowest point.[14] Cutbacks in government funding for STD programs in late 1950s and early 1960s was reflected by the rise in the rates of reported STDs.[13]

STD rates continued to rise in the mid to late 1970s, particularly among men having sex with men (MSM).[18] The emergence of gay and bisexual men from the shadows of society in this time period was accompanied by a relaxed sexual standard, particularly in larger cities where there was safety and comfort in numbers.[18,19] The Castro district in San Francisco, parts of West Los Angeles and Hollywood, and Greenwich Village in New York City were but a few well-known neighborhoods where men felt at ease with their sexual orientation.[18] Similarly, in other cities around the world, MSM felt disinhibited from their repressed sexuality of decades past, and this relaxation was accompanied by an increase in STDs.[18-20] The incidence of intestinal parasites such as *Giardia lamblia* and *Entamoeba histolytica*, viral infections such as hepatitis B and herpes simplex virus type II, bacterial infections such as syphilis, anal and oral gonorrhea, and chlamydia, and even unknown conditions rose markedly. The most lethal of these was HIV.

Overview of HIV Epidemic

As described in Chapter 1, HIV has been demonstrated to be a zoonosis of higher primate origin.[21] With economic and political disruptions, large-scale migrations from rural to urban Africa brought HIV to new locations where sexual behaviors were not limited by traditional taboos and family or tribal customs. High partner exchange rates are not uncommon in settings where men are working or fighting in wars far from their families and where female prostitutes (ie, commercial sex workers, professional sex workers) are available. The rapid spread of HIV to Europe, the Caribbean, and North America in the 1970s with the explosive incidence among persons with high risk exposure (MSM, high risk women, blood and blood product recipients, intravenous drug users [IDUs], and infants born to HIV-infected mothers) all occurred in the context of high partner exchange rates, particularly among MSM and IDUs.[24]

In the 1980s, HIV spread virtually unchecked in Africa resulted in the world's highest urban and rural HIV rates, with rising rates of death,[25,26] orphans,[27] and economic chaos from loss of economically productive age groups.[28] In the late 1980s, the pandemic had spread to Asia, where it spread at a rate similar to that in Africa a decade earlier. The highest rates in the Americas were reported from Haiti and Guyana, the poorest nations in the Western Hemisphere.[29] Industrialized nations experienced large HIV epidemics compared with neighboring countries, including Brazil, the United States, Spain, and Italy.[26]

By the 1990s, the epidemic had leveled somewhat in many countries, in part due to the impact of prevention messages and programs, many promulgated by community-based organizations in peer education formats. Thailand turned the corner on its massive epidemic with programs targeting sex workers and sexual behaviors among young men, advocating 100% condom use in brothels.[30] In Uganda, educational programs likewise reduced reported seroincidence in both urban Kampala and rural areas.[31] In a clinical trial in northwest Tanzania, the control of STDs was shown clearly to reduce HIV transmission.[32] In Rwanda, the use of counseling and testing among couples whose infection status was discordant seemed to cut HIV transmission rates in half.[33]

Lessons learned worldwide in HIV control include relearning tried and true measures of STD control. Availability of STD preventive and curative services correlated inversely with degree of risk for HIV seroconversion in Zaire.[34] Active contact tracing in North Carolina worked much better than a passive partner-referral approach to inform sexual contacts that they had been exposed to HIV, with the former permitting counseling, testing, and, when needed, early treatment.[35] Colorado used contact tracing for HIV and HIV reporting in the 1980s, which correlated with the epidemic being kept to a minimum.[36] Other reports from around the world suggested that peer outreach education, STD control measures (including partner reduction and condom use), protection of the blood supply, use of sterile syringes and needles for medical use and among substance abusers, drug and alcohol treatment programs, and, in some settings, counseling and testing (particularly of discordant couples) all helped to reduce HIV seroincidence.[37,38]

Based on the past 20 years of epidemic spread, projections can be made for trends worldwide. The incipient epidemic of HIV in Eastern Europe will expand from IDUs to their sexual contacts and to infants of pregnant women, expanding the HIV problem into the general population. Tuberculosis, already on the rise in parts of Eastern Europe and Russia, will extend its reach, including multiple drug-resistant strains, in parallel with the spread of HIV. The African epidemic will continue at the highest seroprevalence in the world, replenished by young people entering the at-risk pool. The Asian epidemic will continue to expand with spread into subgroups that experience high-risk exposure but have not demonstrated many HIV cases to date, including Nepal, Bangladesh, Pakistan, and parts of India and Sri Lanka.[38-40] Based on rising STD rates, China and Mongolia will also experience a heavier HIV burden.[41-45] The epidemic in Latin America will continue to expand, particularly into areas with high STD rates, such as parts of Central America and the Amazon Basin.[45]

Governments where HIV is not a burden will continue to fund other priorities until AIDS is clearly a problem. Given the long incubation period of AIDS, this means substantial action will be taken only after many years of HIV spread. HIV in Europe and North America will continue to diminish in many communities while expanding in others; the advent of Highly Active Antiviral Therapy (HAART) may diminish the infectiousness of infected persons, but may also discourage high-risk sexual practices.[46] Given the equilibrium established in HIV seroprevalence in most Western countries, new cases will occur largely among young people.[47,48]

Despite the ongoing spread of HIV, politicians and policy makers stubbornly avoid investing in prevention. One exception is in northern Europe, where the Swedes have nearly wiped out incident, autochthonous STDs.[49,50] Despite the lessons of STD control learned in the late 19th and early 20th centuries, the current lack of insight and political courage to promote control of STDs, including HIV, has contributed directly to the magnitude of the world HIV pandemic. This links directly with the difficulty that Americans and others worldwide have with sexual issues. Progress and even success in global eradication of diseases like smallpox, dracunculiasis, and polio show what can be accomplished when public health control measures are supported, and worldwide political and economic commitments are made. Even when eradication is biologically implausible, global control measures like oral rehydration for infant diarrhea can result in measurable impact. However, many governments continue to treat STDs, including HIV, as a topic unworthy of such substantial attention.

Interaction of HIV and Other STDs

Unprotected sexual contact in the presence of other sexually transmitted infections (STIs) enhances the probability of HIV transmission.[34,51-53] Sexual transmission of HIV may be greatly enhanced by several additional cofactors, including the HIV load in the infectious partner, the phenotype of the HIV isolate, the immunogenetic profile of the exposed person, the interface of virus type with secondary and primary cell receptors of HIV, and the activation state of the immune system during and after the infectious event (see Chapter 3 for details).[54-56] The increased HIV risk associated with STIs is due to damage that these infections produce in the integrity of the epithelial lining of the cervix, vagina, urethra, vulva, penis, and anus.[34,57-59] The efficiency of HIV transmission increases with STI co-infection of either ulcerative or inflammatory type.[58] Mucosal ulceration, inflammation, or exudation is likely to increase the frequency of viral contact with target cells through macroscopic or microscopic breaks in mucosal integrity and to recruit immune cells that are readily infected (eg, dendritic cells, macrophages, CD4+ lymphocytes) into the genitourinary tract.[60] Lack of male circumcision may exacerbate the risks.

STIs not only increase susceptibility in the uninfected, exposed individual but also increase the infectiousness of HIV-infected persons who are co-infected with other STIs.[55,60] Viral load in genital secretions rises markedly with co-existing urethritis/STIs. In both semen and vaginal secretions, HIV load is higher with co-existing gonococcal and chlamydia infections. In women with a cervical or vaginal ulcer, HIV is higher in genital secretions. Most notably, treatment of these STDs results in a decrease of genital shedding.[55,61] The concentration of HIV in genital secretions is likely to be a key determinant of the efficiency of HIV transmission in many parts of the world; treatment with antibiotics among persons with STIs can reduce genital shedding of HIV, a finding with marked implications for HIV-prevention programs.[62]

Sexual transmission of HIV can be diminished by STI treatment and restoration of the integrity of the normal mucosal barriers. It is postulated that the restoration of a normal vaginal ecology dominated by hydrogen peroxide–producing lactobacilli may also inhibit the sexual spread of HIV. Similarly, mother-to-child HIV transmission may be reduced with antibiotic treatment of mothers who have bacterial vaginosis.[63] This concept is based on the association of lower genital tract bacterial vaginosis with risk of histologic chorioamnionitis and the increased risk of HIV transmission among mothers with chorioamnionitis. Bacterial vaginosis has been associated with HIV, suggesting this causal pathway to be plausible and worthy of investigation for both sexual and perinatal transmission reduction.[64]

Ulcerative STDs have the strongest association with seroconversion,[34,57,58] with relative risk estimates in the 5- to 10-fold excess risk range in cross-sectional studies.[60] Frank genital ulcers are common with chancroid, herpes, syphilis, genital ulcer diseases, and genital warts.[34,57,58] Ulcerative STDs disrupt the integrity of the epithelial mucosa, facilitate HIV contact with the lymphatic and circulatory systems and recruit CD4+ lymphocytes and macrophages to the site of injury/infection,[60] aiding sexual transmission of HIV.[59]

Non-ulcerative STDs are also important risk factors for sexual transmission of HIV.[34,54,65] Relative risk estimates for HIV with non-ulcerogenic STDs have been in the 2- to 5-fold range.[60] Inflammatory and exudative reproductive tract infections such as gonorrhea, chlamydia, trichomoniasis, bacterial vaginosis, or candidiasis are less disruptive of the epithelial tissues than ulcerative STDs. However, the exudate may recruit large volumes of cervical or urethral discharge filled with susceptible cells. Inflammation may result in micro-ulcerations and superficial capillaries, thus facilitating virus-cell contact with vulnerable cells in the mucosal epithelia of the rectum, cervix, vagina, or oral cavity.[60,66] Furthermore, the recruitment of infectious lymphocytes, macrophages, or other cells into seminal or vaginal secretions may increase transmissibility.[66]

The population burden of HIV that can be attributed to STIs differs from the relative risk or risk ratio (RR) of the association. For example, smoking kills about as many people per year from heart disease (RR=1.5) as from lung cancer (RR>12) merely because heart disease is much more common than lung cancer. Similarly, more people are likely infected with HIV each year due to the mucosal disruption of an inflammatory STI than due to an ulcerogenic one because the former is far more common than frank ulcers. The public health implications of this observation must be highlighted: ulcerogenic STDs, despite having the strongest association with HIV seroconversion,[54] should not be the sole target of intervention. Instead, all STIs, including the common inflammatory and exudative conditions, should be targets of public health control in the service of

HIV prevention and in the reduction of adverse reproductive consequences of STDs themselves.

Co-infection with systemic viruses, many of which are transmitted
sexually, may activate the immune system. An activated immune system is
easier to infect with HIV than a quiescent one, with up-regulated primary
and secondary target molecules presented to infectious particles. In
addition, systemic co-infection may stimulate higher HIV production, thus
increasing infectiousness.[60] Organisms studied for such effects include
STIs such as cytomegalovirus, Epstein-Barr virus, HTLV types I and II,
and human herpes viruses types 6, 7, and 8. While in vitro studies and
case reports are often intriguing, epidemiologic data are much less
convincing with *Mycoplasma fermentans*.[67] In addition, co-infection may
reflect the duration of risk behavior and HIV infection. For example, an
HIV-infected sex worker infected 15 years ago with HIV and 12 years ago
with HTLV-I can expect to be sicker than a sex-worker infected with HIV
alone for 2 years.

The interactions between STIs and HIV have contributed to the AIDS
epidemic, particularly when HIV prevalence is low.[66] Among high-risk
populations such as STD patients who commonly report high-risk activities and high-risk partners, HIV transmission can be quite efficient.[66] In
simulations of the initial 10-year period of the HIV epidemic (1981-1990),
more than 90% of HIV infection worldwide was attributed to STD co-
infections.[68] Even given more conservative assumptions about the
prevalence of STDs and about their enhancing effects on HIV transmission, STDs can be shown to play a critical role in the rapid and extensive
spread of HIV infection in diverse settings.[69] The identification and treatment of STDs as risk factors for HIV transmission must be a crucial factor
in the prevention of HIV.[66,68,69]

One topic linked to sexual risk in as yet undetermined ways is the
association of cervical ectopy with HIV risk.[70] Cervical ectopy is the
exocervical exposure of the normally endocervically located columnar
epithelium. The result of this condition is the exposure of the transformation zone (point at which the columnar epithelium transitions to
squamous epithelium) to the vagina, where sperm and potential
pathogens can bathe it in high concentrations. Since the transformation
zone is more susceptible to STD/HIV infection than the squamous or
columnar epithelia (both of which have physical and vascular protective
features, respectively), cervical ectopy may also increase HIV susceptibility in the uninfected.[60] Bleeding during intercourse occurs more often

among young women with cervical ectopy; hence, an HIV-infected woman with cervical ectopy may be more infectious than one without this normal cervical variant. An outstanding question is whether oral or injectable contraceptive hormones increase HIV risk since they are thought to increase cervical ectopy.[60] Unfortunately, we are largely ignorant of the risk factors for cervical ectopy, other than young age (adolescence). Since it is thought that frequent and early exposure to semen may accelerate squamous metaplastic changes in the cervix with the consequent involution of the transformation zone into the endocervix, these relationships of sexual risk behavior, age, contraception, and STDs with HIV risk may prove to be quite complex.[60,66]

Public Health Measures to Reduce HIV Sexual Spread

In the absence of affordable treatment and an effective vaccine against HIV, prevention is the only hope for controlling the worldwide HIV pandemic. Influencing personal behavior is not easy, but established strategies have succeeded in controlling STDs and HIV. Knowledge about the HIV infection levels and transmission patterns in a given population, and awareness of local attitudes towards infection and protection can guide design of public health programs to promulgate safer sexual practices.[37]

Behavior Change

Some politicians and religious populists advocate that strict monogamy or abstinence and drug-free lifestyles are the only acceptable behavioral goals, arguing that working towards "half measures" validates the high-risk lifestyle.[71] This point of view opposes needle exchange for infection drug users and condom provision for adolescents. Abstinence and mutual monogamy are realistic goals for a large segment of the population, particularly when it comes to maintaining these behaviors among persons already practicing these lifestyles. Among younger, sexually naive adolescents, abstinence-oriented education is the appropriate strategy, while risk reduction is the best approach for youth who are already sexually active and unmotivated to abandon their sexual relationships.[60] For a heterosexual or homosexual couple, faithfulness to one another will reduce risk of STD/HIV. However, changing human sexual behavior toward mutual monogamy or celibacy can be difficult as many persons are not motivated to achieve these goals.[72]

The promotion of condom use, partner reduction, and careful partner selection should not be discarded for a more limited message of abstinence and mutual monogamy, though this approach is being legislated in the United States to qualify for federal support. Reliance on abstinence campaigns is deemed the only moral option by some while being perceived as ineffectual by others. Provision of public health services, including condom distribution, is seen as encouraging promiscuity by some and as life-saving by others. Recurrent debates about school-based sexual education and preventive health services for adolescents epitomize these strategic differences.[73] Our failure to pursue aggressively more effective risk reduction has likely contributed to the high proportion of recent HIV seroconversions estimated to occur in America's youth.[47] Both approaches of risk reduction and risk elimination should be highlighted, taking into account community risks and norms.

Most behavioral scientists and public health professionals recognize that considerable progress in prevention can be made among persons who are not ready to give up their high-risk behaviors all at once. The Trans-theoretical or Stages of Change model of prevention science holds that persons may be able to change high-risk behavior in increments, reducing their risks of acquiring or transmitting HIV/STD even when they do not live a risk-free lifestyle.[74-76] This is analogous to a doctor helping a smoker reduce the daily number of cigarettes smoked or choose lower tar and nicotine tobacco at a time when the smoker cannot or will not quit tobacco use altogether. While tobacco risk reduction is seen as desirable to reduce risk even when risk is not being eliminated, this tolerance of risk reduction is rarely extended by public policy makers and moralists to sexual or illicit drug use activities.[71] US policy makers would do well to consider progress in northern Europe, which promulgates sexual and drug use–related risk reduction messages and has lower HIV seroprevalence.[50]

Persons engaged in high-risk behaviors are often motivated to learn about HIV. However, knowledge does not correlate with reduced-risk behavior in all circumstances.[76-78] Informed persons in denial may continue to engage in high-risk activity, underscoring the need to go beyond increasing HIV awareness through conventional educational efforts and implement novel public health measures to foster and maintain behavior change. Creative social marketing could employ the same media and style of advertisement used by commercial clients.[37] Peer counseling and sustained outreach support can also be exercised to sustain behavior change over time.[37] Insights from psychological theory and social marketing experience have led to the rational design of programs that encourage safer sexual practices and overall risk reduction.[79] Safer sex efforts include education for reduction in the number of sexual partners, selection of lower risk partners, use of condoms, prompt recognition and treatment of STDs, and reduction in drug and alcohol use.[60]

The potential for STD/HIV reduction is greatest among young women, who are at increased risk for STD and HIV infection due to both behavioral and biological mechanisms.[60] Younger women are at comparatively higher risk of HIV infection over a given number of exposures. Immature vaginal mucosa in adolescents, with large cervical ectopy zones, may be more susceptible to trauma during sexual relations and may be especially prone to infection with STDs due to the large transformation zone and exposed columnar epithelia. HIV transmission may be facilitated by sexual activity at times when blood exposure is expected (eg, menses, rape, or first coital experience).[60]

Special attention should be given to this highly neglected group of patients, many of whom are adolescents, in terms of comprehensive reproductive health education and delivery of services. Recent interest in integrating STD services in family planning and maternal and child health may work well for older women, but unmarried adolescents often do not feel welcome and often make little use of such facilities. Offering a non-judgmental and accessible service to vulnerable populations such as sex workers and adolescents could have a considerable impact on HIV prevention.[80,81] Among the innovative approaches already being used with some success in the United States and internationally are peer education, social marketing, school-based sexual education for youth, community-based programs to reduce drug experimentation in adolescents, programs for alcohol risk reduction in high-risk groups (including the military), risk reduction for active sex workers, and street outreach for runaways and the homeless, targeting populations at highest HIV risk.[82-85] Chapter 6 offers additional suggestions for developing interventions capable of reaching vulnerable women at high risk for HIV infection.

Behavioral and community-based educational and co-factor reduction efforts can be successful. In Thailand, condom promotion has been successful, especially in the sex work industry.[86,87] In Tanzania, community-based STD control has achieved short-term reductions in HIV seroincidence.[88-90] Long-term impact of STD control on HIV is unknown, but the 2-year follow-up data reveal that a relatively straightforward syndromic management approach, without use of laboratory diagnostics, reduced HIV seroincidence by 42%. In Zaire, STD and condom services for sex workers reduced HIV risk in proportion to the frequency with which the services were utilized.[34] Comprehensive services for drug users has lowered risk in the Netherlands.[93] In the United States, peer counseling among gay men and intensive counseling among runaway adolescents have proved effective in reducing high-risk behavior.[91,92] In addition, needle exchange programs to reduce contaminated injections among IDUs demonstrate efficacy and can be expected, in turn, to affect sexual transmission from IDUs to their sexual partners and offspring.[94]

Barrier Methods

Male condoms are highly effective in preventing HIV transmission, both by blocking HIV and by reducing the transmission of other STDS.[95,96] In Rwanda, HIV testing and counseling, AIDS education, and free condoms and spermicides distributed to women of childbearing age had significant effects on condom use and HIV seroconversion rates prior to the 1994 genocide.[33,97] Thailand launched a nationwide campaign to reach a goal of 100% condom use among commercial sex workers.[30,86] The campaign included condom distribution in brothels and a mass advertising campaign promoting condom use.[86,87] As a result, condom use dramatically increased (more than 90%) among commercial sex workers, STD prevalence was lowered, and HIV prevalence declined among several groups with high rates of partner change.[30,86,87,98-100] Similar success have been achieved in programs involving commercial sex workers in Kenya[101,102] and in Bolivia.[103]

In Kinshasa, Laga et al. suggested that the willingness of the male clients to use condoms would need to be raised to ensure the success of any such program.[34] Although condom use increased markedly among female sex workers, condom use with all clients never exceeded more than 60%. The main obstacle cited was the male client's refusal to use a condom.[34] This illustrates the urgent need for additional chemical or physical barrier methods that are under women's control.[104] It also highlights the need to address male behavior and risk reduction as has been done in Thailand. In Thailand, the growing use of condoms among commercial sex workers prior to the large-scale condom programs is attributed to awareness in government and military circles of the high prevalence of HIV in this population.[99,100] In the United States, an increase in condom use among young adults in the 1980s was attributed to the growing perceived risks of acquiring HIV, reflecting a growing awareness of the impact of the HIV epidemic and the messages of HIV prevention programs.[105] Absolute numbers do not tell the whole story, however, since the lowest condom uptake is often among the highest risk persons.

A controlled clinical trial of condom use for HIV prevention is not feasible for ethical reasons, though available data nonetheless demonstrate that regular condom use protects against HIV infection.[106] In the United States, use of condoms in the heterosexual population remains relatively low, especially among adolescents, but is increasing in some surveys.[105] Thus, promotion of condoms as a means of safe sex practice should form an essential component of any public health measure for HIV prevention. Public awareness of the risks of HIV and of the protective benefits of condoms is not yet sufficient to convince persons at highest risk to use them. Factors inhibiting the use of condoms include their price, potential inconvenience, embarrassment resulting from their purchase and use, and perceived reduced sexual pleasure. Policies that overcome these barriers by lowering the price of condoms, improving their availability, and increasing their social acceptability could increase condom use and reduce HIV transmission.[91]

Some studies suggest that condom use is associated with higher HIV seroconversion risk. In fact, high-risk men and women may use condoms more often than mutually monogamous married persons. However, sporadic condom use by high-risk persons with repetitive exposures merely reduces the transmission efficiency for the given encounter in which the condom is used. Studies that ensure 100% condom use, as occurred in studies of spouses of men with hemophilia, prove that condom efficacy is high.[106]

Unfortunately, available female-controlled barriers (eg, female condoms, spermicides) do not have convincing data showing that these modalities are successful.[104,107] These innovative and important tools for potential HIV control could empower women to protect themselves without the cooperation of their sexual partners[108] and should remain the topic of intense research investigation as to their efficacy. Definitive field trials of microbicide and female condom must be designed and implemented quickly.[104,107]

STD Control

The causal link between classic STDs and HIV transmission has been demonstrated through in vitro, clinical, and epidemiologic studies.[51,66] The increase in STD prevalence has implications for the evolution of the HIV epidemic and should be addressed effectively by strengthening STD control programs. Evidence clearly shows that interventions targeting vulnerable persons at the individual or at the community level can produce substantial reductions in high-risk sexual behaviors and reduce HIV transmission. In addition, "classic" STD control approaches such as partner notification can be helpful in reaching persons at risk.[35,109]

Despite our knowledge of the impact of STDs on HIV, STD control remains limited by several issues, including cost of diagnosis and treatment in settings with poor access to health care.[96] Syndromic management refers to the treatment of possible associated STDs based on the symptoms displayed by the patient, with or without laboratory confirmation. Syndromic management is a more feasible STD control strategy in resource-poor settings and has been endorsed by the World Health Organization (WHO) and United Nations AIDS (UN AIDS).[96] Disadvantages include the cost and risk of over-treatment with antibiotics and suboptimal identification of chlamydial and gonococcal cervical infection in women with vaginal discharge. Nonetheless, syndromic approaches offer a marked improvement over current practices for treating symptomatic STDs in most parts of the developing world.[110] In many settings, training of health care workers in STD syndromic management, making available effective antibiotics for STDs, and promoting health care-seeking behavior can decrease STD/HIV incidence.[111]

In Rakai, Uganda, a rural region near Lake Victoria, a periodic population "sweep" with curative antibiotics, independent of individual diagnosis, was implemented in the hopes it might be a cost-effective approach to HIV control.[112] This approach failed to control HIV.[112,113] In a carefully designed and conducted study, the investigators could find no HIV-related benefits for the mass chemotherapy program, though other health benefits were noted.[112] Perhaps treating STDs every tenth month was insufficient to prevent transmission compared with immediately available syndromic management as in Mwanza. Alternatively, the HIV epidemic may have been so mature that a suboptimal STD control campaign did little to change transmission dynamics.[113] The lesson learned may be that "STD control can help prevent HIV, though the techniques and the intensity of the STD control program must be adequate to alter HIV transmission dynamics in a given setting."[113]

HIV-infected persons with untreated genitourinary tract infections are likely to be far more infectious than those receiving treatment for such infections.[51] Treatment of the HIV infection itself with antiretroviral chemotherapy reduces HIV plasma virus load and almost certainly reduces genital tract viral load as well.[114] While a treated individual is less infectious early in the course of antiretroviral chemotherapy, the prolonged survival in a relatively healthy AIDS-free state may permit a longer span of high-risk sexual activity. The population consequences of widespread antiviral chemoprophylaxis and chemotherapy—net benefits to society in reduced transmission from reduced infectiousness or net increased transmission due to longer lifespan of infected individuals—remains unknown.[115,116] This issue highlights the urgency of effective behavior change programs focused on HIV-infected persons.[46]

Conclusions

It is encouraging to see successful pilot projects and progress where sound public health policy has overcome political objections in an effort to reduce transmission by all reasonable and feasible routes. Converting these individual successes into sustained worldwide disease control remains elusive.[28] Given the rapid recognition of the modes of transmission of HIV (risky behavior was a recognized factor prior the discovery of HIV in 1983), the failure of subsequent control activities serves as a discouraging reminder of the difficulties faced in translating knowledge into practice. Treatment-oriented health care systems have little incentive to invest money in prevention; effective prevention targets the highest risk groups in community-based programs rather than in the health care system settings per se.

In the realm of public policy and behavior change, the AIDS epidemic requires political and community leaders to take risks within their leadership positions to educate and advocate for effective though sometimes controversial strategies for control of HIV transmission. Development and testing of novel, female-controlled barrier methods ranks among the highest research priorities. Assessment of the impact of STD control in reducing HIV should be emphasized in both industrialized and developing nations. Rapid, cheap STD diagnostics, low-cost broad-spectrum antibiotics effective against all STDs in single dose regimens, and STD vaccines are likewise needed.

A partially effective HIV vaccine could be helpful if coupled with other prevention strategies.[117] Drug abuse and risk reduction among drug users remains among the highest priorities in the United States, Europe, and parts of Asia. This topic is integrally linked to STDs as drug users often support their addiction with sexual services. The impact of alcohol and recreational drugs on sexual disinhibition further heightens HIV/STD risk (see Chapter 7 for an in-depth review).

Success in reducing perinatal transmission will depend fully on our approach to universal testing of pregnant women to permit them to choose antiretroviral chemoprophylaxis if they are seropositive (see Chapter 10 for discussion of universal testing and privacy issues). Novel approaches to perinatal risk reduction are needed to complement drugs, particularly in parts of the world where drugs and HIV testing are very costly in the local economy. These approaches include STI control in pregnant women.[63]

Finally, creativity in behavioral interventions must be highlighted. Sophisticated marketing techniques sell concepts and encourage consumption. These same strategies could be used to address social concerns and could work even better if left unshackled by political constraints.

Summary Points

• The straightforward statement that HIV is a sexually transmitted infection has proven controversial when traditional STD control measures are proposed.

• Historical efforts to control STDs have focused on female prostitution and the threat of STDs to military efficiency during world wars.

• In the United States, the Venereal Disease Control Division focused on case reporting, contact tracing, widespread availability of testing, promotion of condom prophylaxis, establishment of treatment facilities, and public education programs conducted at the level of state and local health departments.

• Lessons learned worldwide in HIV control include relearning these tried and true measures of STD control. Additional measures include peer education, protection of the blood supply, use of sterile syringes and needles (medical use and for IDUs), testing of pregnant women, and partner counseling. Both approaches of risk reduction and risk elimination should be highlighted, taking into account community risks and norms.

• Sexually transmitted infections both increase the probability of HIV transmission and increase the infectiousness of HIV-infected persons. Sexual transmission of HIV can be diminished by treating the infection and restoring the integrity of the normal mucosal barriers.

• Co-infection with systemic viruses may activate the immune system, which in turn is more easily infected with HIV. In addition, systemic co-infection may stimulate higher HIV production, thus increasing infectiousness.

CHAPTER 9

The Changing Face of AIDS: Implications for Policy and Practice

Paul E. Farmer, David A. Walton, Jennifer J. Furin

D ecember 1999. End of a millennium and, according to a recent magazine cover, "The End of AIDS." But prospects do not look so rosy if one is running what is termed, in an urban teaching hospital, "the AIDS service." In the latter part of this month, we admitted fewer patients—only six—than we might have a decade ago, and the patients were different in many ways. Only three were men; two were homeless. Three were women. All were people of color. Most did not have private insurance, and most, at the time of their admission, took neither anti-HIV therapies nor appropriate prophylaxis for opportunistic infections. Yet HIV infection can be suppressed. Why, then, does HIV continue to grow at an impressive rate in some regions, even as it contracts in others?

In both industrialized and developing nations, HIV has rapidly become entrenched among the poorest and most disenfranchised populations. Ignored for more than a decade, this relentless concentration of disease has had a number of implications. First, communities already burdened by excess rates of disease and premature death now have another, growing problem. Second, those most in need of new therapies are those least able to obtain them. Third, even the clinical presentation of HIV disease is changing over time. HIV alters the course of pre-existing diseases ranging from tuberculosis to cervical neoplasia. (See Chapter 6 for a discussion of the delay in recognizing HIV and AIDS in women.)

Trends reported in the epidemiological and public health literature have obvious if often unexamined implications for clinical practice, just as new developments in diagnosis and treatment of HIV have obvious if unrealized promise for millions now living with HIV. This chapter discusses the limitations of conventional epidemiological and clinical studies of AIDS, including those relying on the concepts of "risk categories" and "risk groups," and provides a dynamic view of the rapidly changing global pandemic. (See Chapter 1 for a review of epidemic patterns according to HIV subtype.) We will also evaluate trends in the epidemiology of HIV-related opportunistic infections and explore implications of these trends for clinical practice and public health policy.

Epidemiology of HIV: Principles and Pitfalls

Histories of AIDS and HIV have already been written from several points of view and with varying degrees of success.[1,2] In the early years of the epidemic, most accounts discussed AIDS risks in terms of "risk groups" or "risk behaviors." The risk groups most commonly cited in epidemiological research on AIDS then included homosexual and bisexual men, intravenous drug users (IDUs), people who receive blood products, and children born to HIV-infected mothers. As noted in Chapter 4, the early years of the epidemic were notable for a large number of speculations about both the origin of AIDS and the nature of risks. Indeed, the inclusion in US commentaries of Haitians as a risk group and the ensuing public controversies led to the rethinking of the nature of risk and risk analysis.[3] Researchers came to recognize that HIV infection was not limited to social groups bound by language, ethnicity, or sexual preference.

As the epidemic advanced, the expansion of risk led researchers away from the concept of risk group to one of risk behaviors. Risk behaviors were held to include anal or vaginal intercourse without the use of a condom, sexual intercourse with multiple partners, and the sharing of needles among IDUs. In more recent years, the concept of risk behaviors has also been questioned; increasingly, people diagnosed with HIV infection are unable to identify any agreed-upon risk behavior. For example, in a study of anonymous HIV testing of US women attending an urban prenatal clinic, researchers found that 43% of the women who tested positive for HIV reported no "traditional" risk behaviors.[4] In another study conducted among US blood donors, nearly half of the women found to be seropositive for HIV could not identify a risk factor for their infection.[5] This is because social conditions, rather than certain behaviors or membership in some discretely bonded group, account for a significant proportion of risk for HIV as a sexually transmitted disease (STD).

Large-scale serosurveys suggest that the nature of HIV risk is changing. Although interpretive chaos reigned initially, the 1984 development of serologic tests for HIV led to an ever expanding, if difficult to decipher, database. In looking at the global patterning of HIV early in the pandemic, epidemiologists discerned three "patterns" of transmission based on the groups perceived to be at risk and on the timing and rate of spread of HIV:

• Pattern I countries were defined as those that saw extensive spread of HIV in the late 1970s and early 1980s, with most cases of HIV infection occurring in gay men and IDUs. Examples included the United States, Canada, Australia, and most countries in Western Europe.

• Pattern II countries were those with extensive spread of HIV in the mid to late 1970s and early 1980s and in which heterosexual transmission was the dominant pattern of spread. Haiti and most sub-Saharan African nations were held to be examples.

• Pattern III countries began to register extensive spread of HIV in the 1980s; some called this pattern "mixed," since both heterosexual and homosexual transmissions were documented, but seroprevalence remained at low levels even among many of those designated as "at-risk" in other countries. At the time the framework was advanced, Eastern Europe, the Middle East, and Asia were said to be representative of Pattern III epidemiology.[6]

This classificatory scheme is no longer in wide use, since it presents a static picture of a rapidly changing pandemic. Again, life conditions—the social circumstances of entire populations—sculpted the contours of risk, as Mann and coworkers noted: "Other influencing factors, such as social evolution, political unrest, and economic disruption or success, also modified over time the social context within which risk behaviors flourished or receded."[7] This interaction between a virus and a human population in which modes of potentially infectious contact are constantly shifting is the phenomenon to which risk assessment must now direct its attention. The schedule of "risk groups" and "risk behaviors" will necessarily vary from setting to setting, as it is a consequence of economic flaws, configurations of political and military power, social adaptations to the environment, and the availability of medical and social services.

In fact, the global AIDS pandemic comprises several changing "subepidemics" in which certain groups find themselves confronted with high-risk situations, while others living in the same regions are shielded from risk. Furthermore, analyses of risk based on geography (eg, country-wide profiles) miss the local social inequalities so central to the spread of HIV. In many settings, steep grades of inequality, including gender inequality (see Chapter 6 for details), serve as the leading cofactor in the spread of HIV.[8] Thus, both serosurveys and studies of self-reported risk show that it is increasingly difficult to deploy conventional concepts of risk, risk categories, and risk behaviors.[9-14]

Global Epidemiology of HIV

By December 1999, approximately 33.6 million people worldwide were living with HIV. More than 95% of prevalent cases and 95% of all deaths from advanced HIV disease occur where medical services are scarce or substandard.[15] The estimated prevalence of HIV in various regions is presented in Table 1.

TABLE 1. Cumulative Cases of HIV Infection Throughout the World (December 1998 data)*

Region	Cases
North America	920 000
Western Europe	520 000
Eastern Europe and Central Asia	360 000
Latin America	1 300 000
Sub-Saharan Africa	23 300 000
Caribbean	360 000
North Africa and Middle East	220 000
East Asia and Pacific	530 000
South and Southeast Asia	6 000 000
Australia and New Zealand	12 000
Total	33 600 000

* Data from UNAIDS/WHO.[15]

Appreciating the dimensions of the global burden of HIV disease is important, as are estimations of national burdens. However, although country-wide data are essential for public health officials, the notion of nationally shared risk can obscure the dynamics of HIV spread. National data do not account for regional variations in HIV incidence and prevalence. In the United States, for example, almost 90% of all women with HIV come from only eight states.[16,17] HIV distribution can be strikingly uneven within endemic regions in which individuals are erroneously considered to share a homogeneity of risk. AIDS in Africa is often discussed as though "Africa is a country and not one continent composed of more than 50 sovereign nations."[18] Within these sovereign states, some people are at exceptionally high risk of HIV disease, while others are shielded from risk. (See Chapter 1 for an overview of differences in HIV subtype and subsequent risk throughout Africa.)

Another issue of importance is the incomplete nature of case reporting. Underreporting of HIV/AIDS and of deaths due to HIV is a significant problem for resource-poor nations. Even in the United States, a country with enormous (though unevenly distributed) health resources, the Centers for Disease Control and Prevention (CDC) estimates that "deaths for which HIV infection was designated the underlying cause represent approximately two-thirds to three-fourths of all deaths attributable to HIV infection."[19]

United States and Canada

An estimated 920 000 North Americans are infected with HIV. In other words, only 0.26% of the global burden of HIV is felt in North America.[15] The nature of the North American epidemic is changing rapidly. Between 1981 and 1987, 64% of US AIDS cases occurred among men having sex with men (MSM). During the same period, injection drug use accounted for 17% of AIDS cases and heterosexual contact for 3% of cases.[20] In the period between 1993 and 1998, however, the proportion of AIDS cases among MSM decreased to 45%, while the proportion of AIDS cases attributable to injection drug use and heterosexual contact increased to 28% and 16%, respectively.[17] The US epidemic is thus a moving target, with seroprevalence studies offering a glimpse of a future in which AIDS will play a major part. Table 2 illustrates data from 1996 statistical models of estimated seroprevalence of 96 cities in the United States.

TABLE 2. Prevalence of HIV among IDUs, MSM, and Heterosexual Adults*

City	IDU	MSM	Heterosexual
Los Angeles	3.8%	22.6%	1.3%
Miami	21.9%	31.4%	5.1%
Newark	38.0%	17.9%	6.4%
New York City	41.0%	29.2%	4.3%

* *Data from Holmberg.*[21]

Social inequalities are central to the US epidemic. In a national survey conducted between 1988 and 1991, a weighted seroprevalence of 0.39% was found for the entire national population. Black study participants were four times more likely to be HIV-positive than were white or Mexican-American participants.[22] In 1994, the death rate for HIV among black men was almost four times as high as for white men; for black women, the death rate for AIDS was nine times as high as for white women. Unlike the early days of the epidemic in the United States, when the infected population consisted primarily of homosexual men, today new cases of HIV infection result predominately from intravenous drug use and heterosexual contact. Also, the incidence of AIDS among women is increasing more rapidly than the incidence of AIDS among men in the United States, although MSM still account for the largest number of AIDS cases. (For more on this topic, see Chapters 5 and 6.)

As HIV has settled in among the urban poor, including an increasing proportion of women, the nature of presenting complaints has changed as well. Among patients with HIV disease, rates of Kaposi's sarcoma have declined significantly; rates of invasive cervical cancer have risen.[23] Bacterial infections and tuberculosis have been important opportunistic infections among the US urban poor. Because these trends have enormous implications for the practitioner, it is important to underscore the role of poverty and other social inequalities in determining both disease distribution and outcomes. (Chapter 6 reviews gender inequities in more depth.) Many activities central to the practice of medicine—for example, assessing risk, predicting likely opportunistic infections in the HIV-

Figure 1. The proportion of AIDS cases by race/ethnicity shows a shift in the at-risk populations over the 13 years examined.

Reprinted with permission from the Centers for Disease Control and Prevention.[17]

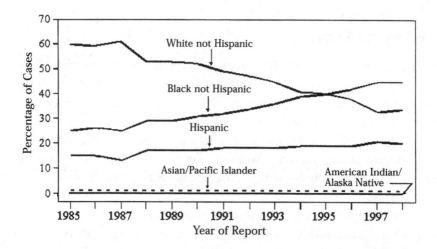

Figure 2. This figure shows the 12-year rise in both the incidence of AIDS among US women (line graph) and the percentage of AIDS cases (bar graph).

Reprinted with permission from the Centers for Disease Control and Prevention.[17]

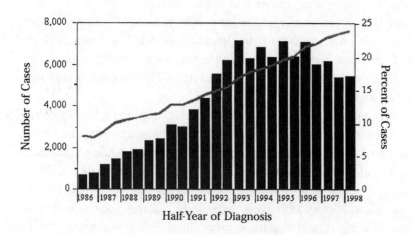

infected, predicting patients' ability to acquire and adhere to expensive and difficult regimens, and access to increasingly important laboratory testing—are tightly linked to socioeconomic and insurance status. These problems are even more daunting in the most gravely affected regions of the world, which are also the poorest.

Sub-Saharan Africa

To date, nearly 70% of all HIV infection is thought to have occurred in sub-Saharan Africa, even though the continent is home to only 10% of the world's population. An estimated 23.3 million people are infected,[15] with 1.2 women infected for every infected man.[24] In certain parts of Uganda and Tanzania, infection rates are significantly higher among women than among men.[25,26] Women tend to be infected at a younger age than do male counterparts,[27] a trend also registered elsewhere in the world.[28]

Heterosexual contact is the primary risk factor associated with infection in sub-Saharan Africa. Rates of HIV infection are high among African commercial sex workers, most of whom are poor; in cities across the continent, between 35% and 88% of prostitutes surveyed were found to be infected with HIV.[29] Migrant labor and disruption of stable sexual unions continue to predict risk for HIV infection. One study of male truck drivers in Kenya found that over 27% tested positive for HIV.[30] As elsewhere in the world, however, it is increasingly difficult to discern clearly bounded "risk groups." Fisher and Toko found that 6.9% of ostensibly healthy blood donors in northeastern Zaire were HIV-positive.[31] A national seroprevalence study in Uganda conducted between 1987 and 1988 found that overall seroprevalence was about 5%. The same researchers later reported an infection rate of 16% among rural women and 12% among rural men.[32]

Many hypotheses have been proposed to explain high rates of HIV in Africa. These have ranged from biological explanations regarding the subtypes of HIV found on the continent[33] to the existence of unique cultural and sexual practices.[34] (See Chapter 1 for a more thorough review.) To date, none of these hypotheses has adequately explained variations in risk. Factors left largely unexplored address socioeconomic status, power differential, and structured inequality.[35,36] War and social dislocation also appear to be closely linked to increased transmission of HIV. Sero-surveys conducted among young urban Rwandan women revealed an HIV seroprevalence of 32%.[37] Increasingly, then, African patients with HIV disease are young women, many of whom present with "slim disease," one of a series of common bacterial or mycobacterial infections.[38,39]

Latin America and the Caribbean

Approximately 4% of HIV infection in the world is registered in Latin America and the Caribbean, where 1.3 million people are estimated to be infected. Table 3 provides estimates for various countries throughout the region.

TABLE 3. Total HIV/AIDS Cases by Country (December 1998 data)*

County	Cases
Argentina	120 000
Bahamas	6 300
Brazil	400 000
Chile	16 000
Colombia	72 000
Dominican Republic	83 000
El Salvador	18 000
Haiti	190 000
Honduras	43 000
Jamaica	14 000
Mexico	180 000
Trinidad and Tobago	6 800

* Data from UNAIDS/WHO.[15]

In the first years of the Latin American epidemic, HIV/AIDS was seen primarily among homosexual and bisexual men; in several countries, a history of sexual contact with a North American predicted risk for HIV/AIDS.[3] Sharing of contaminated injection equipment among IDUs accounts for a substantial proportion of HIV infection in certain settings. In a study of IDUs in Argentina, seroprevalence ranging from 20% to 62% has been reported; seroprevalence as high as 29% has been reported among IDUs in Mexico City; 73% of IDUs living in Santos City, Brazil, are reported to be HIV-infected.[27] In one area of Port-au-Prince, Haiti, as many as 50% of female sex workers were infected with HIV by 1990.[40]

As the Latin American epidemic progressed, however, more and more patients diagnosed with HIV had no history of prostitution, IDU, or homosexual contact. Incidence has increased dramatically among heterosexuals. In Brazil, 4% of reported AIDS cases were registered among heterosexuals in 1985, compared with 20% in 1990 and 33% in 1997.[41,42]

The case of Haiti is also instructive. In contrast to theories positing Haiti as the source of the global AIDS pandemic, HIV was probably introduced to the country only within the past two decades. Careful review of clinical records and pathologic specimens has revealed no likely case of AIDS until 1979, when Kaposi's sarcoma was diagnosed in two previously well young adults. By December 1990, Haiti had reported 3086 cases of AIDS to the Pan American Health Organization; most observers felt that the actual number of cases was significantly higher. By 1992, in a Port-au-Prince STD clinic, HIV infection had become as common as more well-established STDs such as syphilis.[43,44] Complications of HIV infection have become the leading cause of young adult death in urban Haiti.[45]

How has HIV infection become so widespread, at least in urban Haiti, in such a short period of time? In the early 1980s, the epidemic seemed to have an epicenter in the city of Carrefour, a center of poverty and prostitution bordering the south side of Port-au-Prince. Of the potential risk factors, bisexual activity was by far the most significant according to studies conducted in urban Haiti in the early 1980s; a high percentage of the homosexual contact had been with North Americans.[46] The rate of transfusion-associated transmission was at the time higher in Haiti than in the United States. By 1986, however, heterosexual transmission—or, in the language of the day, "no risk factor"—was demonstrated or strongly suspected in approximately 70% of Haitian AIDS cases (see Table 4).[47] These trends became more pronounced over the subsequent decade.[48] Additional evidence for heterosexual transmission of HIV are the high

TABLE 4. Changing Risk Factors in Haitians with AIDS, 1983-1987

Risk Factor	1983 (N=38)	1984 (N=104)	1985 (N=132)	1986 (N=185)	1987 (N=100)
Bisexuality	50%	27%	8%	4%	1%
Transfusion	23%	12%	8%	7%	10%
IDU	1%	1%	1%	0%	1%
Heterosexual	5%	6%	14%	16%	15%
Undefined	21%	54%	69%	73%	73%

* Data from Pape and Johnson.[49]

rates (over 50%) of infection among sex workers in the Port-au-Prince area, the ever decreasing male-to-female ratio among Haitians with AIDS, and the growing number of pediatric AIDS cases.[3,40,49]

During 1986 and 1987, sera from several cohorts of ostensibly healthy urban adults were analyzed for antibodies to HIV; rates of seropositivity were high. In a group of individuals working in hotels catering to tourists, HIV seroprevalence was a sobering 12%. In a group of 502 mothers of children hospitalized with diarrhea and among 190 urban adults with a comparably low socioeconomic background, seroprevalence rates were 12% and 13%, respectively. Among urban factory workers, 5% were found to have antibodies to HIV. In all series, rates were comparable for men and women, which suggested to many observers that the high attack rate in Haitian men would slowly give way to a pattern like that seen in parts of Africa.[50]

Large numbers of urban Haitians have been exposed to HIV, mainly through heterosexual transmission. Scant research has been conducted in rural Haiti, but one study of diagnoses made in an ambulatory clinic revealed that almost 70% of all patients with symptomatic HIV disease were women.[51] A small case-control study revealed that none of these women had a history of prostitution, none had used illicit drugs, and none had a history of transfusion. None of the women had had more than six sexual partners. In fact, several of the afflicted women had had only one sexual partner (see Table 5). Although women in the study group had (on average) more sexual partners than did controls, the difference was not striking: the average for each group was still less than three lifetime partners per woman.

The chief risk factor in this small cohort involved not the number of partners but rather the profession of these partners. Most of the women with HIV disease had a history of sexual contact with soldiers or truck drivers, comparatively well-off men whose profession involves a great deal of travel and (in the case of soldiers) the ability to coerce unwilling partners. Of the women diagnosed with HIV disease, none had a history of sexual contact exclusively with peasants. Among the seronegative controls, none reported contact with soldiers, and most had only had

TABLE 5. Case-Control Study of AIDS in Rural Haitian Women*

Patient Characteristics	Patients with AIDS (N=25)	Control Group (N=25)
Average number of sexual partners	2.7	2.4
Sexual partner of a truck driver	12	2
Sexual partner of a soldier	9	0
Sexual partner of a peasant only	0	23
Ever lived in Port-au-Prince	20	4
Worked as a servant	18	1
Average number of years of formal schooling	4.5	4.0
Ever received a blood transfusion	0	2
Ever used illicit drugs	0	0
Ever received more than 10 intramuscular injections	17	19

* Data from Farmer.[48]

sexual relations with peasants from the region. Histories of extended residence in Port-au-Prince and work as a domestic were also strongly associated with a diagnosis of HIV disease. This and complementary studies led us to conclude that social inequalities—here, gender inequality and poverty—serve as powerful cofactors for the transmission of HIV in rural Haiti. Conjugal unions with nonpeasants—salaried soldiers and truck drivers who are paid on a daily basis—reflect poor women's quest for economic security. In this manner, truck drivers and soldiers served as a "bridge" to spread infection among the rural population, just as North American tourists seem to have served as a bridge to the urban Haitian population. But just as North Americans are no longer important in the transmission of HIV in Haiti, truck drivers and soldiers will soon no longer be necessary components of the rural epidemic. Poverty and gender inequality will serve to mainstream a steady, growing rate of HIV transmission.

Asia

HIV and AIDS were not known in Asia until relatively late in the global pandemic. A late start did not preclude, however, an important surge in transmission. HIV infection rates are currently soaring in Southeast Asia, particularly in Thailand but also in Burma, Vietnam, Laos, Cambodia, China, and the Philippines. Nearly 18% of HIV infections in the world occur in South and Southeast Asia, where an estimated 6 million people have HIV/AIDS.[15] Projections suggest that by 2014, one million Thai people will have died of HIV/AIDS.[52,53]

Ten years ago, almost no cases of HIV were reported in India. Recent estimates place the number at approximately 4 million,[54] and experts predict that India will have more new cases of HIV infection each year than any other country in the world.[55,56] As elsewhere, the disease is strikingly patterned in its distribution. Rates among IDUs are as high as 64%, and as many as 30% of commercial sex workers are infected with HIV.[55,56] In Pune, 47% of commercial sex workers tested positive for HIV; the same study found 14% of the women who had never been commercial sex workers to be HIV-positive.[57] Among female sex workers in Thailand, one study found that HIV seroprevalence had increased from 3% in 1989 to 29% in 1993.[27] Surveys have revealed rates as high as 66%.[58] Seroprevalence of 15% has been documented among IDUs in urban China and of 30% among Malaysian IDUs.[59,60] Recent estimates suggest that, among total AIDS cases registered in China, the percentage of IDUs exceeds 75%.[61]

In attempting to explain the explosive epidemic in Asia, researchers and popular press alike have tended to blame female prostitutes for spreading the disease to the "general population." However, few data support this perception. HIV is more readily transmitted from men to women than from women to men, and[62,63] HIV is most significant as an "occupational risk" of commercial sex workers. Furthermore, the vast majority of Asian women who are sex workers are poor and have few other means of supporting themselves and their families. For example, one study of Calcutta sex workers found that 49% became commercial sex workers to escape extreme poverty; more than 84% were illiterate, and more than 21% reported family disturbances that pushed them into prostitution.[64] It has been estimated that up to 50% of Bombay's prostitutes were recruited through trickery or abduction.[65]

As in Haiti, poverty and gender inequality are at the root of risk for exchanging sex for money, just as they are at the root of risk for HIV. (See Chapter 6 for an in-depth review of this topic.) Since hundreds of millions of women living in Asia are living in poverty and with gender inequality, clearly a broad swath of vulnerability to HIV exists in the region. Again, the encroachment of HIV into populations already living with high burdens of infection and parasitic diseases will mean increased incidence of these as well. (This is also discussed in Chapter 8.)

Changing Profiles in Opportunistic Infections

Although few attempts have been made to understand how these changing risk profiles affect the practice of HIV care, seldom has the link between a population-based approach and clinical management been so crucial, as both regional and temporal variations in AIDS-related opportunistic infections suggest. Variations in opportunistic infections are largely of two types: regional variations in the prevalence, and changes in incidence registered over the history of the pandemic. From the outset, different patterns of opportunistic infections were seen in Africa and the United States. The most common among North Americans with AIDS has long been *Pneumocystis carinii* pneumonia (PCP), a diagnosis only rarely made in Africa. Early in the pandemic, researchers reported that only 14% of Africans were diagnosed with PCP, compared with 67% of HIV-positive people in the United States and Europe.[66] More recent studies continue to report low rates of PCP in Africa, even in those rare instances in which patients with pulmonary symptoms went to bronchoscopy,[67-71] although PCP rates as high as 33% have been reported among some study populations.[72]

It is tempting to speak of a phenomenologically distinct "tropical AIDS," but it is also necessary to exclude the possibility that many Africans with HIV disease simply succumb earlier and to more virulent pathogens. One of these is clearly *Mycobacterium tuberculosis* (TB). HIV and TB exhibit a synergy that is particularly noxious to their human hosts. In patients who carry quiescent TB infection—nearly 2 billion persons, or roughly one third of the world's population, are thought to fall into this category[73]—subsequent infection with HIV often means that dormant TB "reactivates," as cell-mediated immunity wanes. In much of the world, reactivation TB heralds previously unsuspected HIV infection.[74]

TABLE 6. Estimated Distribution of Persons with HIV/TB Coinfection (1997 data)*

Region	HIV/TB Coinfection
North America	60 000
Western Europe	65 000
Eastern Europe and Central Asia	20 000
Latin America and the Caribbean	450 000
Sub-Saharan Africa	7 300 000
North Africa and Middle East	107 000
East Asia and Pacific	307 000
South and Southeast Asia	2 400 000
Australia and New Zealand	1000
Total	10 7000 000

* Data from UNAIDS/WHO.[15]

TB may, in fact, be the world's most common AIDS-associated opportunistic infection: recent surveys suggest that of the 1.86 billion persons estimated to be infected with HIV, 10.7 million of them are coinfected with *Mycobacterium tuberculosis*.[75] Table 6 shows the estimated prevalence of HIV/TB coinfection in each of the WHO regions.

Tuberculosis is the most important opportunistic infection in Haitians with HIV, a finding noted as early as 1993. In our research in Haiti, TB is the most common presenting illness among patients diagnosed with HIV (see Figure 3).[76] Although most Haitians with AIDS are coinfected with *M. tuberculosis*, the converse is not true. Data from urban Haiti suggest that a majority of those hospitalized for tuberculosis are seropositive for HIV,[40,77] but in more rural areas the majority of TB-infected patients only have TB. In the country's central plateau, only 5% of our TB patients are coinfected with HIV.[78]

High rates of TB among patients with HIV disease have been registered elsewhere in Latin America. In a study of 177 AIDS patients in Mexico, the most common infections were cytomegalovirus (69% of patients), TB (25% of patients), and PCP (24% of patients).[79] In Brazil, 87% of AIDS patients in one study had oral candidiasis, 32% had TB, and 24% had PCP. The authors of this study concluded that "the clinical spectrum of opportunistic infections more closely resembled that reported in Africa and Haiti, with a greater frequency of fungal and mycobacterial infections than PCP and viral infections."[80] A study done in Rwanda found that among patients with HIV who present with symptoms of pulmonary disease, the most common underlying pathogen was *M. tuberculosis*.[70] In an autopsy study from Côte d'Ivoire, 53% of all AIDS deaths could be attributed to one of three conditions: tuberculosis, bacteremia (primarily with gram-negative rods), or cerebral toxoplasmosis. As the authors note, "the three major underlying pathologies (TB, toxoplasmosis, and bacteremia) are either preventable or treatable."[69]

Within the United States, differential distributions of opportunistic infections also occur. Significant differences exist between men and women, between IDUs and gay men, and even between cities, such as Miami and San Francisco. In a study of AIDS-indicative diagnoses among cases reported to the CDC, Kaposi's sarcoma was less likely to be reported among women than among men who acquired HIV infection through homosexual contact. In general, the study found that esophageal candidiasis, herpes simplex virus, and cytomegalovirus were more likely to be reported among women than men.[81] An autopsy study of 565

Figure 3. The pie chart below shows the presenting diagnoses for 200 patients with HIV at the Clinique Bon Sauveur from 1993 to 1995.

Reprinted with permission from *AIDS Clinical Care.*[76]

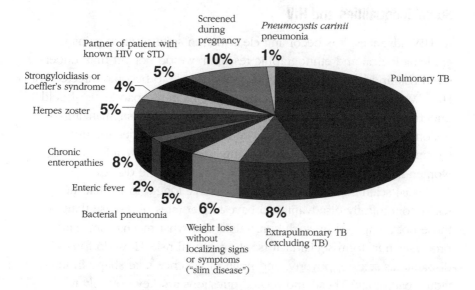

adults in Los Angeles who died of AIDS also demonstrated that women were less likely to have Kaposi's sarcoma then were men who had acquired HIV infection through homosexual transmission.[82] Sexually transmitted infection, cervical cancer, pelvic inflammatory disease, and recurrent vaginal candidiasis continue to be documented at extraordinarily high rates among women with HIV, and the natural history of these conditions seems to be worsened by HIV.[83-86] (Chapter 8 reviews in detail the interactions between HIV and other STDs.)

Finally, many have noted shifts in the incidence of opportunistic infections within a given population. In 1981, Kaposi's sarcoma was seen in most patients with AIDS and was the most common AIDS-defining diagnosis among gay men in New York and San Francisco; 6 years later, fewer than one third of those diagnosed with AIDS were found to have this cancer.[87,88] On the other hand, the incidence of serious infections with *Salmonella* species, *Streptococcus pneumoniae*, *Staphylococcus aureus, Campylobacter* species, and *Haemophilus influenzae* is significantly higher among HIV-infected patients compared with seronegative controls.[89] Atypical presentations, including higher rates of bacteremia, are common, as are relapses after standard courses of antibiotics.[90] As the epidemic settles in on the urban poor, these diseases are registered more frequently.[91,92]

Social Inequalities and HIV

As HIV advances, it is becoming clear that, in spite of great gains in epidemiological and ethnographic research, we do not yet fully under-stand risk and how it is structured. Who is likely to become infected with HIV? Who is shielded from risk? Recent trends in the pandemic should undermine the falsely reassuring—and inappropriately stigmatizing—notion of discrete "risk groups" to be identified by epidemiologists. Groups not previously viewed as being "at risk" for HIV infection (eg, women living in poverty) are being devastated by the disease.

Social scientists and physicians alike have long known that the socioeconomically disadvantaged have higher rates of disease than do those not hampered by such constraints. But what mechanisms and processes transform social factors into personal risk? How do forces as disparate as sexism, poverty, and political violence take shape in indi-vidual pathology? These and related questions are key not only to epidemiology but to clinical practice as well. These questions are posed acutely in considering HIV infection, as AIDS has become in many settings the leading cause of young adult deaths throughout the world.

Although many observers would agree that social forces are the strongest enhancers of risk for infection, this subject has been neglected in both the biomedical and public health literature on HIV. "To date," note Krieger and coworkers in an important review of the epidemiolog-ical literature, "only a small fraction of epidemiological research in the United States has investigated the effects of racism on health." They report a similar dearth of attention to the effects of sexism and class differences; inclusive studies examining the conjoint influence of these social forces are simply nonexistent.[93] Navarro, noting growing class differentials in mortality rates in the United States, deplored "a deafening silence on this topic."[94] In another review of changes in mortality rates, Marmot observes wryly that such trends are "of much interest to demog-raphers but, judging by papers in the major medical journals, of little interest to doctors."[95]

In Canada, Hogg and coworkers found an association between lower socioeconomic status and shorter survival following infection with HIV among a group of gay men.[96] In a US study of HIV-positive patients who presented to a hospital with pulmonary symptoms, Medicaid patients were more likely to die in the hospital than were privately insured patients.[97] Another study found that uninsured HIV-patients were less likely to participate in clinical trials, and this was associated with a higher risk of death.[98] Women living in poverty are particularly vulnerable to inequalities of access to antiretroviral therapy.[99]

Physicians need to be aware of the growing impact of poverty and inequality not only in enhancing risk for HIV infection but also in affecting the course of the disease. Poverty is a tremendous obstacle to receiving adequate HIV treatment, even in countries where these therapies are available. For example, in a 1993 US study examining HIV-related expenditures, Weiss and coworkers found that the cost of medications for a one-month period for people with CD4 counts between 200 and 299 per mm^3 was $488. For those whose CD4 counts were between 100 and 199 per mm^3, the monthly cost of medications rose to $548 per month. When CD4 counts fell below 99 per mm^3, the average monthly cost of medications rose to $1,043.[100]

In 1998, Perdue and colleagues demonstrated the mean cost for patients with a CD4 count greater than 500 per mm^3 as $538 per month. For patients with CD4 counts less than 200 per mm^3, the mean was as high as $1,268 per month.[101] The protease inhibitors, which have revolutionized the treatment of HIV, cost between $4,320 and $8,010 per year of treatment. Combination regimens that include protease inhibitors cost about $10,000 per year of life saved.[102] Many residents of a wealthy country such as the United States find these costs prohibitive; in poor countries in Africa, the Caribbean, Latin America, and Southeast Asia the high cost of these medications often means they are not options at all.

The underuse of both prophylactic and antiretroviral therapy by US women has been documented repeatedly.[103-105] The HIV epidemiology research study (HERS) indicates that less than 58% of enrolled women with CD4 counts of less than 200 per mm^3 were receiving PCP prophylaxis.[106] Furthermore, many studies have documented differential survival between men and women, with women living for shorter periods of time after becoming infected with HIV.[107-111] (For a comprehensive discussion of gender inequities and HIV infection, see Chapter 6.)

Conclusions

Increasingly, the HIV pandemic is patterned so that "AIDS cases are clustered in areas with high levels of poverty and poor access to medical care."[112] One implication is that it is difficult to dissociate the battle against HIV disease from broader efforts addressing the social, political, and economic factors that put many people at risk of acquiring HIV infection in the first place. At the same time, such understandings must not lead to paralysis, since much remains to be done on both the clinical and health policy level. In 1992, the World Health Organization proposed a "global strategy" for preventing and treating HIV. Among their recommendations were the following:

• Prevention of transmission of HIV through education, the provision of health and social services, a reduction in the demand for psychoactive drugs and injectable drugs, and by "providing a supportive social and economic environment."[113]

• Provision of services to people living with HIV as well as to affected families and communities. These services should include medical care, counseling, clinical management, and social and economic support for people with HIV and for their families.

• Mobilization of national and international efforts for prevention and treatment of HIV, including advocacy, the work of nongovernmental organizations, international coordination of research, and financing the costs of the AIDS pandemic worldwide.

Each of these goals will demand careful and regular review of public health policies, as other contributions to this volume have noted.

In spite of public health slogans such as "AIDS is for everyone," AIDS has always been strikingly patterned in its distribution. However, the nature of that patterning has changed. The changing epidemiology of the disease has many implications for clinical practice, both within the United States and throughout the world. Although the effort necessary to prevent HIV transmission is daunting, primary care providers can intervene in a manner that might alter some of the unwelcome trends described above. For those caring for patients with and at risk for HIV infection, one of the most important implications of the AIDS-outcomes literature is that very often, prophylaxis works. In a study of gay men with CD4 cell counts of less than 100 per mm^3, the incidence rate of PCP among those receiving no chemoprophylaxis was 47.4 per 100 person-years; among men receiving antiviral therapy, the rate was 21.5 per 100 person-years; and the rate dropped to 12.8 per 100 person-years if the patient was receiving both antiretrovirals and PCP prophylaxis.[114,115]

So what is to be done? Among persons potentially at-risk for HIV, primary care providers could:

• Maintain a high index of suspicion of HIV infection and recognize the growing significance of high-risk situations (eg, poverty and gender inequality). Several investigations reveal the under-recognition of HIV infection among poor women living in the United States. For example, Schoenbaum and Webber demonstrated that in one Bronx emergency room serving a population with very high rates of HIV infection, only 11% of women were assessed for HIV risks.[116]

• Assess HIV risk factors in a non-judgmental fashion and engage adolescent and adult patients in discussions about AIDS and other STDs. Studies have shown that many physicians do not routinely assess the HIV risk factors of their patients. For example, Ferguson, Stapleton, and Helms found that only 11% of the residents and staff physicians they surveyed routinely screened for high-risk behaviors.[117] A national survey conducted in 1990 found that HIV transmission counseling was given in fewer than 1% of patient visits.[118] Gerbert and colleagues found that only 15% of the patients surveyed had discussed AIDS with their physicians in the past five years, and three-fourths of these discussions were initiated by the patients themselves.[119]

• Assess, prior to testing, the environment of the person at risk and how knowledge of HIV serostatus might affect his or her physical and emotional safety. Although data are lacking, a recent survey in the urban United States suggests that, in one large cohort, most women did not have housing security; almost 20% stated that they had "no safe place to live."[106]

• Assess the mechanisms by which economic and other constraints interfere with behavioral risk reductions. Once these impediments are identified, help to devise strategies to overcome these personal and social barriers.

For persons already living with HIV infection, clinicians could:

• Recognize that differential distribution—geographically and socially—of endemic parasitic, bacterial, and viral infections will determine risk for many opportunistic infections in a given patient population. Most of these infections, though potentially fatal, can readily be prevented or effectively treated early in their course.

• Stay abreast of new therapeutic developments. Studies continue to reveal significant variation in the knowledge of AIDS management in the United States, with the expected attendant results.[120,121] A study done in Holland shows that continuing education for general practitioners can also lead to better communication with patients regarding HIV.[122]

• Identify barriers to optimum health-care utilization and design systems to overcome these barriers. Coordination of care on both a hospital and community level appears to be key and often involves a team approach to management.

• Provide proven therapies to all people with HIV. As Moore and coworkers note, "the challenge now appears to be to increase the use of that therapy in all segments of the population infected with HIV."[123]

Although existing treatment strategies are imperfect, scrupulous attention to these matters would, in principle, prolong the lives of millions already infected. One of the most important studies of the AIDS era comes from Baltimore, where in the 1980s, significant race-based differences in survival helped to reveal how social inequalities become embodied as poor outcomes.[124] In more recent years, extraordinary efforts were made to erase such inequality. Chaisson, Keruly, and Moore suggest that if first-rate HIV care is provided to a cohort of poor persons, then "access to medical care is a more important predictor of survival" than are sex, race, and income level."[125] This is a remarkable claim and, if true, heartening news for physicians and other providers.

Much remains to be done. In the space of a single generation, complications of HIV infection have become the leading cause of young adult deaths in much of the world. As HIV spreads, the biological characteristics of the pandemic are changing rapidly. But, as we have tried to show, these transformations are not simply reflections of the advent of HIV to new populations and shifts in the incidence of opportunistic infections. Rather, the nature of HIV risk is changing. Although the complete history of the pandemic's course has yet to be written, it has long been clear that HIV is most deeply entrenched among the poor and marginalized; social inequality has served as a powerful cofactor for HIV transmission.

As HIV settles into the world's urban slums and works its way into poorer rural regions, traditional notions of "risk groups" and "risk factors" are of increasingly limited utility. The emergence of AIDS has generated a vast amount of research, but our understanding of disease dynamics has not kept pace with the disease, nor have our therapeutic and preventative efforts managed to slow the pandemic's progress. In each of these arenas—clinical, research, policy, and preventive—we have already tools that could avert millions of deaths. What we lack most, it seems, is the will to apply them.

Summary Points

• The modes of potentially infectious contact are constantly shifting, and social inequality, political unrest, and economic disruption all modify the ecology of risk. These multiple and diverse factors prevent researchers from establishing clearly defined distribution patterns and risk groups.

• Distribution of AIDS varies widely around the globe and within countries and within narrow regions or subpopulations of the same country. Social and political factors have altered transmission patterns and distribution over time, particularly where economic and gender inequalities exist.

• Regional and temporal variations in AIDS-related opportunistic infections require a population-based approach to clinical management of disease. Clinical manifestations also differ between men and women, especially in developed countries.

• Physicians must be aware of the growing impact of poverty not only in enhancing risk for HIV infection but also in affecting treatment and ultimately the course of the disease. Public health policy must embrace and address the fact that HIV is most deeply entrenched among the poor and marginalized.

CHAPTER 10

Privacy and the Public Health: Conflict and Change in the AIDS Epidemic

Ronald Bayer

During the early years of the AIDS epidemic, a powerful movement emerged in both the United States and in other democratic nations to protect the privacy of those with, or at risk for, HIV. It was a remarkable movement because it joined together those who spoke in the name of the most socially vulnerable and those who spoke in the name of public health. For AIDS activists, respecting the claims of privacy in the context of an epidemic was crucial to protecting those with the disease against irrational fears and deeply embedded hostilities. For public health officials, respecting privacy was crucial to engaging those most at risk for acquiring and transmitting disease. All the more striking was the extent to which the movement for the protection of privacy was able to guide public policy in the United States at a time when the national political leadership was unconcerned with AIDS and hostile to those who were most at risk—gay men and intravenous drug users (IDUs).

During the epidemic's first years, advocates of those with AIDS, public health officials, and promoters of civil liberties frequently asserted that the claims of civil liberties and public health did not clash. They noted that good public health required the protection of civil liberties, and that restrictions on civil liberties would be counterproductive from the perspective of public health. From this vantage, much of the ideology of public health, with its focus on the common good and the subordination of claims of the individual to those of the collective, seemed distinctly old fashioned. AIDS, it was sometimes said, would be instrumental in compelling a rethinking of the ethos of public health in ways that were more rights-sensitive.

What has been the lasting impact of the policy decisions made during the epidemic's first years? Have the exacting commitments to privacy endured? Has the vision of AIDS serving as a driving force for refashioning of public health proved itself?

In this chapter, these questions will be examined through two issues that have been at the center of controversy for many years: the conditions under which testing for HIV infection should occur, and the question of whether those with HIV infection should be reported by name to public health registries. The analysis will reveal that by the end of the 1990s, the effort to uphold the exceptionalist perspective, so focused on individual rights, had lost its vitality. In the end, it was the traditions of public health that would come to inform and shape policies involving AIDS.

The Politics and Ethics of Informed Consent

From the outset, the test developed to detect antibody to the AIDS virus—first used on a broad scale in blood banking—was mired in controversy.[1] Uncertainty about the significance of the test's findings and about its quality and accuracy led to disputes that inevitably took on a political and ethical character. Issues of privacy, communal health, social and economic discrimination, coercion, and liberty were always at the forefront.

Out of these controversies emerged a broad voluntarist consensus. Except for clearly defined circumstances, testing was to be done under conditions of voluntary informed consent, and the results were to be protected by stringent confidentiality safeguards. To underscore the importance of protecting the privacy of tested individuals, the option of anonymity was made broadly available. This consensus was supported by gay leaders,[2] civil libertarians,[3] bioethicists,[4] public health officials,[5] and professional organizations representing clinicians.[6]

As the importance of identifying those with asymptomatic HIV infection became a matter of clinical concern, in the late 1980s the political context of the debate over testing underwent a fundamental change. Gay organizations began to urge homosexual and bisexual men to have their antibody status determined under confidential or anonymous conditions. Physicians pressed for AIDS to be "returned to the medical mainstream" and for the HIV-antibody test to be treated like other blood tests—that is, given with the presumed consent of the patient (see Chapter 3 for a discussion of HIV testing in the context of health care practitioners in the workplace).

In a national survey of physicians, 66% approved the proposition that doctors should be able to order the antibody test for patients without their informed consent; 74% supported mandatory testing of pregnant women.[7] In December 1990, the House of Delegates of the American Medical Association called for HIV infection to be classified as a sexually transmitted disease (STD). Although the delegates chose not to act on a resolution that would have permitted testing without consent, their decision regarding classification had clear implications for a more routine approach to HIV screening, one in which the standard of specific informed consent would no longer prevail.[8] However, questions about the testing of newborns led to the greatest pressure for an abrogation of maternal privacy that would follow from mandatory newborn testing.

HIV Screening for Newborns and Pregnant Women

Despite the indeterminacy of HIV status of seropositive newborns and the absence of a therapeutic intervention for asymptomatic HIV seropositive infants, many pediatricians—notably those who were responsible for the care of babies with AIDS—became strong advocates for the early identification of seropositive newborns. Among the most forthright advocates for early identification was Dr. Margaret C. Heagarty of New York's Harlem Hospital. While reluctant to embrace the language of mandatory newborn testing in public settings, she repeatedly underscored the terrible cost of failing to identify all of those who might be infected:[9(p92)]

> Antibody positive newborns that represent potentially infected children must be identified to their physicians at birth, because the content of their medical care differs from that provided the normal child. For example, the management of a normal six-month-old with fever of unknown cause may very well be expectant, but the management of the same child, known to be antibody positive, must be much more aggressive. In short, at present pediatricians of the city [of New York] are forced to care for children with no tools beyond a high index of suspicion and their clinical skills to determine which infant or child is an immunological time bomb and which is not.

Several physicians were less circumspect about the implications of the push to identify all potentially infected children at the earliest possible moment. In 1990, the chairman of pediatrics at Downstate Medical Center in Brooklyn described the case for screening as "compelling." "For a physician to be prevented from making an accurate diagnosis of his

patient is an abridgment of both the child's rights and the physician's."
To protect a woman's anonymity at the expense of the child was "unrea-
sonable." Then, pointing to the limitations imposed by the special
considerations for privacy evoked by the AIDS epidemic—by HIV "exceptionalism"[10]—he concluded that "we would not permit this in any other
medical situation."

What is so striking in these calls was the readiness with which a
number of clinicians had come to equate early identification and aggressive intervention with the best interest of the child. From that perspective,
the mother's opposition or disinclination to accede to the testing of her
child was a barrier to crucial care. Given the priority accorded to the
interest of the child and the pediatrician's self-perception as the child's
advocate, these physicians considered it an ethical and professional
responsibility to override those obstacles.

The Institute of Medicine (IOM) report HIV *Screening of Pregnant
Women and Newborns,*[11] published in 1991, most clearly demonstrates
the depth of the divide between opinions. The report challenged the
assumptions of those who had begun to argue that the child's interest
necessitated the creation of programs that could identify, at the earliest
possible moment, those born to mothers with HIV infection. Not simply a
rejection of mandatory screening, which the IOM report found ethically
unacceptable under any circumstances, the report cast doubt on voluntary
efforts as well. "The magnitude of benefit derived from such intensive
primary care and early medical intervention is still uncertain."[11] (p27)

Recognizing that advances in diagnostic and therapeutic capacity
might well render its caution obsolete, the IOM panel underscored the
conditions under which a voluntary screening program would be found
acceptable:[11]

> If safe, effective, anti-retroviral therapy or prophylactic treatment
> for opportunistic infection and a definitive diagnostic screening
> tool for newborns were available, the argument for voluntary
> newborn HIV screening with a "right of refusal" to ensure that all
> infants who would benefit from early intervention were identified
> would be compelling.

Thus, a change in therapeutic options might yield an important
departure from the exacting standards of specific informed consent so
central to the demands of privacy. The severe criteria for a voluntary

screening program enunciated by the IOM panel was apparently met in early 1991 when the *Morbidity and Mortality Weekly Report* published "Guidelines for Prophylaxis against *Pneumocystis carinii* Pneumonia for Children Infected with Human Immunodeficiency Virus."[12] The guidelines urged that oral doses of Bactrim be administered to children whose CD4 count has dropped below 1500 as a prophylaxis against *Pneumocystis carinii* pneumonia (PCP). Although the consensus statement did not call for routine or mandatory testing, it did underscore the critical importance of identifying all such babies.

The need to identify at-risk children did not, in and of itself, dictate the conclusion that the testing of newborns take place without the prior consent of their mothers. For those who had long believed that such testing was in the interest of infected children, the new recommendations strengthened the case for mandatory HIV testing at birth. Most babies born with HIV infection were born to mothers who had become infected by intravenous drug use. They were born in understaffed, overextended obstetrical services of inner city hospitals. The experience of pediatricians serving large numbers of babies with AIDS in the prior 2 years indicated to them that the majority of infected women chose not to be tested even when counseled about the importance of knowing their own HIV status or that of their babies. Thus, these clinicians believed only mandatory HIV testing could define the class of babies who would require follow-up at 3 months of age for PCP prophylaxis.

The argument was made forcefully by Dr. Louis Cooper, chair of pediatrics at New York's St. Luke's-Roosevelt Hospital Center:[13(p7)]

> We don't have the person power to provide intensive care and follow-up for all the 130 000 kids born in New York City every year and their mothers. I can deploy the resources to provide such care for those that are positive. The problem is I don't know which they are. It's ridiculous that you aren't allowed to screen for something that runs in an incidence of 1 out of 50 babies in our hospital.

The divisions within the pediatric community over newborn screening—over the relationship between the evolving scientific evidence and public policy—were reflected in the sharp disputes that characterized the deliberations of the task force on AIDS of the American Academy of Pediatrics. When at last it issued its report[14] on HIV testing in early 1992, the document detailed the benefits as well as the risks and burdens associated with such screening. With its commitment to the tenets of voluntarism, the report nevertheless urged clinicians to recommend HIV testing for infants whose mothers were known to have engaged in high-risk behavior or who came from high seroprevalence areas. However, the task force's final recommendation—clearly a political compromise—held out the possibility that changed but undefined circumstances could result in a modification of the commitment to voluntary testing with informed consent: "The American Academy of Pediatrics opposes mandatory (involuntary) maternal and/or newborn testing at this time."

It was in this context that the move for mandatory newborn testing shifted to the political arena.

In late spring 1993, New York State, which together with California had pioneered the enactment of stringent informed consent requirements for HIV testing, gave serious consideration to legislation that would have mandated the screening of newborns for HIV infection. Had the legislation been enacted, it would have entailed the mandatory screening of all childbearing women.

The proposed amendment to the state's testing regime was introduced into the State Assembly by Nettie Mayersohn, a Democrat with a generally progressive voting record. She focused on the risk that infected mothers could transmit HIV to their uninfected infants through breast-feeding and the prospect of initiating early therapeutic intervention for those who were infected. Mayersohn challenged the morality of the state's ongoing blind seroprevalence study of newborns that could identify the number of newborns who carried maternal antibody but could not, by definition, identify which babies were potentially infected. In a press release entitled "It's a Baby, Not a Statistic, Stupid," she declared:[15]

> We cannot [be charged with] an invasion of the mother's privacy
> if we attempt to get that child into treatment as quickly as
> possible, and indeed in 75% of the cases to give those babies
> who are not infected a chance at life. ... Those babies, if they
> were able to give consent, would be pleading for protection
> from the AIDS virus, just as adult AIDS victims are insisting on
> state-of-the-art medical treatment. We here, in the State legislature,
> have to make the determination that we stand in the place of that
> infant, and that our highest priority has to be the life of that
> infant. The secret is out that the State of New York has been

using babies for statistical purposes but has been denying them treatment and the protection they need to save their lives.

Stunningly, Mayersohn's effort won the support not only of the local newspaper *New York Newsday*[16] but also of two of the three New York branches of the American Academy of Pediatrics.[17]

When at last the *New York Times* spoke out on the issue, the editors made clear their stand on how the task force and ultimately the legislature should decide the issue:[18(p64)]

> No doubt privacy is vital for many AIDS campaigns. But in applying it to newborns the experts are following their theology over a cliff. ... From the evidence at hand, a strong case can be made for exempting newborns from the general policy of voluntary testing after informed consent. It seems cruel and misguided to protect parental privacy when the welfare of tiny babies is at stake.

For those locked in conflict, the 1993 controversy in New York, which reported more HIV-infected newborns than any other state, represented a critical moment in the conflict over newborn testing. Were politically liberal New York to abandon its commitment to voluntarism, it might well set the stage for similar action in other jurisdictions. However, women AIDS activists argued passionately that the pending legislation would represent an affront to the dignity and rights of black and Hispanic women and an unwarranted politicization of the practice of pediatrics that would threaten the well-being of women and children. Their extraordinary mobilization helped forestall legislative approval.

Although this initial effort to mandate newborn testing was thwarted in the past because the state health commissioner opposed the move as an unwarranted intrusion on maternal rights, the picture changed radically 3 years later. In 1996, by which point early intervention was known to be crucial for infected newborns, Governor George Pataki introduced legislation mandating newborn screening "to ensure that those who are born exposed to HIV receive prompt and immediate care and treatment that can enhance their lives."[19] With the support of the chief health official, Barbara De Buono, MD, and the organization representing New York's county health officials,[20] opposition crumbled, and the measure passed with an overwhelming majority in both houses of the legislature.[21]

Ironically, the passage of the newborn testing legislation occurred at a time when interest had begun to shift to the question of screening pregnant women. Three pediatricians long associated with the care of newborns infected with HIV noted:[22(p284)]

> This is another example of scientific progress leaping over the stalled engine of public policy. The inescapable issue is that mothers should undergo testing for HIV infection during pregnancy, not that newborns should undergo testing after delivery [when it may already be too late to make the most significant difference].

The shift toward the question of maternal screening had begun in early 1994 following the remarkable finding of clinical trial 076[23] that the administration of zidovudine during pregnancy could reduce the rate of vertical transmission by two thirds. Coming at a time when the general clinical picture surrounding antiretroviral therapy appeared gloomy, and when prospects for a preventive vaccine seemed to be less than hopeful, these were striking findings. In the aftermath of the study, pressure has mounted to ensure that infected women be identified early in pregnancy.

Although women's rights advocates and the American College of Obstetrics and Gynecology[24] fought hard to preserve the right of pregnant women to undergo HIV testing only after specific informed consent, the prospect of saving newborns from HIV infection proved stronger. That routine or mandatory testing for hepatitis B and syphilis was a matter of policy or practice in many states made the exceptionalist demand for specific informed consent in the case of HIV seem increasingly anomalous. A survey[25] of California obstetricians done in the aftermath of clinical trial 076 found that 64% supported mandatory testing of pregnant women. Even some who had long defended the rights of pregnant women began to modify their position.

Howard Minkoff, MD, an obstetrician in Brooklyn, NY, and Anne Willoughby, MD, of the National Institute of Child Health and Human Development, suggested that the principle of informed consent be supplanted with an "informed right of refusal." The purpose was clear. "When an informed right of refusal ... is used ... a psychological burden is shifted from those who would choose the test to those who would refuse."[26] Requiring a special effort to say "no" would dramatically increase that percentage of persons testing, they believed. Others[27] have called for routine HIV testing during pregnancy, citing data suggesting that pregnant women themselves supported such a move. In 1998, the IOM, in its report *Reducing the Odds: Preventing Perinatal Transmission of HIV in the United States,*[28] recommended the routine testing of all pregnant women in the United States, with an informed right of refusal. Reflective of the changes that have occurred, two members of the panel making the recommendation had long opposed any deviation from the requirement of specific informed consent before testing for HIV.

More striking was the decision of the House of Delegates of the American Medical Association, which in June 1996 passed a resolution calling for mandatory testing of pregnant women. Commenting on that decision, a past president of the Association said:[29(p1)]

> The Association opposed testing early on because society had little to offer victims of HIV other than discrimination. But now that we can offer treatment and alter the course of the disease, and hopefully prevent it in the unborn child, we can embrace a more scientifically oriented position that might benefit all.

Finally, in that same year, the US Congress expressed its discontent with the requirement that the testing of pregnant women and the newborn be based on specific informed consent. Both houses endorsed an amendment to the reauthorization of the Ryan White Care Act (Public Law 104-147), which supports local AIDS treatment efforts. The reauthorization was ultimately enacted and signed by the President. The new law required each state receiving funds to demonstrate that it had achieved a 50% reduction in new pediatric AIDS cases, initiated a program of mandatory newborn screening, or attained a 95% testing rate of pregnant women by the year 2000.[30]

The move toward mandatory perinatal testing and the rejection of the privacy-based perspective that shaped the epidemic's early years reflected the reassertion of the primacy of public health and clinical traditions. In the case of newborns, there is a well-established tradition of mandates screening for inborn errors of metabolism on grounds of efficacy and the medical interests of the child. In the case of pregnant women, hepatitis B and syphilis screening are routine during pregnancy and are often mandated by law or regulation. As the prospects increased for clinical intervention with clear benefit to infected but asymptomatic children, it became increasingly difficult to sustain the claim that a mother's primary interests should take precedence.

How the loosening of the privacy-informed standard of specific informed consent for newborns and pregnant women ultimately might affect testing policy and practice more generally is difficult to predict. Clearly the integration of HIV testing into general medical practice will produce a tendency to treat HIV screening like other diagnostic blood tests. In early 1999, the Centers for Disease Control and Prevention (CDC) tentatively suggested that specific informed consent for HIV testing be replaced by a right of refusal. Drawing on arguments made by the IOM in *Reducing the Odds*, the CDC noted that such a change "may be preferable as a means of increasing acceptance of HIV testing and identifying HIV-infected persons in settings in which testing is routinely offered (eg, drug treatment centers, TB clinics, correctional facilities) as part of the standard of care."[30]

Name-Based Reporting

If the history of perinatal HIV testing illustrates how a changed clinical and political climate have affected privacy in the clinical setting, the issue of name-based reporting of AIDS and HIV reveals how the reassertion of traditional public health perspectives has affected public policy over the course of the epidemic.

As the dimensions of the threat posed by AIDS became increasingly apparent, state and local health departments moved to require that physicians and hospitals report by name those diagnosed with the new syndrome. Only such reporting would permit health officials to have an accurate epidemiological picture of the disease with which they were confronted. Only such reporting would permit the application of other appropriate public health measures to the sick. The public health required this abrogation of the principle of confidentiality, as had always been the case when epidemic threats were involved.

It is thus remarkable, given the salience of concerns about the privacy of individuals with AIDS, that efforts to mandate case reporting by name met little resistance. Indeed, an appreciation that only accurate epidemiological information could unlock the mysteries associated with the transmission of the new disease led the Board of the American Association of Physicians for Human Rights in 1983 to call upon local health authorities to make the names of AIDS cases reportable.[31]

Controversy did emerge, however, when the CDC called upon local
health departments to forward to Atlanta full case reports, including the
names of those about whom they had been informed. For the CDC, such
identified reports were essential if an accurate, unduplicated record of
cases was to be developed for the nation as a whole. Distrust of the
intentions of federal authorities and anxieties about how such a national
list might be abused led gay leaders to oppose such efforts. Ultimately,
the CDC was compelled to agree, albeit reluctantly, to reporting by a
unique coding mechanism—Soundex.

However, the relative ease with which AIDS was incorporated under
state and local health requirements governing the reporting of communicable diseases did not extend to efforts to make results of the HIV
antibody tests reportable.

The first successful attempt to mandate public health reporting of HIV
antibody test results came in Colorado. In August 1985, Thomas Vernon,
executive director of the Department of Health, proposed that his state
require such reporting.[32] Drawing on the scientific understanding of the
test's significance—federal health officials had just reported very high
rates of viral recovery from those who were "strongly reactive" to the
ELISA test—he noted that positive findings were "a highly reliable
marker" for infection with HTLV-III and "probably for infectiousness as
well."[33] As a result, he argued, reporting could alert responsible health
agencies to the presence of persons likely to be infected with a
dangerous virus.

Name-based reporting would permit public health agencies to
ensure that infected persons were properly counseled about the significance of their laboratory tests and about what they needed to do to
prevent further transmission of the virus. Those charged with monitoring
the prevalence of infection with the AIDS virus would be better able to
accomplish their tasks, and infected persons could be expeditiously
notified when effective antiviral therapeutic agents became available.
Every traditional public health justification for reporting applied,
according to Vernon, to infection with the AIDS virus. Responding to
concerns about breaches in confidentiality that could result in social
ostracism, loss of insurability, and loss of employment, Vernon and his
deputy for STDs asserted that the system for protecting such public
health records had been effective for decades. There was no reason
to believe that in the case of infection with the AIDS virus, the department's record would be tarnished.

Following efforts by Colorado and other state officials with an aggressive public health posture to require name-based reporting of those infected with HIV, James Mason, director of the CDC, wrote to state health officials asking them to consider the possibility of requiring "some kind of reporting."[34] Such a move, Mason stressed, would necessitate the existence of confidentiality protections, including legislative shields for health department records against disclosure. But while noting the public health benefits that might follow from the adoption of mandatory reporting, Mason warned that such a move had to be "weighed against the possibility that such a requirement might discourage persons from agreeing to non-anonymous testing."

During the very first years of the epidemic, a broad alliance of AIDS activists, civil libertarians, and public health officials from high-prevalence states successfully resisted calls for the name-based reporting of HIV infection. It was thus a great setback for those who opposed reporting that the Presidential Commission on the HIV Epidemic—appointed by President Reagan—urged in its mid-1988 final report the universal adoption of a policy first chosen by Colorado 3 years earlier.[35] More significant were the fissures that had begun to appear in the alliance opposing named-based reporting, particularly in those states where the prevalence of HIV infection was high and where gay communities were well organized.

In an address that was met with cries of protest, Stephen Joseph, commissioner of health in New York City, told the Fifth International Conference on AIDS that the prospect of early clinical intervention necessitated "a shift toward a disease control approach to HIV infection along the lines of classic tuberculosis practices."[36] A central feature of such an approach would be the "reporting of seropositives" to assure effective clinical follow-up and the initiation of "more aggressive contact tracing." Joseph's proposals opened a debate that was only temporarily settled by the defeat of New York's Mayor Edward Koch in his bid for reelection. When newly elected Mayor David Dinkins selected Woodrow Myers, formerly commissioner of health in Indiana, to replace Joseph, his appointment was almost aborted, in part because he had supported named reporting.[37] The festering debate was ended only by a political decision on the part of the mayor, who had drawn heavily on support within the gay community, to stand by his appointment while promising that there would be no name-based reporting in New York.

In New Jersey, which shared with New York a relatively high level of

HIV infection, the commissioner of health also supported named reporting, and the politics surrounding the issue were very different. Both houses of the state legislature endorsed without dissent a confidentiality statute that included named reporting of cases of HIV infection.[38] New Jersey simply exemplified a national trend. Although at the end of 1989 only nine states required named reporting without any provision for anonymity, states were increasingly adopting policies that required reporting in at least some circumstances.[39] The arguments were always the same: new therapeutic possibilities provided the warrant for reestablishing a standard of traditional public health practice.

At the end of November 1990, the CDC declared its support for HIV reporting, which it asserted could "enhance the ability of local, state and national agencies to project the level of required resources" for case and prevention services.[40] Within a week, the House of Delegates of the American Medical Association endorsed the reporting of names as well, thus breaking with the traditional resistance of medical practitioners to such intrusions on the physician-patient relationship.

In the following years, the CDC continued to press for named reporting of HIV cases, an effort that eventually assumed the dimensions of a campaign. During the mid to late 1990s, a growing number of public health officials supported the effort. Indeed, the Council of State and Territorial Epidemiologists adopted resolutions in 1989, 1991, 1993, and 1995 encouraging states to consider the implementation of HIV-case surveillance. Central to their arguments was the assertion that AIDS-case reporting captured an epidemic that was as much as a decade old, and that an accurate picture of the incidence and prevalence of HIV infection required a surveillance system based on HIV-case reporting.

Nevertheless, resistance on the part of AIDS activist organizations and their political allies persisted, and as a consequence, HIV cases typically became reportable by name only in states with relatively few cases of AIDS, which were typically states that did not have large cosmopolitan communities with effectively organized gay constituencies. By 1996, although 26 states had adopted HIV-case reporting, they represented jurisdictions with only 24% of reported AIDS cases.[41] By October 1998, the figure had risen to 32 states (3 states reported only pediatric cases), involving about 33% of AIDS cases. But it was clear that support for anonymous reporting was weakening. Florida, with its large case load, had become a reporting state, and Texas, which together with Maryland, had experimented with a unique identifier system of HIV-case reporting as an alternative to the use of names, had come to the conclusion that such an approach was unworkable.[42]

Nothing more forcefully underscores the changes occurring at the end of the 1990s than the events that transpired in New York. In 1997, the state with the largest concentration of AIDS cases began, for the first time, to consider name reporting. Although a task force charged with the responsibility of advising the commissioner of health on the matter remained bitterly divided, the lines of cleavage were clear. Only representatives of community-based organizations opposed name reporting. Public health officials on the committee and throughout the state supported HIV-case reporting by name. That deadlock only paved the way for final action in the legislative arena. On June 19, 1998, in the waning hours of the legislative session, the Democratic Party–controlled assembly voted 112 to 34 for a bill that would mandate case reporting by name and a more aggressive approach to partner notification. In so doing, it joined the Republican-dominated senate, which had already passed the bill. For advocates of name reporting, the significance of the New York decision could not be overstated.

The New York decision is best understood in terms of the effects of therapeutic advances on the national policy debate about name reporting. That effect is made clear in an editorial published in late 1997. Jointly authored by Larry Gostin, a well-known proponent of civil liberties, John Ward, MD, of the CDC, and Cornelius Baker, the African American President of the National Association of People With AIDS, the editorial represented a new alliance. Locating the argument for named reporting in the context of the remarkable therapeutic achievements represented by the protease inhibitors and the advent of HAART, the authors declared:[43(p11,62)]

> We are at a defining moment of the epidemic of HIV infection and AIDS. With therapy that delays the progression to AIDS, mental illness, and death, HIV infection or AIDS is becoming a complex clinical disease that does not lend itself to monitoring based on end state illness. Unless we revise our surveillance system, health authorities will not have reliable information about the prevalence of HIV infection. ...To correct these deficiencies, we propose that all states require HIV case reporting.

HIV-case reporting would also give public health authorities a greater ability to "ensure timely referrals for health and social services."

Most AIDS-service organizations remained adamantly opposed to name reporting, arguing instead for the use of unique identifiers. For example, the National Minority AIDS Council (NMAC) declared:[44]

> NMAC is firmly opposed to HIV name reporting because it poses significant social risks, particularly for people of color—including women, immigrants, gay men and substance abusers. Name reporting may serve to hinder rather than promote important public health goals by deterring individuals from seeking HIV testing in the first place, and for those who test positive, delaying early entry into treatment.

Despite such opposition, the decade-long battle to define the realm of confidentiality in a way that would preclude the reporting by name of those with HIV infections was drawing to a close. The CDC, which had long quietly supported name reporting, had become an ardent advocate for such efforts. Public health officials, who at the outset had opposed name reporting as counterproductive, had also switched ground. Here, as in the case of HIV screening, the traditional values and practices of public health were again imposing themselves. The vision of the early 1980s of a public health policy committed to privacy as a preeminent value became a relic of the epidemic's first years.

Conclusions

It would be a mistake to view the move from the privacy-defining commitment of the epidemic's dawn as reflecting nothing more than a conservative and traditionalist impulse within public health. Public health professionals, constrained as they are by the political context within which they operate, are driven by an ideology of pragmatism. To the extent that opposition to name reporting of HIV or a commitment to exacting standards of informed consent were viewed as enhancing the overarching goals of HIV prevention, then an alliance with those ideologically or politically committed to privacy was easy to forge. But when it became increasingly clear that public health goals could be impeded by a strict adherence to privacy, the foundations of the alliance that so defined the epidemic's first years was subject to strain and ultimately was torn asunder.

Nothing more clearly underscores the extent to which public health pragmatism can result in a sustained commitment to radical reforms instead of a return to more traditional practices and policies than the issue of needle exchange for IDUs. First proposed by those who had come to appreciate the strategy of harm reduction adopted in Europe, needle exchange met with skepticism and political hostility in the United States. Ultimately, however, public health officials saw in proposals to provide drug users with sterile injection equipment an approach that could radically reduce the incidence of infection.

In Oregon, New York, and New Jersey, for example, public health leaders who had become critics of privacy-informed exacting HIV testing policies and who were early advocates of HIV name reporting became ardent defenders of needle exchange. New York City health commissioner Stephen Joseph and New Jersey's Molly Coye exemplified this pattern. Ultimately, despite the opposition of a conservative Congress and a fearful administration, public health officials rejected both assertions about the dangers of needle exchange and underscored its potential benefits in impeding the spread of HIV.

The disjunction between elected officials and their appointed public health officials on needle exchange also makes clear why shifting positions on HIV reporting and testing cannot be reduced to political responsiveness on the part of the latter. While examples abound of capitulation to the demands of those with political power, it would be a mistake to minimize the role of the pragmatic public health world view in shaping the response to AIDS. In this instance, the initial commitment to exacting standards of privacy came to be viewed as counterproductive to the overriding commitment to AIDS prevention.

Inclusion, Representation, and Parity: The Making of a Public Health Response to HIV

Jean McGuire

"Inclusion, representation, and parity" are threshold planning and programmatic requirements for states and localities accessing almost $300 million dollars each year in HIV prevention funds from the Centers for Disease Control and Prevention (CDC).[1] No phrase more aptly marks the most critical changes in US public health practice brought on by the HIV epidemic. In summary fashion, these words reflect an evolved response to the multifactoral challenges of AIDS: a once unknown and still unpredictable infectious agent; considerable mortality now reduced by promising but burdensome treatments; the troubling and underanalyzed intersections of sex, drugs, race, gender, and culture; and the ongoing obstacles posed by the lack of universal access to health care.

Inclusion, representation, and parity have emerged as the necessary philosophical and structural responses to an enigma that continues to test the limits of expert knowledge with the realities of lived experience. This chapter will focus on the products of that struggle as seen in the development of new frameworks, partners, and roles in US[2] public health practice in HIV disease and, potentially, beyond.

Background

In CDC guidance for HIV prevention cooperative agreements, "inclusion" refers to the need for stakeholders—ranging from infected patients to clinical and behavioral scientists—to participate in decision-making regarding HIV prevention needs and resource allocation. "Representation" addresses the expectation that partnerships will reflect the demographic profile of the local epidemic, matching the race, sex, sexual orientation, transmission risk, age, and geographical characteristics of affected communities.[3] "Parity" refers to the creation of equitable access to meaningful participation by all constituencies. This requirement simultaneously imparts to states and local jurisdictions the obligation to address power differentials among individuals and communities involved in service planning and to assure that the decision-making in which these groups participate is both evidence-based and cost-effective.[4]

The principles of inclusion, representation, and parity similarly guide federal requirements for state and local HIV health care planning and service delivery funded under the Ryan White CARE Act.[5] More than $1.3 billion of HIV care is delivered through this statutory mechanism on an annual basis. Additionally, HIV clinical and behavioral research activities funded through the National Institutes of Health (NIH) have, for almost a decade, actively incorporated consumers and multidisciplinary providers in the agency's specification of research goals, protocols, outcome measures, and monitoring.[6] Diverse participatory processes have become both the threshold for and the hallmark of HIV-related prevention, research, and care.

How did the principles of inclusion, representation, and parity come to shape and be articulated within HIV public health policy, administration, and practice? In part, they were the inevitable products of intersecting necessities, opportunities, and histories, some of which will be briefly referenced here.

The identification of a deadly new illness[7] within an ostracized community created an unusual circumstance for both public health officials and gay men: one needed the other, if the cause and cure for this new plague were to be discovered. Epidemiologists had to suspend normative judgments and expand their understanding of behavior and environment as facilitators of risk. Clinicians and public health practitioners had to address barriers posed by stigma and fear when promoting care and assuring access. Gay men and their communities had to learn to trust people and institutions that had, at times, vilified their lifestyles.[8] From the beginning, uncertainty and risk were the backdrop for this mutuality of need.

HIV-related collaborations were most notable for two reasons: the multiplicity of disciplines that came together in often novel partnerships, and the centrality of affected individuals and communities. AIDS emerged at a time when public health practice was becoming increasingly multidisciplinary.[9] However, uncertainty about the correlates of both risk and recovery in this new disease created a particular urgency regarding the integration of diverse technologies, skills, and perspectives.

While infectious disease and other specialists struggled to manage the manifestations of deadly opportunistic infections, palliative care and social service providers shaped a humane system of support that formed the bedrock of the first decade's public health response. Community-organizing efforts provided a basis for voluntary care and support as well as incipient prevention efforts. Developing diagnostic[10] tools improved the possibility of disease detection but amplified opportunities for discrimination, demanding the incorporation of legal analyses in evolving AIDS public health practices. Rapidly changing disease profiles required the coordinated attention of such medical specialties as virology, hematology, oncology, gynecology, and neurology.[11]

Like other arenas in which multiple disciplines are both required and have laid claim, HIV/AIDS has often been burdened by conflicting lenses, technologies, interests, and resources. Lawyers struggled with public health practitioners over privacy protection and case identification. Bench scientists competed with drug developers for primacy in research funding. Psychologists challenged sociologists and educators over models for sustainable behavior change. The conflict between primary versus specialty disease management continues.

Real and perceived parity issues among various domains sometimes delayed or distorted needed coordination and collaboration.[12] Simultaneously, however, the fight against AIDS has successfully and inclusively engaged historically unrelated groups in difficult initiatives, including antidiscrimination protection, testing policies, drug and vaccine development procedures, clinical care delivery, and reimbursement solutions.[13]

If the degree of multidisciplinary public health planning in AIDS was without precedent, so much more so was the incorporation of consumers and others from affected communities in deliberative service and policy planning. This did not occur as a matter of course. Angry and fearful gay community members organized in the face of minimal responsiveness from many public health and medical institutions. The resulting resistance, demonstrations, and analytic contributions of ACT/UP and other AIDS activists[14] greatly shaped the HIV drug development and approval process as well as prevention and care support. Persons with AIDS (PWA) and other affected community members claimed and were accorded more central roles in public health policy and program planning than had been previously seen in other arenas.

Their extraordinary visibility and success depended in part on past histories of struggle. The path for PWA and their advocates was paved by prior mobilizations, including labor, women's, and civil rights movements; gay liberation; birth control and abortion rights efforts; and, most recently, the extraordinary health care and civil rights activism of the disability community. In each of these arenas, the voices of differentially affected individuals had become both legitimate and central in the articulation of litigated and legislated policies.[15]

The disability community, in particular, had set the standard for the primacy of consumers in the determination of rights, resources, and services.[16] Their struggles shaped a holistic view of the service needs of people with handicapping and other health conditions.[17] People living with HIV/AIDS, the new consumer group with disabilities, entered an established framework for making claims regarding accessible, comprehensive care. As women and people of color became more affected by and more involved in the epidemic, they further expanded the expectations of competent and comprehensive HIV prevention and care; sex, race, culture, and language became critical variables in developing and assessing effective interventions and support.[18] These prior social and health movements inspired and provided the basis for the recent mobilization of public health practices. In summary, the lack of clear behavioral or biological correlates of protection, the limitations of available therapeutics, the disenfranchisement of affected people, and the deadly infectiousness of HIV required inclusive, representative, and participatory processes that bridged multiple disciplines and various communities.

Evolving Frameworks

Antidiscrimination Protection as a Public Health Response

Although the role of discrimination in health care access had, by the time of the AIDS epidemic, been well recognized in the context of sex, race, class, and disability,[19] it had only been minimally addressed with regard to disease prevention and control. HIV presented a truly novel conundrum: identification and interruption of this new infectious agent depended heavily on the cooperation of marginalized individuals who participated in activities that were both deeply stigmatized and often illegal.[20] In fact, the police arms of public health had actively engaged in restrictive and punitive interactions with gay communities, sex workers, and intravenous and other drug users. Building trust was necessary to create the epidemiological and clinical profiles needed for developing a preventive and therapeutic knowledge base.

For affected communities, stigma and discrimination previously related only to their outlawed behaviors quickly expanded into active disenfranchisement based on their disease status. By 1986, discrimination in access to health care, housing, and other basic needs had been well documented; by 1988, the Presidential Commission on the Human Immunodeficiency Virus Epidemic had made antidiscrimination protections a centerpiece of its national blueprint to fight the epidemic.[21] That same year, the first federally authorized protections regarding HIV status were encoded in the Fair Housing Amendments Act, and, by mid 1990, enactment of the Americans with Disabilities Act offered broad protections against HIV discrimination in public accommodations, employment, and access to care. Since that time, more than 25 states have also passed HIV antidiscrimination laws and related public health and administrative regulations.

These developments signaled a new understanding of the role of discrimination in public health: ie, the cooperation of and the care for individuals affected by an infectious disease requires the proactive assurance of their safety and well-being. Moreover, fear and discrimination affect more than epidemiological investigations; the ability to develop and deliver effective prevention messages and services, the capacity to test promising therapeutics, and the need to provide compassionate care require both reducing the uncertainties of affected communities and improving the responses of clinical, social, and other caregivers, as well as the general public.[22] Voluminous HIV antidiscrimination litigation, legislation, and legal analyses attest to the ongoing evolution of this framework and suggest the development of important corollary applications to other disease processes.[23]

Harm Reduction as a Prevention Approach

Like antidiscrimination concerns, harm (or risk) reduction[24] practices emerged in public health well before the advent of AIDS. The earliest government condom distribution activities actually date to the First World War (as described in Chapter 8). Seat belt promotion, alcohol and tobacco control, and bicycle helmet requirements all rely on reducing possible harm[25] in the face of an ongoing, potential risky behavior. However, in the arenas of sexual health and drug use, interventions rarely went beyond abstinence messages, diagnosis, and clinical treatment. Inadequate understanding of both the profile and the promoters of sexual and drug-related behaviors had left public health poorly positioned to deal with the emergence of HIV/AIDS (as reviewed in Chapter 5). Even as gross correlates of HIV infection became generally known—anal sex, multiple partners, concurrent sexually transmitted diseases (STDs), contaminated injection devices—the ecologies of sexual and drug use risk remained unclear, requiring the development of intermediate levels of intervention.[26]

HIV-related harm reduction frameworks grew out of community-based initiatives that subsequently acquired more thorough analytic and programmatic understanding. By 1986, gay men in New York, San Francisco, and Los Angeles began actively promoting the reduction of sexual partners, the use of condoms, and the eroticization of safer sex as mechanisms for interrupting a still poorly understood viral transmission process. Within a year, bleach kit distributions among intravenous drug users (IDUs) had begun in San Francisco, Boston, Baltimore, and New York. Shortly thereafter, Yolanda Serano and other New York City activists began dispensing clean needles. By 1988, other countries with fewer social prohibitions developed more expansive models. Academic research here and abroad began to profile the effectiveness of these and other HIV harm reduction interventions.[27] Increasingly, the diverse risks and needs of differently affected communities became reflected in the variety of interventions that evolved: eg, group masturbation parties for gay men, surreptitious condom application training for sex workers, and instructions on cleaning works and cookers for drug users.

Alternative harm reduction strategies continue to evolve as the nature of relative risks, the reality of individual readiness, and the availability of support necessary for behavior change become clearer. "Smorgasbord" and "hierarchy" approaches have emerged in an effort to present nonjudgmental options to affected communities and individuals. These mixtures of behavioral and device-based alternatives often lack complete efficacy data but nevertheless represent acceptable alternatives in various populations at risk for HIV.[28] One interesting example was the *Harm Reduction Hierarchy for Women* published by the New York AIDS Institute in 1993. Incorporating interventions as diverse as abstinence, female and male condom use, foam and other barrier methods, and oral and nongenital sex play, the list provoked praise for its women-led development and derision for the uncertain safety profile of some of the proposed alternatives.

Beyond efficacy concerns, HIV-related harm reduction efforts are problematic to government administrators because of the degree to which these approaches toward sexual and drug behavior appear to contravene other public health and legal imperatives. Additionally, they provide ample opportunity for political grandstanding by moral and fiscal conservatives. Public disputes regarding condom promotion and distribution early in the epidemic limited not only the meaningful availability of barrier protection but also the development of effective prevention messages. Behind this debacle lay historic tensions regarding the role of the state in matters of sexual intimacy and contraception. These unresolved tensions continue to constrain condom-related information and access, particularly for adolescents who now account for the highest rates of new infections in the United States.[29]

No politicization of harm reduction has been more problematic than that surrounding needle exchange in the United States. Ambivalence concerning drug use, interdiction, and treatment has kept Americans from experiencing the benefits seen elsewhere following early intervention in HIV needle-related transmission.[30] Government-sponsored reviews and endorsements of the efficacy of clean needle distribution programs languish in bureaucratic limbo, unable to secure either effective program development or federal and local funding streams.[31] The resulting credibility gap for state and local public health officials has further augmented citizen resistance to siting and supporting needle exchange programs.

HIV-related risk reduction activities thus pose several challenges to public health practitioners. The strategies appear to countenance negative social and public health behaviors. The uncertainties about efficacy and the politicization of the issues and interventions create challenging leadership, administrative, and fiscal concerns. The lack of a national consensus toward harm reduction undermines local initiatives for change. In spite of these obstacles, progress in developing harm reduction programs has occurred, testimony to the compelling work of affected community members, behavioral and clinical practitioners, and often courageous public health officials.

Ecology of Risk as a Framework for Prevention

Increasing appreciation of ecology of risk has advanced understanding and acceptance of harm reduction strategies. Although disease prevention and health promotion efforts have historically focused on the determinants of individual behavior change, the HIV pandemic has given rise to a large body of knowledge addressing the broader context of risky sexual and drug-related behaviors. Economists, geographers, anthropologists, and other professionals have contributed to this promising effort, with some of the most important analyses emerging first from work in developing countries.

For example, economic and epidemiologic understanding of demographics along truck routes in Uganda and in mining towns in South Africa demonstrated the impact of forced displacement of married men on regional profiles of HIV spread.[32] In Thailand, limited financial opportunities for rural families fueled a sex trade in adolescent girls whose high rates of HIV have been closely linked with transmission rates among the military and other cohorts of men frequenting urban brothels.[33] (Chapter 9 reviews such merged epidemiological and socioeconomic data with regard to the spread of the pandemic around the world.)

In the United States, Fullilove, Fullilove, and Wallace, among others, have described the correlation of eroding social, economic, and structural supports with increased rates of HIV in devastated urban cores.[26, 34] Recognizing the source of HIV risk as well beyond the circumstances of individual behavior, comprehensive prevention interventions now include efforts as diverse as community mobilization, economic opportunity development, literacy training, and voter registration.[35] (Chapter 6 examines these wider complex needs and needed innovative responses in depth.)

Appreciating the ecology of sexual and drug-related risks creates a dilemma for public health practitioners and for publicly funded services. "We can't take on all of the implications of poverty, racism, and disenfranchisement" is an oft-heard refrain in HIV prevention and care planning. The expansive nature of the sociological and economic contributors to HIV risk fuels great concern regarding the appropriate use of limited public health resources. Moreover, few empirical data validate the protective effects of mobilization and other empowerment-related interventions, though nascent efforts at measurement are underway (see Chapter 6 for suggested measures).[36]

In spite of these challenges, however, it is readily apparent that articulating ecology of sexual and drug risks—from histories of child abuse through the burdens of neighborhood blight—is significantly affecting public health theory and practice.

Contributions of Existing Theories of Caring

The HIV field has relied on and contributed to the expansion of older frameworks of care in public health practice. For example, the concept of "least restrictive environment,"[37] well developed in disability-related services, became the underpinning of much of the early HIV support efforts. In the absence of effective treatments and in the face of considerable discrimination, particularly in hospital and long-term care settings, keeping people with HIV at home or in community-based facilities offered the hope of humane and compassionate support for loved ones as they died. As more treatment alternatives evolved, the least restrictive care paradigm paved the way for competent HIV medical support in familiar, local primary care settings versus more distant, academic tertiary care facilities.

Palliative, hospice, and home-based care had become an area of increasing theoretical, programmatic, and financial interest prior to HIV primarily because of the efforts of cancer patients and their providers. HIV expanded the need for, the visibility of, and the challenges within this underdeveloped arena of care.[38] In particular, HIV gave credence to the contributions of trained volunteers, the benefits of complementary and alternative therapies, and the importance of spiritual modes of healing. Touch became particularly important in a disease where uninformed fears of transmission led to the physical distancing of loved ones and caretakers alike. Massage, acupuncture, and other healing practices that involved the laying on of hands provided crucial support to patients struggling with physical pain and social isolation. Public health was thus faced with new questions regarding policy, programs, and resource allocation responsibilities for nonallopathic forms of care.[39]

As AIDS acuity has diminished, the roles of nonallopathic interventions have expanded to address wellness and secondary prevention. Acupuncture serves as a mechanism for relieving treatment-induced neuropathy and other side effects and for improving psychological well-being. Peer and other emotional support services have shifted their focus from the challenges of death and dying to the complex treatment decision-making process, unpredictable illness trajectories, possible job re-entry, and status disclosure for sexual partners. Exercise, yoga, nutrition planning, and stress reduction practices have become components of comprehensive care planning, even among poorer populations whose basic primary care and life support needs appear to disallow wellness concerns.[40]

Public health HIV planning efforts have been stressed by the changing nature of the HIV disease profile and the emerging response and support systems. In many respects, public health systems found it easier to address the initial periods of greater mortality and fewer treatment options because the course of disease was more predictable and the necessary service mix more familiar. The recent success of combination therapies has created challenging dilemmas for public health planners. They are simultaneously uncertain about how much long-term and palliative care capacity must be sustained for increasingly fewer dying individuals and how much nonclinical emotional and other support services can be provided for growing caseloads of individuals living with both HIV and AIDS. The increasingly complex and expensive treatment of the disease strains the commitment to social, emotional, voluntary, and nonallopathic support mechanisms important for maximizing health and preventing further transmission. The resolution of this conflict will determine the extent to which the early holistic approaches to HIV affect response to wellness and health maintenance in this and other acute and chronic illness.

Treatment Adherence Support

The final arena in which HIV-related care has newly shaped public health practice is medication compliance. Early in the advent of HIV combination therapies, researchers and clinicians identified serious efficacy problems associated with even minor deviations from the new protocols. Drug failure and resistance development greatly impact patients' health status and future treatment options; at the same time, the resulting increased risk of transmitting resistant virus creates broader public health concerns.

Medication compliance concerns had been chronicled in clinical and public health literature addressing the treatment of asthma, psychiatric illness, and hypertension. Lack of patient compliance in completing antibiotic regimens is a cause of lower treatment efficacy and emerging antibiotic resistance. In asthma, increased hospitalizations and deaths are associated with inappropriate inhalant use. In hypertension, increased morbidity is attributed to insufficient drug regimen adherence. Most research about compliance in these areas focuses on individual patient behavior as the source of the problem.[41]

A similar victim-blaming construct emerged early in the history of the use of highly active antiretroviral therapy (HAART). However, people with HIV and advocates refocused concerns about patient behavior onto the clinical and social support needed to assure compliance. As in many other HIV venues, language has been deemed symbolically important: patient "compliance" concerns have now been re-framed as treatment "adherence" problems. Furthermore, public health responsibility for providing adherence support has been articulated through research, policy making, and resource allocation mechanisms. The goals for adherence support include maximizing the well-being of each patient and reducing potential resistant virus transmission.

Summarizing Emerging Frameworks

Across the spectrum of HIV prevention and care, new and revised frameworks of public health practice have responded to the changing nature of the epidemic. Most notably, public health has embraced:

- the centrality of antidiscrimination assurances in infectious disease case-finding, prevention, and care;

- the preventive role of ecological and harm reduction theories of risk and behavior change;

- new applications of least restrictive environment, wellness, and palliative care models; and

- the public health interest in adherence support.

These shifts in public health practice have resulted from the activism of affected communities and the multidisciplinary coalitions of practitioners and researchers who joined forces with their patients. New approaches have been made possible by the most significant change wrought by the epidemic: the ongoing commitment to inclusion, representation, and parity in HIV public health policy and program development.

New Partners

The tripartite forces of lethality, uncertainty, and stigma shape the experience of HIV. In addition to demanding new frameworks of prevention and care, they also require new partnerships across the borders of disciplines, practice, and experience. The best-known partnership formed as a result of these converging forces has been the collaboration of consumers and researchers in HIV drug development and experimental drug access.[42] This section will focus on new relationships developed between epidemiology and the law, between clinical research and primary care, and between prevention and clinical services.

Disease Surveillance, Epidemiology, and the Law

Disease surveillance has a long history in the United States (see Chapter 8). Public epidemiological and field investigation capacity at the CDC allowed the contours of the US HIV epidemic to be recognized early. However, epidemiologists could not have been successful in mapping this new disease without the collaboration of affected people, many of whom understood that they had much to risk in terms of their outlaw status and their stigmatized condition.

Public health surveillance has enjoyed a privileged status in terms of its access to private, personally identifying information, often about potentially stigmatizing behaviors. Protection of the public's health has accorded state and localities the right to acquire information about both index cases and their contacts and has similarly permitted quarantine and other restrictions for individuals who pose ongoing risks of disease transmission. Other histories of punitive state action toward gay men, drug users, immigrants, and people of color have, not unexpectedly, made many fearful of the investigatory authority of state HIV surveillance and reporting programs.[43] Actions within some states have additionally spurred concerns that public health data may be used spuriously by law enforcement and judicial agencies.[44] As a result, legal theorists, litigators, and advocates undertook what were novel challenges to state disease surveillance early in the epidemic.[45] (Chapter 10 reviews in depth name reporting, contact tracing, and other surveillance activities that became the focus of legislative and litigated battles.)

For both lawyers and surveillance personnel, these debates were new and largely dichotomized by the privacy concerns of individuals and the public health responsibility of the state. Initially very adversarial, public health planners and legal advocates have since found themselves working with many shared goals: to maximize consumer use of HIV testing, to enhance state agency collection of HIV/AIDS epidemiologic information necessary for prevention and care planning, and to assure the privacy and safety of infected individuals. Consumers and service providers were critical in bridging the prior divide. The development of anonymous and confidential testing models was one pragmatic result of these joint efforts. Similarly, joint challenges to mandatory testing proposals over the last two decades represent another area of effective partnership. The inclusion of antidiscrimination recommendations in the National and Presidential AIDS Commissions of the 1980s and the passage of the Americans with Disabilities Act (1990) would not have been possible without the broad collaboration of public health planning organizations like the Council of State and Territorial Epidemiologists.

In spite of these developments, HIV surveillance remains a contested domain. Most recently, the initiation of required state-based HIV reporting systems has tested relationships among legal, epidemiological, clinical, and consumer domains (see Chapter 10 for details). Old arguments regarding privacy and need-to-know have resurfaced especially in the face of CDC recommendations for name-based systems. Indeed, ongoing development of detection and surveillance mechanisms, as well as the continually shifting contours of the epidemic, will likely prompt more challenges and new partnerships for those seeking to balance confidentiality concerns and disease tracking requirements. However, the lessons from prior struggles in HIV offer great promise for the resolution of this and other medical information and disease surveillance debates.

Researchers and Primary Care Practitioners: Novel Collaborations
The integration of clinical research and primary care grew out of several developments in HIV disease. First, the advocacy of gay men, other consumers, and many of their practitioners forced changes in Food and Drug Administration (FDA) and National Institutes of Health (NIH) regulations governing access to experimental therapies.[46] They argued that the risk-benefit assessment for research participation and experimental drug use should shift in the face of significant lethality. With no therapies available, physicians treating this new illness collaborated with researchers to gain compassionate use or other access to developing drug regimens. Patients wanted both options for themselves and for the possibility of helping others.

Also contributing to the integration of research and care was the development of the community-based research movement. Many treating physicians grew frustrated with the difficulties of accessing academic-based trials and with the narrow focus of many of those research protocols. Begun almost simultaneously in San Francisco, New York, and Boston, community-based research efforts relied on the involvement of private and clinic-based practitioners working mostly in primary care settings. Within their first 2 years, community research sites proved their capacity for rigor as well as access by producing the first critical data regarding PCP prophylaxis.[47]

Further bolstering the intersection of research and care was the growing understanding of discriminatory practices in research settings. By 1990, the National AIDS Commission, among others, had noted the lack of participation in HIV clinical trials by women and people of color (reviewed in Chapter 7). Among their recommendations was the colocation of HIV clinical research efforts in primary care institutions serving the poor (discussed in Chapter 6). By 1991, memorandums of agreement between NIH and the Health Resources and Services Administration (HRSA) affirmed from a federal policy perspective the utility and appropriateness of locating research in community health centers and other poverty-based care sites. Beyond the funding of community-based research sites, NIH required its academic-based trials to diversify trial participants by linking to clinics and other local care settings. HRSA also provided resources to augment those linkages.[48] Research access had become a standard of care in a disease for which there was no cure.

The colocation and integration of HIV research and primary care presented public health entities with the opportunity to make treatment options available to consumers and their providers while also addressing the barriers to clinical trial participation historically faced by women and people of color. However, it also situated public health agencies and their representatives in what are still unresolved administrative and ethical dilemmas surrounding the multiple interests of health care settings and providers involved both in caring for patients and managing research protocols and productivity.[49] Of particular concern in some settings has been the apparent commodification of patients as cash-poor clinics recognize the financial benefits of becoming a part of research efforts.

Since the formation of HIV research and primary care collaborations, NIH and HRSA have sponsored other research and care linkages outside of HIV/AIDS.[50] Many patients will benefit from the infusion of expertise and treatment options that will occur as a result of these collaborations. Nonetheless, it will be critical to monitor and evaluate the further development of this partnership—and of public health's role within it.

Prevention and Care: Removing False Dichotomies

As with most of public health, HIV services have been rigidly delineated in terms of preventive versus therapeutic and supportive care due to divergent funding streams and often-balkanized professional disciplines. However, these functions cannot be dichotomized in an infectious disease for which early identification and care is critical and prevention of future transmission relies on the individuals knowing their status and being treated. Fortunately, effective linkages have developed between these domains, and these efforts are expanding, due to the encouragement of consumers and providers, the leadership of public health officials, and the growing expectations of federal agency partners.

Federal support for HIV-related prevention and care flows to states and jurisdictions primarily through three mechanisms.[51] Cooperative agreements with CDC have funded HIV counseling, testing, and prevention education efforts since 1988. Clinical and social support services have been funded by HRSA through demonstration programs in the 1980s and through the formula-driven Ryan White CARE Act since 1990. The federal Medicaid program has been paying, through its state-matched entitlement, increasing proportions of the clinical care for poor people with HIV.

As these funds flow from different federal administrative structures, they are similarly bifurcated at state departmental and programmatic levels,[52] further reinforcing the distinctions between domains that should be better integrated. In some states, HIV counseling and testing services are located with other STD activities but not with HIV prevention or care; in other circumstances, Ryan White CARE resources may find themselves segregated from prevention, counseling, and testing on the one hand and from Medicaid resources on the other. Dollars are distributed within communities in similarly segmented ways, with prevention resources often going to community-based social service programs and care funding to hospital outpatient and other primary care settings.

Beyond the funding divide, HIV prevention and care efforts are conceptually distant both because their target populations are treated as distinct and because their relative interventions are seen as discreet. For most of the last 2 decades, prevention has focused almost entirely on seronegative people, while care-related efforts have targeted only infected individuals. Prevention has asserted education and behavior change as its primary agenda, and care programs have focused on HIV clinical and social service support. HIV counseling and testing has been situated precariously between these 2 domains, alternatively embraced as an opportunity for prevention intervention, assaulted for its limitations as an agent of behavior change, and heralded for its ability to bring people into care.

Disciplines have differentially distributed themselves across these arenas, further circumscribing the vision of either prevention or care delivery. Educators, sociologists, and anthropologists have been associated primarily with the province of prevention, while medical practitioners and social workers have predominated in care. Psychologists have been present in both domains, concentrating on the tools of behavior change in the one and emotional support in the other. These distinctions have meant that the critical lenses of prevention and care have not been easily accessible to one another.

Preventive clinical services such as STD screening and treatment have failed to be incorporated adequately into community-based prevention programming (the importance of which is discussed in Chapter 8). Similarly, risk assessment and harm reduction prevention tools have been almost nonexistent in HIV care environments. Although both arenas embrace empowerment models, care has produced more clearly identified roles for infected individuals and their families; prevention, on the other hand, has struggled with adequately engaging and supporting participation from affected communities.[53]

Some of the challenges faced within HIV prevention and care are quite similar. While practitioners and advocates in both have actively promoted interdisciplinary efforts, each arena has seen those efforts seriously limited by internal and external political, fiscal, and ideological disagreements.[54] Both have faced the difficulties posed to their early community mobilization efforts by pressures to more narrowly focus prevention and care interventions on the delivery of clinical diagnostic and treatment services.[55] In addition, both prevention and care continue to be challenged by the shifting course of the epidemic and the opportunities and burdens posed by new knowledge, technologies, and treatments (see Chapter 9 for an international perspective). Emerging developments have raised shared concerns in intersecting areas as diverse as the prevention impact of improved health status, the testing and disclosure implications of early treatment efficacy, and the behavioral complexities of treatment adherence.

The divide between prevention and care has closed somewhat with the advent of more effective combination therapies. The rapid improvement in health status of many patients prompted a new focus on the prevention needs of people who were beginning to live longer with HIV infection. Consumers themselves have greatly contributed to articulating this concern. Providers and funders at all government levels began to require the integration of HIV prevention services in care arenas,[56] and federal guidelines specifically address some of these issues.[57] Obstacles to realizing change include increasing clinical productivity requirements, lack of reimbursement options for behavioral services, and attitudinal and competency issues among clinical staff. Nevertheless, promising developments have occurred in areas as diverse as innovative clinic-based linkages to drug treatment, harm reduction, and needle exchange programs for individuals who relapse and emerging clinic-based and linked prevention case management services for individuals facing safe sex challenges.

Innovative diagnostic technologies and local and federal program design requirements have furthered the integration of clinical and prevention efforts. FDA approval of oral mucosal HIV testing has made possible significant expansion of HIV counseling and testing in such nonclinical settings as crack houses, drop-in centers, and bars. This success prompted some HIV prevention programs to begin integrating other STD testing, including urine screening for chlamydia, into outreach and drop-in settings. The coordination and integration of HIV and other STD prevention, testing, and treatment efforts is likely to expand considerably, given recent program requirements from both CDC and HRSA.[58]

HIV is not the only disease arena in which integration of prevention and care is evolving.[59] However, for HIV, such integration relies on the effective coordination of many diverse behavioral and clinical disciplines and is necessary for reducing morbidity and mortality both among infected individuals and among the broader population.

Summarizing New Partners

Responses to the threat of HIV demand not just new understandings of risk resiliency and remediation but also new models of partnership and collaboration. This section has reviewed three examples of novel partnerships evoked by the public health response to HIV. All three represent new domains of inclusion, representation, and parity across distinct disciplines and intersecting community and individual relationships. Each also presents conundrums to public health administration, practice, and financing, the resolution of which will shape the likelihood of these partnerships enduring not just in HIV but also beyond.

New Roles

Developments in HIV prevention and care have also produced new roles for lay and professional collaborators in the struggle against AIDS. Some were addressed in the previous section. For example, primary care doctors found themselves becoming co-principle investigators on research protocols. Preventionists have been increasingly involved in creating access to clinical screening and treatment services. Visiting nurses and Red Cross health educators have, especially in more rural areas, found themselves at the leading edge of sexual and drug behavior harm reduction and prevention service delivery. Case managers have been challenged to develop models that integrate social, emotional, practical, and clinical monitoring and support.

This section will focus on public health roles that emerged or expanded during the first two decades of the US epidemic: consumers and peers as expert collaborators and educators; volunteers as critical prevention and care service delivery adjuncts; and government as convener and consensus builder in community planning processes.

Being Is Knowing: the Contributions of Consumers

Two things propelled PWA into central public health roles early in the epidemic: strategic, forceful activism and mutuality of need. Historically, other health-related consumers have come together. In fact, the characterization of "people with..." came from the mobilization of consumers with developmental disabilities in the 1970s who asserted that they and others with handicapping conditions were people first. By the time HIV emerged, consumers in several disease and disability arenas had successfully claimed central roles in determining their health care access and support needs. For example, consumers or their representatives became required members of interdisciplinary teams responsible for active treatment plan development under Medicaid's intermediate care program for people with mental retardation.[60] Children with disabilities and their parents became mandated members of individual educational plan development teams under the Education for All Handicapped Children Act of 1975 (Public Law 94-142). Consumer-directed personal care assistance became a hallmark of vocational rehabilitation and other federal support mechanisms by the early 1990s. Consumers demanded respect for their autonomy and individualized needs such that education, public health, and medical care gradually embraced their claims for client-centered services.

Similar concerns shaped the ways in which persons with HIV came to be critical participants in the development of research, care, and prevention related to their needs. Additionally, the lethality and the uncertainty associated with HIV compelled early consumer activism and prepared clinicians and researchers to welcome infected individuals as informed experts in the development of prevention and treatment models. Finally, prior experiences of being marginalized and the power of this new stigma created early community demands for visibility, input, and self determination.

A 1983 meeting of primarily gay activists and PWA produced a manifesto called the Denver Accord, which asserted the rights of those living with AIDS and created the National Association of People with AIDS, an advocacy and information organization focused on consumers' needs.[61] These early activists were compelling and courageous spokespeople and effectively championed the role of consumers in local and national struggles for compassionate and humane care. The recognition of PWA as necessary partners in public policy deliberations was recognized as early as the first Congressional hearing held by Rep. Henry Waxman (D-CA) on what in 1983 was still known as Gay Related Immune Deficiency.

Since that time, consumer participation has become a measure of quality assurance in federally funded HIV activities. Consumer advisory boards have been required components of NIH-funded AIDS clinical trial sites since 1990, and consumers have had ongoing representation in NIH's national AIDS research planning groups since that time. Consumer involvement in HIV care planning has been required as a part of compliance with the Ryan White CARE Act since 1991, and HRSA has funded technical assistance to support this effort. Site visits to CARE programs across the country generally involve review of consumer participation and often include meetings with consumer representatives. Finally, infected consumers as well as other representatives from affected communities are mandated participants in state and local HIV prevention, cooperative agreement planning groups supported by CDC.

Consumer participation in the planning, development, and monitoring of HIV programs has enriched service delivery. People living with HIV/AIDS have inspired energy and creativity, demanded accountability, and required responsiveness in programs, policies, and providers—private and public alike. PWA have reframed research policies and protocol designs to maximize the likelihood of successful recruitment and retention. Consumer need and consumer demands helped shape the extensive array of social, emotional, and voluntary support structures that have proliferated across the country. Consumers are now leading the way in shaping primary and secondary prevention efforts focused on the realities and needs of living longer and more safely with an infectious disease. From the beginning, however, the most important and enduring contribution of visible consumer involvement has been the extent to which it challenges stigma and isolation and promotes participation in care and support.

Consumer involvement in HIV has truly enhanced the focus, quality, and responsiveness of service delivery. However, the presence of vocal and demanding consumers has also made HIV service providers and public health officials uncomfortable and sometimes resistant.[62] An ongoing challenge to the effective involvement of consumers in HIV and elsewhere is the difficulty some face in seeing beyond the limits of their own illness experience to what may be different experiences or needs of others living with the same condition. Here the importance of inclusive and representative processes must be stressed, as they can provide a context for these critical individual experiences to be understood in relationship to many differently affected communities and many competing needs.

Peers: the Imperative of Shared Identity

Peer members of affected communities have been increasingly relevant in public health practices designed to reach marginalized individuals at risk of disease or in need of services. As outreach workers and educators, indigenous community members, or peers, have become one of the largest growing components of the public health workforce, contributing extensively to efforts to increase levels of immunization, control alcohol and substance abuse, and improve maternal and child health. Efforts to formalize peer training, improve their wages, and institutionalize them as critical members of the public health profession has increased in recent years.[63]

Early in the HIV epidemic, community activists and public health practitioners recognized that the mistrust between service providers and communities affected by HIV needed to be overcome, if prevention messages and access to testing and care were to be successful. Peer-based interventions and practices were recognized as critical to achieving those connections. Peers workers in HIV have, as a result, provided considerable support to people seeking to change risky drug and sexual behaviors, to individuals struggling to disclose their status to partners, and to people burdened with the constant therapeutic, mental health, and other challenges of living with the virus. Peer outreach workers distribute condoms and clean needles, provide access to HIV counseling and testing, and bring people into treatment and care. Because of their access, credibility, and influence in arenas where public health practitioners and others may not be welcome, peers have become necessary templates for the support of many HIV service elements.

The urgency and the complexity of HIV and the critical role of the peer connection have brought new credibility to this emerging component of public health work. However, the expanding use of peers in HIV and elsewhere raises several concerns: How extensive does their training need to be? What are appropriate skill requirements for workers going into potentially dangerous areas? What is responsible compensation? What is necessary supervision? Posing additional challenges for many peer workers in HIV are their own histories and experiences of risk. What, then, are the implications for the peer worker who returns to people and settings connected to his or her prior risky behavior? Having been a sex worker or an addict concomitantly provides a peer with particularly valuable insight into the challenges faced by others but may also place peer workers at risk in their new workplace. Further consideration of this issue must be undertaken if peers are to be appropriately supported in the work they do. The implications for public health administration are considerable, and the value of these workers is demonstrable.

Volunteers: the Backbone of the First Decade, a Question for the Future

By 1990, estimates suggested that tens of thousands of individuals had become a part of the unpaid workforce supporting HIV prevention and care efforts.[64] These individuals first responded to the need to provide basic care and support to people dying with AIDS. Shunned in hospitals and in other public health settings, PWA were fed, housed, bathed, and otherwise cared for by friends, lovers, and, eventually, organized armies of community members. Early on, volunteers also joined speakers bureaus and other efforts to disseminate prevention information.

Volunteers were the backbone of what became know as the San Francisco model,[65] an early integrated system of clinical and social support replicated in many of the hardest hit cities. As their roles became more extensive, community groups began to organize, coordinate, train, and supervise the diverse corps of voluntary workers. Unpaid lay individuals were trained to handle complex infusion lines, personal assistance chores, and difficult social, emotional, clinical, and mental health challenges. By the time the Ryan White CARE Act passed, the institutional capacity needed to support so much critical unpaid labor was recognized as an allowable expense under these new discretionary resources. The training, stipends, and emotional support of HIV service volunteers remains an allowable expense under the CARE Act 10 years later. Like consumers and peer workers, volunteers have also helped reduce stigma and isolation, the greatest burdens of this disease. Moreover, they made possible more humane systems of care in the context of a challenging and deadly disease.

The future of voluntary work in the epidemic is in question. Fatigue has set in. Liability and competency concerns have arisen with more complex client support needs. Poor communities increasingly in need of volunteer assistance lack adequate capacity, because the communal burdens of poverty extend well beyond the problems of HIV. Finally, public health agencies are struggling with the appropriateness of financially supporting extensive voluntary systems at a time when per capita service resources are shrinking and when similar resources are not devoted to volunteers working with other needy sick populations.

Despite these familiar conundrums about the appropriate role of public resources in voluntary efforts, the voluntary sector in HIV has been important for more than just its additional service capacity. Volunteers from board members to home health workers have continuously provided a critical base of informed and caring people who are aware of the epidemic, its burdens, and its human toll. They help shape a sympathetic public necessary to the ongoing development of nondiscriminatory, responsive, and humane HIV services.

Government as Convener, Consensus Builder, and Coordinator

The 1990 passage of the Ryan White CARE Act mandated representative HIV care planning and decision-making groups in states and local jurisdictions; later, in 1994, CDC's prevention planning guidance required similar bodies for prevention planning and oversight. Community members were to be empowered with critical fiscal and programmatic authority through planning bodies. Local and state governments were entrusted with the roles of funders, conveners, and coordinators of these processes. Government, in essence, incurred the obligation of maintaining and sustaining the previously voluntary, unfunded, community mobilization effort.

These mandates created clear requirements regarding both the inclusiveness and representativeness of decision-making bodies for resource distribution and program development. Participants are selected who reflect the diversity of the local epidemic and have skills and experiences needed to guide the effort. The funded governmental entity bears the obligation to assure that the planning bodies are appropriately representative and that they are adequately supported in making the decisions required by law. Public accountability is relatively transparent. In many jurisdictions, the result has been innovative and responsive program planning and support.[66]

Mandates, however, do not assure inclusion, representation, or responsiveness. Concerns have risen regarding the extent to which at least some community processes and their outcomes have reflected local needs, particularly in communities of color.[67] With regard to prevention, the capacity of planning groups to engage in evidence-based decision making has been limited, and resources have not always followed the profile of the epidemic.[68] In the care arena, shifting funding to more recently affected communities has been complicated by the complexity of care delivery, the stability and experience of available providers, and the reluctance of previously funded communities to share resources. In many jurisdictions, HIV planning groups have fallen victim to problems faced by prior health care planning bodies, including the regional Health Services Agencies of the 1970s; they have found that pre-existing power relationships tend to prevail in spite of the diversification of community representatives.[69]

Government is an uneasy partner in these collective enterprises. On the one hand, it benefits from a broad range of input. Representative and inclusive processes bring information and other resources to public health deliberations and can assist government agencies by shaping support for potentially difficult choices. On the other hand, public officials can be awkward or even obstructive participants in public consensus building. They have obligations and constraints that go beyond the scope of these planning groups and they face institutional limitations in providing effective leadership for such politically charged policy issues as harm reduction, health care access, and racial disparity.

Summarizing New Roles

New public health roles have emerged in the process of building a response to the challenges of HIV. The evolving functions of consumers, peers, volunteers, and government speak both to the changes required by the demands of the epidemic and to the emergence of collaborative health planning in other complex, poverty-related, public health arenas. Butterfoss and his colleagues maintain that community health coalitions and the diversification of the roles of affected community members and others is an ecological response to "… the severity and complexity of chronic health conditions that are rooted in the larger social, cultural, political, and economic fabric."[70] The developments in HIV thus add to changes in an already shifting public health environment.

Conclusions

This chapter has provided a broad overview of the evolution of the public health response to the HIV epidemic here in the United States. The challenges of HIV demand the "inclusion, representation, and parity" of those living with and responding to the clinical, behavioral, social, emotional, and legal challenges of the epidemic. The ecology of risk and remediation requires diverse, multidisciplinary, and novel responses. These in turn present public health practice with opportunities for inno-vation and growth, while raising new questions about equity, expertise, efficacy, and efficiency. Many of these developments hold promise for affecting public health practice broadly. However, the legacy of HIV in this regard has yet to be realized and will ultimately be shaped by the courage and generosity that informs the development of public health practice in the next century.

Summary Points

- Through their use and definition, the terms "inclusion," "representa-tion," and "parity" reflect major issues raised and addressed by the AIDS epidemic.

- New frameworks created in response to the epidemic were based on antidiscrimination policies, harm reduction practices, ecological factors, expanded care-giving modalities, and treatment adherence support.

- New partnerships between epidemiology and the law, between clinical research and primary care, and between prevention and clinical services optimized disease surveillance, treatment, and prevention efforts.

- New roles arose for various participants in the epidemic. Patients play active and mandated roles in the development, implementation, and monitoring of HIV programs. Peers provide critical insight when designing and carrying out interventions. Volunteers form an essential though weakening force in the response to HIV. Government goes beyond merely providing funds to ensure innovative and responsive program planning and support.

References and Notes

CHAPTER 1

[1] Gottlieb MS, Schroff R, Schanker HM, Weisman JD, et al. *Pneumocystis carinii* pneumonia and mucosal candidiasis in previously healthy homosexual men: evidence of a new acquired cellular immunodeficiency. *N Engl J Med.* 1981;305:1425-1431.

[2] Masur H, Michelis MA, Greene JB, Onorato I, et al. An outbreak of community-acquired *Pneumocystis carinii* pneumonia: initial manifestation of cellular immune dysfunction. *N Engl J Med.* 1981;305:1431-1438.

[3] Siegal FP, Lopez C, Hammer GS, Brown, AE et al. Severe acquired immunodeficiency in male homosexuals, manifested by chronic perianal ulcerative herpes simplex lesions. *N Engl J Med.* 1981;305:1439-1444.

[4] Anonymous. Epidemiologic aspects of the current outbreak of Kaposi's sarcoma and opportunistic infections. *N Engl J Med.* 1982;306:248-252.

[5] Davis KC, Horsburgh CR Jr, Hasiba U, Schocket AL, et al. Acquired immunodeficiency syndrome in a patient with hemophilia. *Ann Intern Med.* 1983;98:284-286.

[6] Poon MC, Landay A, Prasthofer EF, Stagno S. Acquired immunodeficiency syndrome with *Pneumocystis carinii* pneumonia and *Mycobacterium avium*-intracellulare infection in a previously healthy patient with classic hemophilia. Clinical, immunologic, and virologic findings. *Ann Intern Med.* 1983;98:287-290.

[7] Elliott JL, Hoppes WL, Platt MS, Thomas JG, et al. The acquired immunodeficiency syndrome and *Mycobacterium avium*-intracellulare bacteremia in a patient with hemophilia. *Ann Intern Med.* 1983;98:290-293.

[8] Curran JW, Lawrence DN, Jaffe H, Kaplan JE, et al. Acquired immunodeficiency syndrome (AIDS) associated with transfusions. *N Engl J Med.* 1984;310:69-75.

[9] Jaffe HW, Francis DP, McLane MF, Cabradilla C, et al. Transfusion-associated AIDS: serologic evidence of human T-cell leukemia virus infection of donors. *Science.* 1984;223:1309-1312.

[10] Clumeck N, Mascart-Lemone F, de Maubeuge J, Brenez D, et al. Acquired immune deficiency syndrome in Black Africans. *Lancet.* 1983;1:642.

[11] Piot P, Quinn TC, Taelman H, Feinsod FM, et al. Acquired immunodeficiency syndrome in a heterosexual population in Zaire. *Lancet.* 1984;2:65-69.

[12] Van de Perre P, Rouvroy D, Lepage P, Bogaerts J, et al. Acquired immunodeficiency syndrome in Rwanda. *Lancet.* 1984;2:62-65.

[13] Rubinstein A, Sicklick M, Gupta A, Bernstein L, et al. Acquired immunodeficiency with reversed T4/T8 ratios in infants born to promiscuous and drug-addicted mothers. *JAMA.* 1983;249:2350-2356.

[14] Oleske J, Minnefor A, Cooper R Jr, Thomas K, et al. Immune deficiency syndrome in children. *JAMA.* 1983;249:2345-2349.

[15] Scott GB, Buck BE, Leterman JG, Bloom FL, et al. Acquired immunodeficiency syndrome in infants. *N Engl J Med.* 1984;310:76-81.

[16] Francis DP, Curran JW, Essex M. Epidemic acquired immune deficiency syndrome (AIDS): Epidemiologic evidence for a transmissible agent. *J Natl Cancer Inst.* 1983;71:1-4.

[17] Rogers MF, Morens DM, Stewart JA, Kaminski RM, et al. National case-control study of Kaposi's sarcoma and *Pneumocystis carinii* pneumonia in homosexual men: Part 2. Laboratory results. *Ann Intern Med.* 1983;99:151-158.

[18] Essex M, McLane MF, Lee TH, Falk L, et al. Antibodies to cell membrane antigens associated with human T-cell leukemia virus in patients with AIDS. *Science.* 1983;220:859-862.

[19] Gelmann EP, Popovic M, Blayney D, Masur H, et al. Proviral DNA of a retrovirus, human T-cell leukemia virus, in two patients with AIDS. *Science.* 1983;220:862-865.

[20] Barre-Sinoussi F, Chermann JC, Rey F, Jasmin C, Chermann JC. Isolation of T-lymphotropic retrovirus from a patient at risk for acquired immune deficiency syndrome (AIDS). *Science.* 1983;220:868-871.

[21] Poiesz BJ, Ruscetti FW, Gazdar AF, Bunn PA, et al. Detection and isolation of type C retrovirus particles from fresh and cultured lymphocytes of a patient with cutaneous T-cell lymphoma. *Proc Natl Acad Sci USA.* 1980;77:7415-7419.

[22] Ammann AJ, Abrams D, Conant M, Chudwin D, et al. Acquired immune dysfunction in homosexual men: immunologic profiles. *Clin Immunol Immunopathol.* 1983;27:315-325.

[23] Fahey JL, Prince H, Weaver M, Groopman J, et al. Quantitative changes in T helper or T suppressor/cytotoxic lymphocyte subsets that distinguish acquired immune deficiency syndrome from other immune subset disorders. *Am J Med.* 1984;76:95-100.

[24] Lane HC, Masur H, Gelmann EP, Longo DL, et al. Correlation between immunologic function and clinical subpopulations of patients with the acquired immune deficiency syndrome. *Am J Med.* 1985;78:417-422.

[25] Essex M. Adult T-cell leukemia/lymphoma: Role of a human retrovirus. *J Natl Cancer Inst.* 1982;69:981-985.

[26] Essex M. Horizontally and vertically transmitted oncornaviruses of cats. *Advanc Cancer Res.* 1975;21:175-248.

[27] Essex M, McLane MF, Tachibana N, Francis DP, Lee TH. Seroepidemiology of HTLV in relation to immunosuppression and the acquired immunodeficiency syndrome. In: Gallo RC, Essex ME, Gross L, eds. *Human T-Cell Leukemia/Lymphoma Virus.* Cold Spring Harbor: Cold Spring Harbor Laboratory; 1984:355-362.

[28] Kalyanaraman VS, Sarngadharan MG, Robert-Guroff M, Miyoshi I, et al. A new subtype of human T-cell leukemia virus (HTLV-II) associated with a T-cell variant of hairy cell leukemia. *Science.* 1982;218:571-573.

[29] Popovic M, Sarngadharan MG, Read E, Gallo RC. Detection, isolation, and continuous production of cytopathic retroviruses (HTLV-III) from patients with AIDS and pre-AIDS. *Science.* 1984;224:497-500.

[30] Gallo RC, Salahuddin SZ, Popovic M, Shearer GM, et al. Frequent detection and isolation of cytopathic retroviruses (HTLV-III) from patients with AIDS and at risk for AIDS. *Science.* 1984;224:500-503.

[31] Schupbach J, Popovic M, Gilden RV, Gonda MA, et al. Serological analysis of a subgroup of human T-lymphotropic retroviruses (HTLV-III) associated with AIDS. *Science.* 1984;224:503-505.

[32] Sarngadharan MG, Popovic M, Bruch L, Schupbach J, Gallo RC. Antibodies reactive with human T-lymphotropic retroviruses (HTLV-III) in the serum of patients with AIDS. *Science.* 1984;224:506-508.

[33] Hinuma Y, Gotoh Y, Sugamura K, et al. A retrovirus associated with human adult T-cell leukemia: in vitro activation. *Gann.* 1982;73:341-344.

[34] Hinuma Y, Komoda H, Chosa T, Kondo T, et al. Antibodies to adult T-cell leukemia-associated antigen (ATLA) in sera from patients with ATL and controls in Japan: a nation-wide sero-epidemiologic study. *Int J Cancer.* 1982;29:631-635.

[35] Yoshida M, Seiki M, Yamaguchi K, Takatsuki K. Monoclonal integration of human T-cell leukemia provirus in all primary tumors of adult T-cell leukemia suggests causative role of human T-cell leukemia virus in the disease. *Proc Natl Acad Sci USA.* 1984;81:2534-2537.

[36] Gallo RC, Sliski AH, de Noronha CM, de Noronha F. Origins of human T-lymphotropic viruses. *Nature.* 1986;320:219.

[37] Miyoshi I, Yoshimoto S, Fujishita M, Taguchi H, et al. Natural adult T-cell leukemia virus infection in Japanese monkeys. *Lancet.* 1982;2:658.

[38] Saxinger CW, Lange-Wantzin G, Thomsen K, et al. Human T-cell leukemia virus: A diverse family of related exogenous retroviruses of humans and old world primates. In: Gallo RC, Essex ME, Gross L, eds. *Human T-Cell Leukemia/Lymphoma Virus.* Cold Spring Harbor: Cold Spring Harbor Laboratory; 1984:355-362.

[39] Homma T, Kanki PJ, King NW Jr, Hunt RD, et al. Lymphoma in macaques: association with virus of human T lymphotropic family. *Science.* 1984;225:716-718.

[40] Hayami M, Komuro A, Nozawa K, Shotake T, et al. Prevalence of antibody to adult T-cell leukemia virus-associated antigens (ATLA) in Japanese monkeys and other non-human primates. *Int J Cancer.* 1984;33:179-83.

[41] Watanabe T, Seiki M, Hirayama Y, Yoshida M. Human T-cell leukemia virus type I is a member of the African subtype of simian viruses (STLV). *Virology.* 1986;148:385-388.

[42] Alizon M, Wain-Hobson S, Montagnier L, Sonigo P. Genetic variability of the AIDS virus: nucleotide sequence analysis of two isolates from African patients. *Cell.* 1986;46:63-74.

[43] Myers G, Pavlakis GN. Viruses: The Retroviridae. In: Wagner RR, Fraenkel-Cowat H, eds. *Evolutionary potential of complex retroviruses.* New York, NY: Plenum Press; 1995.

[44] Mellors J, Kingsley L, Rinaldo C, Jr., Todd JA, et al. Quantitation of HIV-1 RNA in plasma predicts outcome after seroconversion. *Ann Intern Med.* 1995;122:573-579.

[45] Essex M, Kanki P. The Origins of the AIDS virus. *Sci Am.* 1988;259:64-71.

[46] Kanki P, McLane MF, King NW Jr, Letvin NL, et al. Serologic identification and characterization of a macaque T-Lymphotropic retrovirus closely related to HTLV-III. *Science.* 1985;228:1199-1201.

[47] Barin F, M'Boup S, Denis F, et al. Serological evidence for virus related to simian T-lymphotropic retorvirus III in residents of West Africa. *Lancet.* 1985;2:1387-1390.

[48] Clavel F, Mansinho K, Chamaret S, et al. Human immunodeficiency virus type 2 infection associated with AIDS in West Africa. *N Engl J Med.* 1987;316:1180-1185.

[49] Marlink R, Kanki P, Thior I, Travers K, et al. Reduced rate of disease development after HIV-2 infection as compared to HIV-1. *Science.* 1994;265:1587-1590.

[50] Popper SJ, Dieng-Sarr A, Travers KU, et al. Lower human immunodeficiency virus (HIV) type 2 viral load reflects the difference in pathogenicity of HIV-1 and HIV-2. *J Infect Dis.* 1999;180:1116-1121.

[51] Sankale JL, de la Tour RS, Renjifo B, Siby T, et al. Intrapatient variability of the human immunodeficiency virus type 2 envelope V3 loop. *AIDS Res Hum Retroviruses.* 1995;11:617-23.

[52] Sankalé JL, MBoup S, Essex M, Kanki P. Genetic characterization of viral quasispecies in blood and cervical secretions of HIV-1- and HIV-2-infected women. *AIDS Res Hum Retroviruses.* 1998;14:1473-1481.

[53] Fischinger PJ, Robey WG, Koprowski H, Gallo RC, Bolognesi DP. Current status and strategies for vaccines against diseases induced by human T-cell lymphotropic retroviruses (HTLV-I, -II, -III). *Cancer Res.* 1985;45(9 suppl):4694s-4699s.

[54] Gessain A, Caudie C, Gout O, Vernant JC, et al. Intrathecal synthesis of antibodies to HTLV-1 and the presence of IgG oligoclonal bands in the cerebrspinal fluid of patients with endemic tropical spastic paraparesis. *J Infect Dis.* 1988;157:1226-1234.

55 Zagury D, Bernard J, Leibowitch J, Safai B, et al. HTLV-III in cells cultured from semen of two patients with AIDS. Science. 1984;226:449-451.

56 Goodenow M, Huet T, Saurin W, Kwok S, et al. HIV-1 isolates are rapidly evolving quasi-species: evidence for viral mixtures and preferred nucleotide substitutions. J Acquir Immune Defic Syndr. 1989;2:344-352.

57 Balfe P, Simmonds P, Ludlam CA, Bishop JO, Brown AJ. Concurrent evolution of human immunodeficiency virus type 1 in patients infected from the same source: rate of sequence change and low frequency of inactivating mutations. J Virol. 1990;64:6221-6233.

58 Delassus S, Cheynier R, Wain-Hobson S. Evolution of human immunodeficiency virus type 1 nef and long terminal repeat sequences over 4 years in vivo and in vitro. J Virol. 1991;65:225-31.

59 Myers G, Pavlakis GN. Evolutionary potential of complex retroviruses. In: Levy JA, ed. The Retroviridae. New York, NY: Plenum Press; 1992:1-37.

60 Ou CY, Ciesielski CA, Myers G, Bandea CI, et al. Molecular epidemiology of HIV transmission in a dental practice. Science. 1992;256:1165-1171.

61 Saxinger WC, Levine PH, Dean AG, de The G, et al. Evidence for exposure to HTLV-III in Uganda before 1973. Science. 1985;227:1036-1038.

62 Nahmias AJ, Weiss J, Yao X, Lee F, et al. Evidence for human infection with an HTLV-III/LAV-like virus in Central Africa, 1959. Lancet. 1986;1:1279-1280.

63 Mann JM, Bila K, Colebunders RL, Kalemba K, et al. Natural history of human immunodeficiency virus infection in Zaire. Lancet. 1986;2:707-709.

64 Huet T, Cheynier R, Meyerhans A, Roelants G, Wain-Hobson S. Genetic organization of a chimpanzee lentivirus related to HIV-1. Nature. 1990;345:356-359.

65 De Leys R, Vanderborght B, Vanden Haesevelde M, Heyndrickx L, et al. Isolation and partial characterization of an unusual human immunodeficiency retrovirus from two persons of west-central African origin. J Virol. 1990;64:1207-1216.

66 Zekeng L, Gurtler L, Afane Ze E, Sam-Abbenyi A, et al. Prevalence of HIV-1 subtype O infection in Cameroon: preliminary results. AIDS. 1994;8:1626-1628.

67 Gao F, Bailes E, Robertson DL, Chen Y, et al. Origin of HIV-1 in the chimpanzee Pan troglodytes troglodytes [see comments]. Nature. 1999;397:436-441.

68 Shaw GM, Hahn BH, Arya SK, Groopman JE, et al. Molecular characterization of human T-cell leukemia (lymphotropic) virus type III in the acquired immune deficiency syndrome. Science. 1984;226:1165-1171.

69 Suciu-Foca N, Rubinstein P, Popovic M, Gallo RC, King DW. Reactivity of HTLV-transformed human T-cell lines to MHC class II antigens. Nature. 1984;312:275-277.

70 Hahn BH, Shaw GM, Arya SK, Popovic M, et al. Molecular cloning and characterization of the HTLV-III virus associated with AIDS. Nature. 1984;312:166-169.

71 Hahn BH, Shaw GM, Popovic M, Lo MA, Gallo RC, Wong-Staal F. Molecular cloning and analysis of a new variant of human T-cell leukemia virus (HTLV-ib) from an African patient with adult T-cell leukemia-lymphoma. Int J Cancer. 1984;34:613-618.

72 Robert-Guroff M, Brown M, Gallo RC. HTLV-III-neutralizing antibodies in patients with AIDS and AIDS-related complex. Nature. 1985;316:72-74.

73 Neurath AR, Strick N, Sproul P, Baker L, et al. Radioimmunoassay and enzyme-linked immunoassay of antibodies to the core protein (P24) of human T-lymphotropic virus (HTLV III). J Virol Methods. 1985;11:75-86.

74 Sarngadharan MG, Bruch L, Popovic M, Gallo RC. Immunological properties of the Gag protein p24 of the acquired immunodeficiency syndrome retrovirus (human T-cell leukemia virus type III). Proc Natl Acad Sci USA. 1985;82:3481-3484.

[75] Hardy WD Jr, Essex M. FeLV-Induced feline acquired immune deficiency syndrome: A model for human AIDS. In: Klein ES, Karger B, eds. *Progress in Allergy*; 1986:353-376.

[76] Arya SK, Wong-Staal F, Gallo RC. Transcriptional regulation of a tumor promoter and mitogen-inducible gene in human lymphocytes. *Mol Cell Biol.* 1984;4:2540-2542.

[77] Ratner L, Josephs SF, Starcich B, Hahn B, et al. Nucleotide sequence analysis of a variant human T-cell leukemia virus (HTLV-Ib) provirus with a deletion in pX-I. *J Virol.* 1985;54:781-790.

[78] Weniger BG, Takebe Y, Ou CY, Yamazaki S. The molecular epidemiology of HIV in Asia. *AIDS.* 1994;8(suppl 2):S13-28.

[79] Jain MK, John TJ, Keusch GT. Epidemiology of HIV and AIDS in India. *AIDS.* 1994;8(suppl 2):S61-75.

[80] Nkengasong JN, Janssens W, Heyndrickx L, Fransen K, et al. Genotypic subtypes of HIV-1 in Cameroon. *AIDS.* 1994;8:1405-1412.

[81] Gurtler LG, Hauser PH, Eberle J, von Brunn A, et al. A new subtype of human immunodeficiency virus type 1 (MVP-5180) from Cameroon. *J Virol.* 1994;68:1581-1585.

[82] Charneau P, Borman AM, Quillent C, Guetard D, et al. Isolation and envelope sequence of a highly divergent HIV-1 isolate: definition of a new HIV-1 group. *Virology.* 1994;205:247-253.

[83] Peeters M, Gueye A, MBoup S, Bibollet-Ruche F, et al. Geographical distribution of HIV-1 group O viruses in Africa. *AIDS.* 1997;11:493-498.

[84] Hirsch VM, Olmsted RA, Murphey-Corb M, Purcell RH, Johnson PR. An African primate lentivirus (SIVsm) closely related to HIV-2. *Nature.* 1989;339:389-392.

[85] Robertson DL, Sharp PM, McCutchan FE, Hahn BH. Recombination in HIV-1. *Nature.* 1995;374:124-6.

[86] Artenstein AW, VanCott TC, Mascola JR, Carr JK, et al. Dual infection with human immunodeficiency virus type 1 of distinct envelope subtypes in humans. *J Infect Dis.* 1995;171:805-810.

[87] Evans LA, Moreau J, Odehouri K, Seto D, et al. Simultaneous isolation of HIV-1 and HIV-2 from an AIDS patient. *Lancet.* 1988;2:1389-1391.

[88] Sarr AD, Hamel DJ, Thior I, Kokkotou E, et al. HIV-1 and HIV-2 dual infection: lack of HIV-2 provirus correlates with low CD4+ lymphocyte counts. *AIDS.* 1998;12:131-137.

[89] Travers K, Mboup S, Marlink R, Gueye-Nidaye A, et al. Natural protection against HIV-1 infection provided by HIV-2 [see comments] [published erratum appears in *Science* 1995;268:1833]. *Science.* 1995;268:1612-1615.

[90] Louwagie J, Delwart EL, Mullins JI, McCutchan FE, et al. Genetic analysis of HIV-1 isolates from Brazil reveals presence of two distinct genetic subtypes. *AIDS Res Hum Retroviruses.* 1994;10:561-567.

[91] Bobkov A, Cheingsong-Popov R, Garaev M, Rzhaninova A, et al. Identification of an env G subtype and heterogeneity of HIV-1 strains in the Russian Federation and Belarus. *AIDS.* 1994;8:1649-1655.

[92] Salahuddin SZ, Markham PD, Wong-Staal F, Franchini G, et al. Restricted expression of human T-cell leukemia—lymphoma virus (HTLV) in transformed human umbilical cord blood lymphocytes. *Virology.* 1983;129:51-64.

[93] Nowell PC, Finan JB, Clark JW, Sarin PS, et al. Karyotypic differences between primary cultures and cell lines from tumors with the human T-cell leukemia virus. *J Natl Cancer Inst.* 1984;73:849-852.

[94] Josephs SF, Dalla-Favera R, Gelmann EP, Gallo RC, et al. 5' viral and human cellular sequences corresponding to the transforming gene of simian sarcoma virus. *Science.* 1983;219:503-505.

[95] Sarin PS, Gallo RC. Human T-cell growth factor (TCGF). *Crit Rev Immunol.* 1984;4:279-305.

[96] Robert-Guroff M, Nakao Y, Notake K, Ito Y, et al. Natural antibodies to human retrovirus HTLV in a cluster of Japanese patients with adult T cell leukemia. *Science.* 1982;215:975-978.

[97] Soto-Ramirez L, Renjifo B, McLane MF, Marlink R, et al. HIV-1 Langerhan's cell tropism associated with heterosexual transmission of HIV. *Science.* 1996;271:1291-1293.

[98] Kunanusont C, Foy HM, Kreiss JK, Rerks-Ngarm S, et al. HIV-1 subtypes and male-to-female transmission in Thailand. *Lancet.* 1995;345:1078-1083.

[99] Kanki PJ, Hamel DJ, Sankalé J-L, Hsieh CC, et al. *Human Immunodeficiency Virus Type 1 Subtypes Differ in Disease Progression. J Infect Dis.* 1999;179:68-73.

[100] Letvin NL, Eaton KA, Aldrich WR, Sehgal PK, et al. Acquired immunodeficiency syndrome in a colony of macaque monkeys. *Proc Natl Acad Sci USA.* 1983;80:2718-2722.

[101] Henrickson RV, Maul DH, Osborn KG, Sever JL, et al. Epidemic of acquired immunodeficiency in rhesus monkeys. *Lancet.* 1983;1:388-390.

[102] Chopra HC, Mason MM. A new virus in a spontaneous mammary tumor of a rhesus monkey. *Cancer Res.* 1970;30:2081-2086.

[103] Kawakami TG, Huff SD, Buckley PM, Dungworth DL, et al. C-type virus associated with gibbon lymphosarcoma. *Nat New Biol.* 1972;235:170-171.

[104] Theilen GH, Gould D, Fowler M, Dungworth DL. C-type virus in tumor tissue of a woolly monkey (*Lagothrix* spp.) with fibrosarcoma. *J Natl Cancer Inst.* 1971;47:881-889.

[105] Kanki PJ, McLane MF, King NW Jr, Letvin NL,et al. Serologic identification and characterizatin of a macaque T-lymphotropic retrovirus closely related to HTLV-III. *Science.* 1985;228:1199-1201.

[106] Daniel MD, Letvin NL, King NW, Kannagi M, et al. Isolation of T-cell tropic HTLV-III-like retrovirus from macaques. *Science.* 1985;228:1201-1204.

[107] Biberfeld G, Brown F, Esparza J, Essex M, et al. Meeting report: WHO working group on characterization of HIV-related retroviruses: criteria for characterization and proposal for a nomenclature system. *AIDS.* 1987;1:189-190.

[108] Kanki PJ, Kurth R, Becker W, Dreesman G, McLane MF, Essex M. Antibodies to simian T-lymphotropic retrovirus type III in African green monkeys and recognition of STLV-III viral proteins by AIDS and related sera. *Lancet.* 1985;1:1330-1332.

[109] Kanki P, Kurth R, Becker W, Dreesman G, McLane MF, Essex M. Antibodies to simian T-Lymphotropic retrovirus type III in African green monkeys and recognition of STLV-III viral proteins by AIDS and related sera. *Lancet.* 1985;1:1330-1332.

[110] Georges-Courbot MC, Lu CY, Makuwa M, Telfer P, et al. Natural infection of a household pet red-capped mangabey (*Cercocebus torquatus torquatus*) with a new simian immunodeficiency virus. *J Virol.* 1998;72:600-608.

[111] Essex M. Simian immunodeficiency virus in people. *N Engl J Med.* 1994;330:209-210.

[112] Johnson PR, Fomsgaard A, Allan J, Gravell M, et al. Simian immunodeficiency viruses from African green monkeys display unusual genetic diversity. *J Virol.* 1990;64:1086-1092.

[113] Tsujimoto H, Hasegawa A, Maki N, Fukasawa M, et al. Sequence of a novel simian immunodeficiency virus from a wild-caught African mandrill. *Nature.* 1989;341:539-541.

[114] Allan JS, Short M, Taylor ME, Su S, et al. Species-specific diversity among simian immunodeficiency viruses from African green monkeys. *J Virol.* 1991;65:2816-2828.

[115] Muller MC, Saksena NK, Nerrienet E, Chappey C, et al. Simian immunodeficiency viruses from central and western Africa: evidence for a new species-specific lentivirus in tantalus monkeys. *J Virol.* 1993;67:1227-1235.

[116] Peeters M, Janssens W, Fransen K, Brandful J, et al. Isolation of simian immunodeficiency viruses from two sooty mangabeys in Cote d'Ivoire: virological and genetic characterization and relationship to other HIV type 2 and SIVsm/mac strains. *AIDS Res Hum Retroviruses.* 1994;10:1289-94.

[117] Kirchhoff F, Jentsch KD, Bachmann B, Stuke A, et al. A novel proviral clone of HIV-2: biological and phylogenetic relationship to other primate immunodeficiency viruses. *Virology.* 1990;177:305-311.

[118] Ennen J, Findeklee H, Dittmar MT, Norley S, et al. CD8+ T lymphocytes of African green monkeys secrete an immunodeficiency virus-suppressing lymphokine. *Proc Natl Acad Sci USA.* 1994;91:7207-11.

[119] Lehner T, Wang Y, Cranage M, Bergmeier LA, et al. Protective mucosal immunity elicited by targeted iliac lymph node immunization with a subunit SIV envelope and core vaccine in macaques. *Nat Med.* 1996;2:767-775.

[120] Kanki PJ, Barin F, M'Boup S, Allan JS, et al. New human T-lymphotropic retrovirus related to simian T-lymphotropic virus type IIIAGM (STLV-IIIAGM). *Science.* 1986;232:238-243.

[121] Kanki PJ, Allan J, Barin F, et al. Absence of antibodies to HIV-2/HTLV-4 in six central African nations. *AIDS ResHum Retroviruses.* 1987;3:317-322.

[122] Kanki PJ, M'Boup S, Barin F, et al. The biology of HIV-1 and HIV-2 in Africa. In: Giraldo G, ed. AIDS in Africa New York: Marcel Dekker; 1988:230-236.

[123] Kanki P. HIV-2 infection in West Africa. In: Volberding P, Jacobson M, eds. 1988 *AIDS Clinical Reviews:* Marcel Dekker Publ.; 1989:95-108.

[124] Hardy WD Jr, Zuckerman EE, McClelland AJ, Zuckerman EE, et al. Prevention of the contagious spread of feline leukaemia virus and the development of leukaemia in pet cats. *Nature.* 1976;263:326-328.

[125] Agius G, Biggar RJ, Alexander SS, Waters DJ, et al. Human T-lymphotropic virus type-1 antibody patterns: evidence of difference by age and risk group. *J Infect Dis.* 1988;158:1235-1244.

[126] Sodroski J, Patarca R, Lenz J, et al. Long terminal repeat regions of murine leukemia virus and human T-cell leukemia virus as potential leukemogenic and pathogenic determinants. In: Gallo RC, Essex ME, Gross L, eds. *Human T-Cell Leukemia/Lymphoma Virus.* Cold Spring Harbor: Cold Spring Harbor Laboratory; 1984:149-155.

[127] Towbin H, Staehelin T, Gordon J. Electrophoretic transfer of proteins from polyacrylamide gels to nitrocellulose sheets: procedure and some applications. *Proc Natl Acad Sci USA.* 1979;76:4350-4354.

[128] Draelos M, Morgan T, Schifman RB, Sampliner R. Significance of isolated antibody to hepatitis B core antigen determined by immune response to hepatitis B vaccination. *JAMA.* 1987;258:1193-1195.

[129] Lee TH, McCarty J, McLane MF, Grant CK, Essex M. Feline leukemia virus proteins at the surface of cultured virus-producer cells. In: Rich MA, ed. *Leukemia Reviews International:* New York: Marcel Dekker; 1983:93-94.

[130] Kuga T, Yamsaki M, Sekine S, Fukui M, et al. A gag-env hybrid protein of human T-cell leukemia virus type-1 and its application to serum diagnosis. *Jpn J Cancer Res.* 1988;79:1168-1173.

[131] Smith RG, Nooter K, Bentvelzen P, Robert-Guroff M, et al. Characterization of a type-C virus produced by co-cultures of human leukemic bone-marrow and fetal canine thymus cells. *Int J Cancer.* 1979;24:210-217.

[132] Brown BS, Hickey JE, Chung AS, Craig RD, Jaffee JH. The functioning of individuals on a drug abuse treatment waiting list. *Am J Drug Alcohol Abuse.* 1989;15:261-274.

[133] Mitsuya H, Weinhold KJ, Furman PA, St Clair MH, et al. 3'-Azido-3'-deoxythymidine (BW A509U): an antiviral agent that inhibits the infectivity and cytopathic effect of human

T-lymphotropic virus type III/lymphadenopathy-associated virus in vitro. *Proc Natl Acad Sci USA*. 1985;82:7096-7100.

[134] Donahue RE, Johnson MM, Zon LI, Clark SC, Groopman JE. Suppression of in vitro haematopoiesis following human immunodeficiency virus infection. *Nature*. 1987;326:200-203.

[135] Gendelman HE, Orenstein JM, Martin MA, Ferrua C, et al. Efficient isolation and propagation of human immunodeficiency virus on recombinant colony-stimulating factor 1-treated monocytes. *J Exp Med*. 1988;167:1428-1441.

[136] Ezzell C. US patent for Montagnier. *Nature*. 1989;340:253.

[137] Essex M, Kanki P. The origins of the AIDS virus. *Sci Am*. 1988;259:64-71.

[138] Rey F, Salaun D, Lesbordes JL, Gadelle S, et al. HIV-I and HIV-II double infection in Central African Republic. *Lancet*. 1986;2:1391-1392.

[139] Gallo RC, Montagnier L. AIDS in 1988. *Sci Am*. 1988;259:41-48.

[140] Strom T, Frenkel N. Effects of herpers simplex virus on mRNA stability. *J Virol*. 1987; 61:2198-2207.

[141] Essex M, Sliski A, Cotter SM, Jakowski RM, Hardy WD Jr. Immunosurveillance of naturally occurring feline leukemia. *Science*. 1975;190:790-792.

[142] Saxinger W, Blattner WA, Levine PH, Clark J, et al. Human T-cell leukamia virus (HTLV-I) antibodies in Africa. *Science*. 1984;225:1473-1476.

[143] Broder S, Gallo RC. Human T-cell leukemia viruses (HTLV): a unique family of pathogenic retroviruses. *Ann Rev Immunol*. 1985;3:321-336.

[144] Schupbach J, Kalyanaraman VS, Sarngadharan MG, Blattner WA, Gallo RC. Antibodies against three purified proteins of the human type C retrovirus, human T-cell leukemia-lymphoma virus, in adult T-cell leukemia-lymphoma patients and healthy Blacks from the Caribbean. *Cancer Res*. 1983;43(2):886-891.

[145] Sankalé JL, De La Tour RS, Marlink RG, Scheib R, et al. Distinct quasi-species in the blood and the brain of an HIV-2-infected individual. *Virology*. 1996;226:418-423.

[146] Bakhanashvili M, Hizi A. Fidelity of the RNA-dependent DNA synthesis exhibited by the reverse transcriptases of human immunodeficiency virus types 1 and 2 and of murine leukemia virus: mispair extension frequencies. *Biochemistry*. 1992;31:9393-9398.

[147] Marx PA, Li Y, Lerche NW, Sutjipto S, et al. Isolation of a simian immunodeficiency virus related to human immunodeficiency virus type 2 from a West African pet sooty mangabey. *J Virol*. 1991;65:4480-4485.

[148] Gao F, Yue L, White AT, Pappas PG, et al. Human infection by genetically diverse SIVSM-related HIV-2 in West Africa. *Nature*. 1992;358:495-499.

[149] Marlink RG, Ricard D, M'Boup S, Kanki PJ, et al. Clinical, hematologic, and immunologic cross-sectional evaluation of individuals exposed to human immunodeficiency virus type 2 (HIV-2). *AIDS Res Hum Retroviruses*. 1988;4:137-148.

[150] Poulsen AG, Kvinesdal B, Aaby P, Molbak K, et al. Prevalence of and mortality from human immunodeficiency virus type 2 in Bissau, West Africa [see comments]. *Lancet*. 1989;1:827-831.

[151] Romieu I, Marlink R, Kanki P, M'Boup S, Essex M. HIV-2 link to AIDS in West Africa. *J Acquir Immune Defic Syndr*. 1990;3:220-230.

[152] Anderson RM, May RM. The population biology of the interaction between HIV-1 and HIV-2: coexistence or competitive exclusion? *AIDS*. 1996;10:1663-1673.

[153] Kawamura M, Yamazaki S, Ishikawa K, Kwofie TB, et al. HIV-2 in west Africa in 1966. *Lancet*. 1989;1:385.

[154] Sliski AH, Essex M, Meyer C, Todaro G. Feline oncornavirus-associated cell membrane antigen: expression in transformed nonproducer mink cells. *Science.* 1977;196:1336-1339.

[155] Lee TH, Essex M, de Noronha F, Azocar J. Neutralization of feline leukemia virus with antisera to leukocyte alloantigens. *Cancer Res.* 1982;42:3995-3999.

[156] Shimotohno K, Takano M, Teruuchi T, Miwa M. Requirement of multiple copies of a 21-nucleotide sequence in the U3 regions of human T-cell leukemia virus type I and type II long terminal repeats for trans-acting activation of transcription. *Proc Natl Acad Sci USA.* 1986;83:8112-8116.

[157] Yu X, McLane MF, Ratner L, O'Brien W, et al. Killing of primary CD4+ T cells by non-syncytium-inducing macrophage-tropic human immunodeficiency virus type 1. *Proc Natl Acad Sci USA.* 1994;91:10237-10241.

[158] Wei X, Ghosh SK, Taylor ME, Johnson VA, et al. Viral dynamics in human immunodeficiency virus type 1 infection [see comments]. *Nature.* 1995;373:117-122.

[159] Ho DD, Neumann AU, Perelson AS, Chen W, et al. Rapid turnover of plasma virions and CD4 lymphocytes in HIV-1 infection [see comments]. *Nature.* 1995;373:123-126.

[160] Pantaleo G, Graziosi C, Demarest JF, Butini L, et al. HIV infection is active and progressive in lymphoid tissue during the clinically latent stage of disease [see comments]. *Nature.* 1993;362:355-358.

---

[a] Part of the HIV replication cycle requires the reverse transcription of viral RNA by the virus' reverse transcriptase. This enzyme generates approximately 1 error per 104 nucleotides, or viral genome. Recent estimates of HIV replication in the human host have suggested 1010 to 1012 new viral particles produced per day.[31,55] In retroviruses, the nucleotide sequence drift is most rapid in the *env* gene, where variation occurs at about three times the rate of that seen in other structural genes such as the *pol* gene or the *gag* gene. Within an individual, the average differences between HIV-1 *env* sequences may deviate up to about 1% per year.[59] Yet the variability of viruses between individuals (ie, interpatient variability) is much greater; laboratory error or epidemiologic linkage is considered with viruses that are less than 5% divergent. The higher degree of conservation observed among viruses from a cluster of patients compared with random donors in the same geographical area was used as evidence for a rare case of dental transmission.[60]

[b] That is, gp160, gp120, p55, gp41, p27, p24, and p17.

[c] While some HIVs apparently entered people independently from subhuman primate hosts, others presumably emerged as recombinants from within a single human host.[85] HIV-1 subtype E, for example is a recombinant from a *gag* and *pol* gene region from HIV-1 subtype A, but a distinctly different envelope, presumably from a different human progenitor virus that has not yet been identified. Although rare, dual infections have been described with different clades of HIV-1 in the same human host.[86] Instances of dual infection with HIV-1 and HIV-2 have also been described,[87,88] though infection with one type also appears to offer some protection against subsequent infection with the other.[89] This is not unlike the classic example of Jenner's milkmaids who were protected from lethal smallpox by virtue of infection with the related and attenuated cowpox.

[d] We investigated the possibility that rhesus and related macaque species with SAIDS housed at the New England Regional Primate Research Center might be infected with T lymphotropic retroviruses related to HIV. Several other exogenous retroviruses have been found in subhuman primates, including the Mason-Pfizer type D virus of rhesus,[102] the gibbon ape leukemia virus,[103] and related simian sarcoma virus found in a woolly monkey,[104] and the recently described STLV in numerous Old World species.[37, 39]

[e] At the same time studies were conducted with colonized rhesus monkeys with SAIDS, wild-caught and colony-maintained African green monkeys (*Cercopithicus aethiops*) and other African monkey species were also examined. These studies were undertaken because human AIDS, while clearly present in Africa, had not been recognized in people in Asia. In a serologic survey,

20% to 70% of different groups of wild-caught African green monkeys were found to be seropositive.[108,109] These included monkeys from the eastern region of sub-Saharan Africa—extending from Ethiopia to South Africa—and from Senegal, in the western region of sub-Saharan Africa. Wild-caught African green monkeys were seropositive even more often than colony-maintained animals of the same species.

[f] More recent studies reveal that several African monkey species are infected with different SIVs. These include several species commonly described as African greens, such as vervet, grivet, sabaeus, and tantalus, as well as mona, diana, Sykes', mandrill, and sooty mangabey species.[112-116] Thus far, SIVs have not been described in Asian species or in baboons, though these species can be infected in captivity with some primate lentiviruses. As a group, the SIVs are more closely related to HIV-2s than HIV-1s, although some, such as the mandrill SIV, are evolutionarily distant.[113] The sooty mangabey monkey virus and the Senegalese human HIV-2, on the other hand, are essentially the same at the genetic level.[111,116,117] It is this virus that also apparently accidentally infected the Asian macaques in captivity.[45]

[g] These included the *gag*–encoded p24, the *pol*–encoded p64/53 and p34, and the *env*–encoded transmembrane protein p34.

[h] Because the transmembrane protein of SIV is usually smaller than the comparable protein of HIV-1, this is manifested as the absence of reactivity where it might be expected at gp41 and the acquisition of reactivity with gp32, the carboxy terminus peptide of the *env* gene of SIV.[47]

[i] We designed a quantitative, internally controlled reverse transcriptase-polymerase chain reaction (RT-PCR) that amplifies a portion of the *gag* region of HIV-2 using primers that we have previously shown to be highly sensitive and specific.[140] The assay has a lower limit of detection of 100 copies/ml and is linear over 4 logs.

[j] Although the regulation of viral gene expression in HIV-2 seems to resemble that observed in HIV-1, several differences have been described that may play a role in the differential pathogenicity and in vivo replication of these viruses. Sequence comparisons of HIV-1 and HIV-2 have demonstrated differences in the long terminal repeat (LTR) structure. Whereas HIV-1 has two nuclear factor kappa B (NF-kB) enhancer binding sites, only one can be identified for HIV-2 or most SIVs.[141] The regulation and response to T cell activation via the viral LTR also appears to be distinct in HIV-2 as compared to HIV-1.[27,142,143] Specific and unique elements in the HIV-2 LTR may regulate HIV-2 gene expression independently of the T cell activation signals or cytokines that would normally modulate HIV-1 gene expression.[142-144] Mutational studies of the unique sites in the HIV-2 LTR responsible for inducible enhancer function demonstrate that this function is more readily disrupted in HIV-2 compared with HIV-1,[144] perhaps explaining some of the distinct biological properties of the virus.

CHAPTER 2

[1] Chiasson MA, Berenson L, Li W, Schwartz S, et al. Declining HIV/AIDS mortality in New York City. *J Acquir Immune Defic Syndr*. 1999:21:59-64.

[2] Law MG, de Winter L, McDonald A, Cooper DA, et al. AIDS diagnoses at higher CD4 counts in Australia following the introduction of highly active antiretroviral treatment. *AIDS*. 1999:13:263-269.

[3] Laurence J. The immune system in AIDS. *Sci Am*. 1985:253:84-93.

[4] Brodsky FM. Stealth, sabotage and exploitation. *Immunol Rev*. 1999:168:5-11.

[5] Finzi D, Blankson J, Siliciano JD, Margolick JB, et al. Latent infection of CD4+ T cells provides a mechanism for lifelong persistence of HIV-1, even in patients on effective combination therapy. *Nat Med*. 1999:5:512-517.

[6] Furtado MR, Callaway DS, Phair JP, Kunstman KJ, et al. Persistence of HIV-1 transcription in peripheral-blood mononuclear cells in patients receiving potent antiretroviral therapy. *N Engl J Med*. 1999:340:1614-1622.

[7] Pitcher CJ, Quittner C, Peterson DM, et al. HIV-1-specific CD4+ T cells are detectable in most individuals with active HIV-1 infection, but decline with prolonged viral suppression. *Nat Med.* 1999:5:518-525.

[8] Nash P, Barrett J, Cao JX, Hota-Mitchell S, et al. Immunomodulation by viruses: the myxoma virus story. *Immunol Rev.* 1999:168:103-120.

[9] Piguet V, Schwartz O, Le Gall S, Trono D. The downregulation of CD4 and MHC-I by primate lentiviruses: a paradigm for the modulation of cell surface receptors. *Immunol Rev.* 1999:168:51-63.

[10] Cullen BR. HIV-1 auxiliary protein: making connections in a dying cell. Cell. 1998: 93:685-692.

[11] Zinkernagel RM, Planz O, Ehl S, Battegay M, et al. General and specific immunosuppression caused by antiviral T-cell responses. *Immunol Rev.* 1999:168:305-315.

[12] Laurence J. CD4+ and CD8+ T lymphocyte activation in HIV infection: implications for immune pathogenesis and therapy. *Adv Exp Med Biol.* 1995:374:1-16.

[13] Bucy RP, Hockett RD, Derdeyn CA, Saag MS, et al. Initial increase in blood CD4(+) lymphocytes after HIV antiretroviral therapy reflects redistribution from lymphoid tissues. *J Clin Invest.* 1999:103:1391-1398.

[14] Hellerstein M, Hanley MB, Cesar D, Siler S, et al. Directly measured kinetics of circulating T lymphocytes in normal and HIV-1-infected humans. *Nat Med.* 1999:5:83-89.

[15] Pantaleo G. Unraveling the strands of HIV's web. *Nat Med.* 1999:5:27-28.

[16] Douek DC, McFarland RD, Keiser PH, Gage EA, et al. Changes in thymic function with age and during the treatment of HIV infection. *Nature.* 1998:396:690-695.

[17] Wodarz D, Nowak MA. Evolutionary dynamics of HIV-induced subversion of the immune response. Immunol Rev. 1999:168:75-89.

[18] Miyoshi H, Smith KA, Mosier DE, Verma IM, et al. Transduction of human CD34+ cells that mediate long-term engraftment of NOD/SCID mice by HIV vectors. *Science.* 1999:283:682-686.

CHAPTER 3

[1] Krugman S, Giles JP. Viral hepatitis. New light on an old disease. *JAMA.* 1970;212:1019-1029.

[2] In the case of transfusion-related hepatitis, pivotal studies in the 1970s indicated that a specific circulating antigen (first known as Australia antigen) associated with viral surface particles was correlated with infectiousness, and an antibody to this antigen was correlated with protection from progressive disease. This led to the development of a vaccine against hepatitis B, but clearly other individuals with similar clinical syndromes developed infectious hepatitis due to infections from other transmissible agents. The virological and immunological studies of hepatitis B were greatly abetted by careful epidemiological studies that demonstrated increased prevalence of hepatitis B surface antigen in sexually active gay men, IDUs, health care workers who did invasive procedures, and recipients of blood transfusions from HbsAg+ donors. The development of the screening assay enabled epidemiologists to identify the specific modes and relative efficiencies of hepatitis B transmission.

[3] Openshaw H, Sekizawa T, Wohlenberg C, et al. The role of immunity in latency and reactivation of *Herpes simplex* viruses. In: Nahmias AJ, Dowdle WR, Schinazi RF, eds. *The Human Herpesviruses: An Interdisciplinary Approach.* New York: Elsevier; 1981:289.

[4] The spread of the *Herpes simplex* virus seemed pervasive, but it was unclear why some individuals would have an initial attack and never have recurrences, whereas other individuals had frequent recurrences that could not be controlled. In some cases, the host had an altered immune system, either because of the development of a hematologic malignancy, such as leukemia, or exogenous immunosuppressive drugs or procedures were used to fight cancer or an autoimmune disease. Thus, it was evident by the late 1970s, that viruses like *Herpes simplex,* could be present in the body but inactive for years and would reactivate when the host became immunocompromised. The problem was that in many cases, people who had herpes recurrences did not have obvious signs of, or reasons for, being immunocompromised. So, the reasons

for viral latency and reactivation, and how the human immune system controlled chronic viral infections, were still unclear in the late 1970s.

[5] Allen DW, Cole P. Viruses and human cancer. *N Engl J Med*. 1972;286:70-82.

[6] Vigier P. RNA oncogenic viruses: structure, replication, and oncogenicity. *Progr Med Virol*. 1970;12:240-283.

[7] While training as an infectious disease fellow, I also worked at the Fenway Community Health Center, which began to serve the gay and lesbian community of Boston in 1971. I became increasingly interested in understanding the natural history of the unfolding epidemic of opportunistic infections, neoplasms, and milder manifestations of immunodeficiency, such as the generalized lymphadenopathy, which was common in many of the gay men I saw at the clinic. Unfortunately, I encountered a profound separation at the outset of this epidemic in the approaches used to better understand the evolution of this emerging medical and public health challenge.

[8] As I finished my infectious disease fellowship, I was told that because my interests were more in the realm of clinical epidemiology, I should take an academic position in that area and not attempt to also collaborate with basic scientists trying to isolate the infectious agent or work with immunologists who were trying to understand the immunopathogenesis of the syndrome.

[9] Fields BN, Knipe DM. *Virology*. Vol 1. New York, NY: Raven Press; 1990: 1-1267.

[10] Porter RR. Structural studies of immunoglobulins. *Science*. 1973;180:713-716.

[11] Advisory Committee on Immunization Practices (ACIP). General recommendations on immunization. *MMWR Morb Mortal Wkly Rep*. 1994;43:1-38.

[12] Stevens JG. Latent *Herpes simplex* virus and the nervous system. *Curr Top Microbiol Immunol*. 1975;70:31-50.

[13] Hirsch MS, Schooley RT. Drug therapy. Treatment of herpesvirus infections. *N Engl J Med*. 1983:309:963-970.

[14] Black PH. The oncogenic DNA viruses: A review of in vitro transformation studies. *Annu Rev Microbiol*. 1968;22:391-426.

[15] Coffin JM. Structure and classification of retroviruses. In: Levy JA, ed. *The Retroviridae*. Vol 1. New York, NY: Plenum Press; 1992:19-50.

[16] Haase AT. Pathogenesis of lentivirus infections. *Nature*. 1986;322:130-136.

[17] Poiesz BJ, Ruscetti FW, Gazdar AF, Bunn PA, et al. Detection and isolation of type C retrovirus particles from fresh and cultured lyphocytes of a patient with cutaneous T-cell lymphoma. *Proc Natl Acad Sci USA*. 1980;77:7415-7419.

[18] Krugman S, Overby LR, Mushahwar IK, Ling CM, et al. Viral hepatitis, type B. Studies on natural history and prevention re-examined. *N Engl J Med*. 1979;300:101-106.

[19] Montagnier L, Chermann J, Barre-Sinoussi F, et al. A new human T-lymphotropic retrovirus: characterization and possible role in lymphadenopathy and acquired immune deficiency syndromes. In: Gallo RC, Essex ME, Gross L, eds. *Human T-Cell Leukemia/Lymphoma Virus*. Cold Spring Harbor: Cold Spring Harbor Laboratory; 1984:363-379.

[20] Castiglioni, A. *A History of Medicine*. New York, NY: Alfred A. Knopf; 1969: 1-1013.

[21] Fauci AS. Multifactorial nature of human immunodeficiency virus disease: implications for therapy. *Science*. 1993l262:1011-1018.

[22] Dickler HB, Adkinson NF Jr, Terry WD. Evidence for individual human peripheral blood lymphocytes bearing both B and T cell markers. *Nature*. 1974;247:213-215.

[23] Lucey DR, Clerici M, Shearer GM. Type 1 and type 2 cytokine dysregulation in human infectious, neoplastic, and inflammatory diseases. *Clin Microbiol Rev*. 1996;9:532-562.

[24] Scott P. IL-12: initiation cytokine for cell-medicated immunity. *Science*. 1993;260:496-497.

[25] Davey RT, Chaitt DG, Piscitelli SC, Wells M, et al. Subcutaneous administration of interleukin-2 in human immunodeficiency virus type 1-infected persons. *J Infect Dis*. 1997:175:781-789.

[26] Ho DD, Neumann AU, Perelson AS, Chen W, et al. Rapid turnover of plasma virions and CD4 lymphocytes in HIV-1infection. *Nature*. 1995;373:123-126.

[27] Perelson AS, Neumann AU, Markowitz M, Leonard JM, et al. HIV-1 dynamics in vivo: virion clearance rate, infected cell life-span, and viral generation time. *Science.* 1996;271:1582-1586.

[28] Katzenstein TL, Pedersen C, Nielsen C, Lundgren JD, et al. Longitudinal serum HIV RNA quantification: correlation to viral phenotype at seroconversion and clinical outcome. *AIDS.* 1996;10:167-173.

[29] Mellors JW, Kingsley LA, Rinaldo CR, Todd JA, et al. Quantitation of HIV-1 RNA in plasma predicts outcome after seroconversion. *Ann Intern Med.* 1995;122:573-579.

[30] Mellors JW, Rinaldo CR, Gupta P, White RM, et al. Prognosis in HIV-1 infection predicted by the quantity of virus in plasma. *Science.* 1996;272:1167-1170.

[31] Researchers were surprised to find that the supposedly latent period after acute HIV infection was actually a time of dynamic viral replication with very active cell and viral turnover. More than 10 billion HIV particles are produced daily in most HIV-infected individuals, yet a similar amount may be eliminated from the body of someone with stable infection.

[32] Holmes KK, Sparling PF, Mardh PA, et al. *Sexually Transmitted Diseases.* 3rd ed. New York, NY: McGraw-Hill, Health Professions Division; 1999.

[33] Homeostasis for humans and microbes is a balance between being overwhelmed by microbial invasion and being able to take advantage of some of the powerful effects of chronic microbial colonization. Examples include the ability of gut microflora to process food substrates into vitamin K, and the endogenous defenses in the vagina of chronically colonizing lactobacilli, which are responsible for the low vaginal pH.

[34] DeGruttola V, Seage GR 3d, Mayer KH, Horsburgh CR Jr. Infectiousness of HIV between male homosexual partners. *J Clin Epidemiol.* 1989;42:849-856.

[35] Royce RA, Sena A, Cates W Jr., Cohen MS. Sexual transmission of HIV. *N Engl J Med.* 1997;336:1072-1078.

[36] Szmuness W, Much I, Prince AM, Hoofnagle JH, et al. On the role of sexual behavior in the spread of hepatitis B infection. *Ann Intern Med.* 1975;83:489-495.

[37] An initial problem for investigators was that not all types of transfusion-related hepatitis followed the same pattern in terms of onset, clinical manifestations, and patterns of clinical resolution. The discovery that Australian aborigines tended to have high rates of chronic hepatitis and the isolation of a specific particle (known as the Australia antigen) led to major strides in understanding hepatitis and provided a marker of initial and chronic infection.

[38] Hepatitis B serological testing also facilitated understanding of the natural history of hepatitis B, since at-risk individuals could be tracked prior to infection and for long periods post-infection. If an individual became infected with hepatitis B, they could experience one of several clinical outcomes (eg, acute hepatitis with jaundice, chronic progressive course resulting in debilitation and even death, asymptomatic infection only identified through blood screening). The development of a woodchuck model permitted careful analysis of what hepatitis B actually did to the liver and how it resulted in disease and how the host could potentially clear infection. Subsequently, epidemiologic studies based on the identification of serologic markers established the link between chronic hepatitis B infection and the development of hepatoma.

[39] Sugamura K, Hinuma Y. Human retroviruses: HTLV-I and HTLV-II. In: Levy JA, ed. *The Retroviridae.* Vol 2. New York: Plenum Press; 1993:399-436.

[40] Centers for Disease Control and Prevention. Public Health Service guidelines for the management of health-care worker exposures to HIV and recommendations for postexposure prophylaxis. *MMWR Morb Mortal Wkly Rep.* 1998;47:1-33.

[41] In the late 19th century, increased awareness of the airborne transmission of tuberculosis led to public health movements to decrease urban crowding. Sanitoria—places were tuberculous individuals could be isolated from society, breathe fresh air, and get rest—were built on the presumption that exposure to fresh air and enhanced nutrition would help the individual control and hopefully cure the infection. The recognition of the aerosol spread of tuberculosis also led to enhanced awareness of nosocomial transmission and to the development of pavilion-style hospitals (ie, isolation of patients who were likely to have TB from other patients).

[42] Legislation passed by the Senate in the early 1990s threatened to cut off federal assistance to state AIDS programs if mandatory health care worker HIV screening was not implemented. Fortunately, the bill died in the House of Representatives.

CHAPTER 4

[1] Shilts R. *And the Band Played On*. New York: Penguin; 1988.

[2] Jewell, N. Some statistical issues in studies of the epidemiology of AIDS. *Stat Med*. 1990:9:1387-1416.

[3] Brookmeyer R, Gail M. *AIDS Epidemiology: A Quantitative Approach*. New York, NY: Oxford University Press; 1994.

[4] Lui KJ, Lawrence DN, Morgan WM, Peterman TA, et al. A model-based estimate of the mean incubation period for AIDS in homsexual men. *Science*. 1986:240:1333-1335.

[5] DeGruttola V, Lagakos S. Analysis of doubly-censored survival data with application to AIDS. Biometrics. 1989:45:1-11.

[6] Pagano M, DeGruttola V, MaWhinney S, Tu XM. The HIV epidemic in New York City; projecting AIDS incidence and prevalence. In Jewell N, Dietz K, Farewell VT, eds. *AIDS Epidemiology: Methodological Issues*. Boston: Birkhauser-Boston; 1988:123-140.

[7] Lin D, Fleming T, DeGruttola V. Estimating the proportion of treatment effect explained by a surrogate marker. *Stat Med*. 1997:16:1515-1527.

[8] DeGruttola V, Fleming T, Lin DY, Coombs R. Perspective: validating surrogate markers—are we being naive? *J Infect Dis*. 1997:175:237-246.

[9] Sevin A, DeGruttola V, Nijhaus M, Schapiro JM, et al. Methods for investigating the relationship between drug-susceptibility phenotype and HIV-1 genotype with applications to ACTG 333. Program and abstracts from the Second International Workshop on HIV Drug Resistance and Treatment Strategies; June 24-27, 1998; Lake Maggiore, Italy. Abstract 58.

[10] Kalbfleisch J, Lawless JF. Inference based on retrospective ascertainment: An analysis of the data on transfusion-related AIDS. *JASA*. 1989:84:406, 360-372.

CHAPTER 5

[1] Ostrow DG. Barriers to the recognition of links between drug and alcohol abuse and AIDS. In: Petrakis PL, ed. *Acquired Immune Deficiency Syndrome and Chemical Dependency*. Washington, DC: US Department of Health and Human Services;1987:15-29. DHHS Publication ADM 88-1513.

[2] Program and abstracts of the National Institute of Drug Abuse's Fourth Science Forum Research Synthesis Symposium on the Prevention of HIV in Drug Abusers; August, 3-5 1997; Flagstaff, Arizona.

[3] Centers for Disease Control and Prevention. *HIV AIDS Surveill Rep. 1999;*5(3):4-6.

[4] Stall R, McKusick L, Wiley J, Coates T, Ostrow DG. Alcohol and drug use during sexual activity and compliance with safe sex guidelines for AIDS. *Health Educ Q*. 1986;13:359-371.

[5] Ostrow DG, Van Raden MJ, Fox R, Kingsley LA, Dudley J, Kaslow RA. Recreational drug use and sexual behavior change in a cohort of homosexual men. *AIDS*. 1990;4:759-765.

[6] I remember well the reaction to that presentation. The first was a statement by a well-known pseudo-psychologist that I had proved his assertions that gay men were basically "dirty" and

engaged in coprophilia and other unhygienic practices. The second was Dr. Curran's question as to what I would do with all the money I needed to solve this problem.

[7] Garfein RS, Vlahov D, Galai N, Doherty MC, Nelson KE. Viral infections in short-term injection drug users: the prevalence of the hepatitis C, hepatitis B, human immunodeficiency, and human T-lymphotropic viruses. *Am J Public Health*. 1996;86:655-661.

[8] Vanable PA, Ostrow DG, McKirnan DJ, Taywaditep K, Hope B. Impact of combination therapies on HIV risk perceptions and sexual risk among HIV-positive and HIV-negative gay and bisexual men. *Health Psychol*. 2000;19:134-145.

[9] In fact, as a research psychiatrist, I focused more on the mental health aspects of HIV infection than on the seemingly obvious correlation between substance use and unsafe sex. The newly discovered "AIDS Dementia Complex" needed to be understood so mental health caregivers could be educated as to how to recognize and treat this potentially devastating complication.

[10] Ostrow DG, Eller M, Joseph JG. Epidemic control measures for AIDS: a psychosocial and historical discussion of policy alternatives. In: Corless IB, Pittman-Lindeman M, eds. *AIDS Principles, Practices, and Politics*. New York: Hemisphere Publishing; 1989:301-312.

[11] Patton C. *Sex and Germs: The Politics of AIDS*. Boston: South End Press; 1985.

[12] Shilts R. *And The Band Played On*. New York: St. Martins Press; 1987.

[13] Ostrow DG. Models for understanding the psychiatric consequences of AIDS. In: Bridge TP, AF, Mirsky, Goodwin FK, eds. *Psychological, Neuropsychiatric, and Substance Abuse Aspects of AIDS*. New York, NY: Raven Press; 1988:85-94.

[14] Duesberg PH. AIDS: Non-infectious deficiencies acquired by drug consumption and other risk factors. *Res Immunol*. 1990;141:5-11.

[15] Ostrow DG, Hughes M, Kessler RC. Antisocial personality disorder comorbidity is associated with increased HIV risk-taking in the National Comorbidity Study sample. (unpublished manuscript)

[16] National Institute of Mental Health. *Comorbid Mental Disorders and HIV/STD Prevention*. Request For Applications #MH-99-08. Bethesda, Md.: National Institutes of Health, 1999.

[17] Ostrow DG. Practical prevention aspects. In: Ostrow DG, Kalichman SC, eds. *Psychosocial and Public Health Aspects of New HIV Therapies*. New York, NY: Kluwer-Plenum Press; 1999:151-169.

[18] Ostrow DG, McKirnan D. Prevention of substance-related high-risk sexual behavior among gay men: critical review of the literature and proposed harm reduction approach. *J Gay Lesb Med Assoc*. 1997;1:97-110.

[19] McKirnan DJ, Ostrow DG, Hope B. Sex, drugs and escape: a psychological model of HIV risk behaviors. *AIDS Care*. 1996; 8:655-669.

[20] Critchlow B. The powers of John Barleycorn: beliefs about the effects of alcohol on social behavior. *Am Psychol*. 1986;41:751-764.

[21] Marlatt GA, Rohsenow D. Cognitive processes in alcohol use: expectancy and the balanced placebo design. In: Mello N, ed. *Advances in Substance Abuse: Behavioral and Biological Research*. Greenwick, Conn.: JAI Press; 1980:159-199.

[22] Auerbach JD, Wypijewska C, Brodie HKH, eds. *AIDS and Behavior. An Integrated Approach*. Washington, DC: Institute of Medicine Press; 1994:22-23.

[23] Doll LS, Judson FN, Ostrow DG, O'Malley PM, et al. Sexual behavior before AIDS: the hepatitis B studies of homosexual and bisexual men. *AIDS* 1990;4:1067-1074.

[24] Paul JP, Hays RB, Coates TJ. The impact of the HIV epidemic on US gay male communities. In: D'Augelli AR, Patterson C, eds. *Lesbian, Gay, and Bisexual Identities over the Lifespan: Psychological Perspectives*. New York: Oxford University Press; 1995:347-397.

25 Rofes E. *Dry Bones Breathe. Gay Men Creating Post-AIDS Identities and Cultures.* Binghamton: Harrington Press; 1998:186-197.

26 Sadownick D. *Sex Between Men.* San Francisco: HarperCollins; 1996.27 Hardly a week goes by without someone calling me to ask why the US government does not effectively ban or control sales of poppers, or why there is no crucial body of research on the prevention of HIV infection through sex-drug usage. Just as there is no viable movement to study the legalization of "hard" drugs in the United States, any attempt to seriously study harm reduction approaches to the sex-drug connection would play into the hands of those who feel that to study the situation validates the use and abuse of drugs. Fortunately, there seems to be a new breed of politician emerging who is not afraid to suggest new approaches to the drug problem.

28 Haverkos H, Kopstein AN, Wilson H, Drotman P. Nitrite inhalants: history, epidemiology, and possible links to AIDS. *Environ Health Perspect.* 1994;102:858-861.

29 Wilson H. The poppers-HIV connection. *FOCUS, A Guide to AIDS Research and Counseling.* 1999;14(4):5-6.

30 Owen F. Ecstasy bandits. *Details Magazine* 1998:December:156-161,198.

31 Stall R, Ekdstrand M, Pollack L, McKusick L, Coates TJ. Relapse from safer sex: the next challenge for AIDS prevention efforts. *J Acquir Immune Defic Syndr.* 1990;3:1181-1187.

32 I am very careful whenever I talk about rates of "relapse" to unprotected sex and clearly define what I mean by the term, especially in terms of the psychological sequela of feeling that one has failed in terms of safer sexual precautions. For many men today, engaging in unprotected anal sex is not seen as a risky act, depending on the HIV and treatment status of their partner. This may slow down my presentations or discussions, but is necessary to avoid the otherwise righteous indignation of gay activists and the incorrect use of our research by homophobic conservatives.

33 Dillon B, Hecht FM, Swanson M, Goupil-Sormany I, et al Primary HIV infections associated with oral transmission. Paper presented at: Retrovirus Conference; 2000; San Francisco, Calif.

34 Dax EM, Alder WH, Nagel JE, et al. Amyl nitrite alters human in vitro immune function. *Immunopharmacol Immunotoxicol.* 1991;13:577-587.

35 My primary hypothesis during mechanistic research between 1988 and 1996 was that no single mechanism (but instead a combination of mechanisms along with network interactions) could account for the majority of sex-drug behavior interactions leading to HIV transmission.

36 Friedman SR, Curtis R, Neaigus A, Jose B, et al. *Social Networks, Drug Injectors' Lives and HIV/AIDS.* New York, NY: Kluwer-Plenum Press; 1999.

37 Metzger DS, Navaline H, Woody GE. Drug abuse treatment as AIDS prevention. *Public Health Rep.* 1998;113 (Suppl.1):97-106.

38 Needle RH, Coyle SL, Normand J, Lambert E, et al. HIV Prevention with drug-using populations—Current status and future prospects: introduction and overview. *Pubic Health Rep.* 1998;113(Suppl.1):4-18.

39 Stall, RD, Paul, JP, Barrett, DC, Crosby, GM, Bein E. An outcome evaluation to measure changes in sexual risk-taking among gay men undergoing substance use disorder treatment. *J Stud Alcohol.* 1999;60:837-845.

40 Shoptaw S, Reback C, Freese TE, Ling W. Treatment effects on HIV-related risk behaviors for MSM. Paper presented at: Annual Meeting of the American Psychological Association; 15 August 1998; San Francisco.

41 Ostrow DG, Kalichman SC. Methodological issues in HIV behavioral interventions. In: Peterson JL, DiClemente RJ, eds. *Handbook of HIV Prevention.* New York, NY: Kluwer Academic-Plenum; 2000:67-80.

[42] Kelly JA, St. Lawrence JS, Hood HV, Brasfield TL. Behavioral intervention to reduce AIDS risk activities. *J Consult Clin Psych.* 1989;57:60-67.

[43] Ostrow DG, Vanable PA, McKirnan DJ, Brown LB. Hepatitis and HIV risk among drug-using men who have sex with men: demonstration of Hart's law of inverse access and application to HIV. *J Gay Lesb Med Assoc.* 1999;3:127-135.

[44] Hart JT. The inverse care law. *Lancet.* 1971;1:405-412.

[45] Wyatt G. HIV prevention in minority populations. Panel discussion at: AIDS Symposium of Annual Meeting of the American Psychological Association; 12 August 1998; New York, NY.

CHAPTER 6

[1] Guinan ME, Hardy A. Epidemiology of AIDS in women in the United States: 1981 through 1986. *JAMA.* 1987;257:2039-2042.

[2] Center for Disease Control. Pneumocystis pneumonia - Los Angeles. *MMWR Morb Mortal Wkly Rep.* 1981;30:250-252.

[3] Chu SY, Buehler JW, Berkelman RL. Impact of the human immunodeficiency virus epidemic on mortality in women of reproductive age, United States. *JAMA.* 1990;264:225-229.

[4] Centers for Disease Control and Prevention. *HIV/AIDS Surveillance Rep.* 1999;10(1).

[5] Centers for Disease Control and Prevention. Center for HIV/AIDS Prevention Slide Series L285 (through 1997). Available at: http://cdc.gov/nchstp/hiv.aids/graphics/images/mortality/l285-12.htm

[6] Fee E, Krieger N. Understanding AIDS: historical interpretations and the limits of biomedical individualism. *Am J Public Health.* 1993;83:1477-1486.

[7] Lock M, Gordon D, eds. *Biomedicine Examined.* Dordrecht: Kluwer Academic Publishers; 1988.

[8] Tesh S. *Hidden Arguments: Political Ideology and Disease Prevention Policy.* New Brunswick, NJ: Rutgers University Press; 1988.

[9] Coreil J, Levin JS, Jaco EG. Life style - an emergent concept in the sociomedical science. *Culture Psychiatry Med.* 1985;9:423-437.

[10] Terris M. The lifestyle approach to prevention [editorial]. *J Public Health Policy.* 1980;1:5-9.

[11] Ajzen I, Fishbein M. *Understanding Attitudes and Predicting Social Behavior.* Englewood Cliffs, NJ: Prentice Hall; 1980.

[12] Bandura A. Self-efficacy: toward a unifying theory of behavioral change. *Psychol Rev.* 1977;84:191-215.

[13] Becker MH. The health belief model and sick role behavior. *Health Educ Monogr.* 1974;2:409-419.

[14] Prochaska J, DiClemente C, Norcross J. In search of how people change. *Am Psychol.* 1992;47:1102-1114.

[15] Rosenstock IM, Strecher V, Becker M. Social learning theory and the health belief model. *Health Educ Q.* 1988;15:175-183.

[16] Anastos K, Marte C. Women-the missing persons in the AIDS epidemic. *Health/PAC Bulletin.* Winter:6-15.

[17] Drucker E. Epidemic in the war zone: AIDS and community survival in New York City. *Int J Health Serv.* 1990;20:601-605.

[18] Wallace R. A synergism of plagues: "planned shrinkage," contagious housing destruction, and AIDS in the Bronx. *Environ Res.* 1988;47:1-33.

[19] Wallace R, Wallace D. US apartheid and the spread of AIDS to the suburbs: a multi-city analysis of the political economy of spatial epidemic threshold. *Soc Sci Med.* 1995;41:333-345.

[20] Fife D, Mode C. AIDS incidence and income. *J Acquir Immune Defic Syndr*. 1992;5:1105-1110.

[21] Hu DJ, Frey R, Costa SJ, et al. Geographical AIDS rates and sociodemographic variables in Newark, New Jersey, metropolitan area. *AIDS Public Policy J*. 1994;9:20-25.

[22] Simon PA, Hu DJ, Diaz T, Kerndt PR. Income and AIDS rates in Los Angeles County. *AIDS*. 1995;9:281-284.

[23] Zierler S, Krieger N, Tang Y, Auerbach J, et al. Economic gradients of AIDS incidence in Massachusetts. *Am J Public Health*. 2000;90:1064-1073.

[24] Brown VB, Melchior CR, Huba GJ. Mandatory partner notification of HIV test results: psychological and social issues for women. *AIDS Public Pol J*. 1994;9:86-92.

[25] Barkan S, Deaumant C, Young M, Stonis LF, et al. Sexual identity and behavior among women with female sexual partners in the Women's Interagency HIV Study (WIHS). In: Program and abstracts of the XI International Conference on AIDS; July 7-12, 1996; Vancouver, British Columbia. Abstract.

[26] Moore J, Solomon L, Schoenbaum E, Schuman P, et al. Factors associated with stress and distress among HIV-infected and uninfected women. In: Program and abstracts of the Women and HIV Infection Conference; 1995; Washington, DC. Abstract.

[27] Brown VB, Weissman G. Women and men injection drug users: an updated look at gender differences and risk factors. In: Brown BS, Beschnes GM, with the National AIDS Research Consortium, eds. *Handbook on Risk of AIDS Injection Drug Users and Sexual Partners*. Westport, CT: Greenwood Press; 1993.

[28] Diaz T, Chu SY, Buchler JW, Boyd D, et al. Socioeconomic differences among people with AIDS: Results from a multistate surveillance project. *Am J Prev Med*. 1994;10:217-222.

[29] Lurie P, Fernandes MEL, Hughes V, Arevalo EL, et al. Socioeconomic status and risk of HIV-1, syphilis and hepatitis B infection among sex workers in Sao Paulo State, Brazil. *AIDS*. 1995;9(Suppl):S31-S37.

[30] Farmer P, Conners M, Simmons J, eds. *Women, Poverty and AIDS*. Monroe, ME: Common Courage Press; 1996.

[31] Farmer P, Lindenbaum S, Good MJD. Women, poverty and AIDS: an introduction. *Cult Med Psychiatry*. 1993;17:387-397.

[32] Pivnick A, Jacobson A, Eric K, Doll L, et al. AIDS, HIV infection, illicit drug use within inner-city families and social networks. *Am J Public Health*. 1994;84:271-274.

[33] Schoepf BG. Gender, development, and AIDS: a political economy and culture framework. *Women Int Development Annu*. 1993;3:53-85.

[34] Basset M, Mihloyi M. Women and AIDS in Zimbabwe: the making of an epidemic. In: Krieger N, Margo G, eds. *AIDS: The Politics of Survival*. Amityville, NY: Baywood; 1994:125-139.

[35] Jochelson K, Mothibeli M, Leger J-P. Human immunodeficiency virus and migrant labor in South Africa. In: Krieger N, Margo G, eds. *AIDS: The Politics of Survival*. Amityville, NY: Baywood Publishing Co.; 1994:141-158.

[36] Lurie P, Hintzen P, Lowe RA. Socioeconomic obstacles to HIV prevention and treatment in developing countries: the roles of the International Monetary Fund and the World Bank. *AIDS*. 1995;9:539-546.

[37] Curtis JR, Patrick DL. Race and survival time with AIDS: a synthesis of the literature. *Am J Public Health*. 1993;83:1425-428.

[38] Lucey DR, Hendrix C, Andrzejewski C, Melcher GP, et al. Comparison by race of total serum IgG, IgA, and IgM with CD4+ T-cell counts in North American persons infected with the human immunodeficiency virus type 1. *J Acquir Immune Defic Syndr*. 1992;5:325-332.

[39] Rushton JP, Bogaert AF. Population differences in susceptibility to AIDS: an evolutionary analysis. *Soc Sci Med*. 1989;28:1211-1220.

[40] Cooper R, David R. The biological concept of race and its application to public health and epidemiology. *J Health Polit Policy Law*. 1986;11:97-116.

[41] King JC. *The Biology of Race.* Berkeley: University of California Press; 1981.

[42] Krieger N, Rowley D, Hermann AA, Avery B, et al. Racism, sexism and social class:Implications for studies of health, disease and well-being. *Am J Prev Med.* 1993;9(Suppl 2):82-122.

[43] Polednak AP. *Racial and Ethnic Differences in Disease.* New York, NY: Oxford University Press; 1989.

[44] Airhihenbuwa CO, DiClemente RJ, Wingood GM, Lowe A. HIV/AIDS education and prevention among African-Americans: a focus on culture. *AIDS Educ Prev.* 1992;4:267-276.

[45] Mays VM, Cochran SD. Acquired immunodeficiency syndrome and Black Americans: special psychosocial issues. *Public Health Rep.* 1987;102:224-231.

[46] Dalton HL. AIDS in blackface. *Daedalus.* 1989;115:205-227.

[47] Friedman SR, Sotheran JL, Abdul-Quader A, Primm BJ, et al. The AIDS epidemic among Blacks and Hispanics. *Milbank Q.* 1987;65:455-499.

[48] Friedman SR, Stepherson B, Woods J, Des Jarlais DC, et al. Society, drug injectors, and AIDS. *J Health Care Poor Underserved.* 1992;3:73-89.

[49] Gwinn M, Pappaioanou M, George R, Hannon WH, et al. Prevalence of HIV infection in childbearing women in the United States. *JAMA.* 1991;265:1704-1708.

[49] Holmes MD. AIDS in communities of color [editorial]. *Am J Prev Med.* 1991;7:461-463.

[50] Krieger N, Appleman R. *The Politics of AIDS.* Oakland, Calif: Frontline Publishing; 1986.

[51] Thomas SB, Quinn SC. The Tuskegee Syphilis Study, 1932-1972: implications for HIV education and AIDS risk education programs in the Black community. *Am J Public Health.* 1991;81:1498-1504.

[52] Worth D, Rodriguez R. Latina women and AIDS. *SEICUS Report.* 1987;15:5-7.

[53] Quinn SC. AIDS and the African American woman: the triple burden of race, class, and gender. *Health Educ Q.* 1993;20:305-320.

[54] Essed P. *Understanding Everyday Racism: An Interdisciplinary Theory.* Newbury Park: Sage; 1991.

[55] Friedman SR. Alienated labor and dignity denial in capitalist society. In: Berberoglu B, ed. *Critical Perspectives in Sociology.* Dubuque, IA: Kendall/Hunt Publisher, 1991; 83-91.

[56] Battle S. Moving targets: alcohol, crack and black women. In: White EC, ed. *The Black Women's Health Book: Speaking for Ourselves.* Seattle, WA: Seal Press; 1990:251-256.

[57] Cochran SD, Mays VM. Depressive distress among homosexually active African-American men and women. *Am J Psychiatry.* 1994;151:524-529.

[58] Ickovics JR, Rodin J. Women and AIDS in the United States: epidemiology, natural history, and mediating mechanisms. *Health Psychology.* 1992;11(1):1-16.

[59] Mayer KH, Anderson DJ. Heterosexual HIV transmission. *Infect Agents Dis.* 1995;4:273-284.

[60] Krieger N, Sidney S. Racial discrimination and blood pressure: the CARDIA study of young black and white women and men. *Am J Public Health.* 1996;86:1370-1378.

[61] Williams DR. Black-white differences in blood pressure: the role of social factors. *Ethn Dis.* 1992;2:126-141.

[62] Dressler WW. Health in the African American community: accounting for health inequalities. *Med Anthropol Q.* 1993;7:325-345.

[63] Neighbors HW, Jackson JS, Broman C, Thompson E. Racism and the mental health of African Americans: the role of self and system blame. *Ethn Dis.* 1995;6:167-175.

[64] Levine C. Orphans of the HIV epidemic: unmet needs in six US cities. *AIDS Care.* 1995;7(Suppl 1):S57-S62.

[65] Paone D, Caloir S, Shi Q, Des Jarlais DC. Sex, drugs, and syringe exchange in New York City: women's experiences. *JAMWA.* 1995;50:109-114.

[66] Chiasson MA, Stoneburner RL, Hildebrandt DS, Ewing WE, et al. Heterosexual transmission of HIV-1 associated with use of smokeable freebase cocaine (crack). *AIDS*. 1991;5:1121-1126.

[67] Edlin BR, Irwin KL, Faruque S, McCoy CB, et al. Intersecting epidemics: crack cocaine use and HIV infection among inner-city young adults. *N Engl J Med*. 1994;331:1422-1427.

[68] Fullilove RE, Fullilove MT, Bowser BP, Gross SA. Risk of sexually transmitted disease among black adolescent crack users in Oakland and San Francisco, Calif. *JAMA*. 1990;263:851-855.

[69] Amaro H. Love, sex and power. *Am Psych*. 1995;50:437-447.

[70] Chavkin W, Driver C, Forman P. The crisis in New York City's perinatal services. *NY State J Med*. 1989;89:658-663.

[71] Pivnick A. HIV infection and the meaning of condoms. *Cult Med Psychiatry*. 1993;17:431-453.

[72] Wyatt GE, Dunn KM. Examining predictors of sex guilt in multiethnic samples of women. *Arch Sex Behav*. 1991;20:471-485.

[73] Fisher B, Hovell M, Hofstetter CR, Hough R. Risks associated with long-term homelessness among women: battery, rape, and HIV infection. *Int J Health Serv*. 1995;25:351-369.

[74] Alan Guttmacher Institute. *Sex and America's Teenagers*. New York: Alan Guttmacher Institute; 1994.

[75] Males MA. Adult involvement in teenage childbearing and STD. *Lancet*. 1995;346:64-65.

[76] James J, Meyerding J. Early sexual experience and prostitution. *Am J Psychiatry*. 1977;134:1381-1385.

[77] Ladwig GB, Andersen MD. Substance abuse in women: relationship between chemical dependency of women and past reports of physical and/or sexual abuse. *Int J Addict*. 1989;24:739-754.

[78] Paone D, Chavkin W, Willets I, Friedmann P, et al. The impact of sexual abuse: implications for drug treatment. *J Women's Health*. 1992;1:149-153.

[79] Worth D, Paone D, Chavkin W. From the private family domain to the public health forum: sexual abuse, women and risk for HIV infection. *SIECUS Report*. 1993;21:13-17.

[80] Zierler S, Feingold L, Laufer D, Velentgas P, et al. Adult survivors of childhood sexual abuse and subsequent risk of HIV infection. *Am J Public Health*. 1991;81:572-575.

[81] Zierler S, Witbeck B, Mayer K. Sexual violence and HIV in women living with or at risk for HIV infection. *Am J Prev Med*. 1996;12:304-310.

[82] American Correction Association. *The Female Offender: What Does the Future Hold?* Laurel, Md: American Correction Association; 1990.

[83] De Groot A, Zierler S, Stevens J. Sexual abuse histories among incarcerated women in Massachusetts. Presented at: Women and HIV Infection Conference; 1995; Washington, DC.

[84] Brown VB. HIV infection in women: models of intervention for violence against women. In: Program and abstracts of the Women and HIV Infection Conference; 1995; Washington, DC. Abstract TD2-122.

[85] Deamant C, Cohen M, Markan S, Richardson J, et al. 1996. Prevalence of domestic violence and childhood abuse among women with HIV and high risk uninfected women. In: Program and abstracts of the XI International Conference on AIDS; July 7-12, 1996; Vancouver, British Columbia. Abstract

[86] Vlahov D, Wientge D, Moore J, Flynn C, et al. Violence among women with or at risk for HIV infection. In: Program and abstracts of the XI International Conference on AIDS; July 7-12, 1996; Vancouver, British Columbia. Abstract.

[87] Zierler S. Hitting hard: HIV and violence against women. In: Manlowe J, Goldstein N, eds. *Gender Politics of HIV*. New York: New York University Press; 1997.

[88] Schubiner H, Scott R, Tzelepis A. Exposure to violence among inner-city youth. *J Adoles Health*. 1993;14:214-219.

Dyson J. The effect of family violence on children's academic performance and behavior. *J Natl Med Assoc*. 1990;82:17-22.

[90] Fitzpatrick K, Boldizar J. The prevalence and consequences of exposure to violence among African-American youth. *J Am Acad Child Adol Psychiatry*. 1993;32:424-430.

[91] Taylor L, Zuckerman B, Harik V, Groves BM. Witnessing violence by young children and their mothers. *J Dev Behav Pediatr*. 1994;15:120-123.

[92] Lake ES. An exploration of the violent victim experiences of female offenders. *Violence and Victims*. 1993;8:41-51.

[93] Fullilove M, Fullilove R, Kennedy G, et al. 1992. Trauma, crack and HIV risk. In: Program and abstracts of the VIII International Conference on AIDS; July 19-24, 1992; Amsterdam, The Netherlands. Abstract PoD 5477.

[94] O'Campo P, Gilen A, Faden R, Xue X, et al. Violence by male partners against women during the childbearing year. *Am J Public Health*. 1995;85:1092-1097.

[95] Mills C, Ota H. Homeless women with minor children in the Detroit metropolitan area. *Soc Work*. 1989;34:485-489.

[96] Zorza J. Women battering: a major cause of homeless. *Clearinghouse Rev*. 1991;25:420-429.

[97] Gielen AC, O'Campo P, Faden R, Eke A. Women with HIV: disclosure concerns and experiences. In: Program and abstracts of the Women and HIV Infection Conference; 1995; Washington, DC. Abstract TA1-88.

[98] Rothenberg KH, SJ Paskey. The risk of domestic violence and women with HIV infection: implications for partner notification policy, and the law. *Am J Public Health*. 1995;85:1569-1576.

[99] North RL, Rothenberg KH. Partner notification and the threat of domestic violence against women with HIV infection. *N Engl J Med*. 1993;329:1194-1196.

[100] Padian N, Shiboski SC, Jewell NP. Female-male transmission of human immunodeficiency virus. *JAMA*. 1991;266:1664-1667.

[101] Amaro H, Hardy-Fanta C. Gender relations in addiction and recovery. *J Psychoactive Drugs*. 1995;27:325-337.

[102] Dwyer R, Richardson D, Ross MW, Wodak A, et al. A comparison of HIV risk between women and men who inject drugs. *AIDS Educ Prev*. 1994;6:379-389.

[103] Rosenbaum M. Difficulties in taking care of business: women addicts as mothers. *Am J Drug Alcohol Abuse*. 1979;6:431-446.

[104] Sotheran JL, Wenston JA, Rockwell R, Des Jarlais D, et al. Injecting drug users: why do women share syringes more often than men? Presented at: American Public Health Association; 1992; Washington, DC.

[105] Friedman SR, Jose B, Deren S, Des Jarlais DC, et al. Risk factors for human immunodeficiency virus seroconversion among out-of-treatment drug injectors in high and low seroprevalence cities. The National AIDS Research Consortium. *Am J Epidemiol*. 1995;142:864-874.

[106] Friedman SR, Neaigus A, Jose B, Goldstein M, Curtis R, et al. 1993. Female injecting drug users get infected sooner than males. In: Program and abstracts of the IX International Conference on AIDS; DATE; Berlin, Germany. Abstract PO-DO3-3512.

[107] Solomon L, Astemborski J, Warren D, Munoz A, et al. Differences in risk factors for human immunodeficiency virus type 1 seroconversion among male and female intravenous drug users. *Am J Epidemiol*. 1993;137:892-898.

[108] Beckman L, Amaro H. Personal and social difficulties faced by women and men entering alcoholism treatment. *J Stud Alcohol*. 1986;47:135-145.

[109] Lurie P, Reingold AL, Bowser B, Chen D, et al. *The Public Health Impact of Needle Exchange Programs in the United States and Abroad*. Vol. 1. San Francisco: University of California; 1993.

[110] Wenger L, Murphy S. Barriers to needle exchange: a case for expanded services and legislative reform. Presented at: American Public Health Association; 1995; San Diego, Calif.

[111] Robbins C. Sex differences in psychosocial consequences of alcohol and drug abuse. *J Health Soc Behavior*. 1989;30:117-130.

[112] Karan LD. AIDS perception and chemical dependence treatment needs of women and their children. *J Psychoactive Drugs.* 1989;21:395-399.

[113] Marmor M, Weiss LR, Lyden M. Possible female-to-female transmission of human immunodeficiency virus [letter]. *Ann Intern Med.* 1986;105(6):969.

[114] Monzon OT, Capellan JMB. Female-to-female transmission of HIV [letter]. *Lancet.* 1987;2:40-41.

[115] Perry S, Jacobsberg L, Fogel K. Orogenital transmission of HIV. *Ann Intern Med.* 1989;111:951-952.

[116] Rich JD, Buck A, Tuomala RE, Kazanjian PH. Transmission of human immunodeficiency virus infection presumed to have occured via female homosexual contact. *Clinical Infect Dis.* 1993;17:1003-1005.

[117] Sabatini MT, Patel K, Hirshman R. Kaposi's sarcoma and T-cell lymphoma in an immunodeficient woman: a case report. *AIDS Res.* 1984;1:135-137.

[118] Chu SY, Hammett TA, Buehler JW. Update: epidemiology of reported cases of AIDS in women who report sex only with other women, United States, 1980-1991. *AIDS.* 1992;6:518-519.

[119] Lemp GF, Jones M, Kellogg, TA, Nieri GN, et al. HIV seroprevalence and risk behaviors among lesbians and bisexual women in San Francisco and Berkeley, California. *Am J Public Health.* 1995;85:1549-1552.

[120] *Facts: HIV/AIDS and Women Who Have Sex with Women (WSW) in the United States.* Atlanta, Ga: Centers for Disease Control and Prevention; 1997.

[121] Zierler S, Moore J, Solomon L, Schuman P, et al. Sexuality among a cohort of HIV seropositive and seronegative women. In: Program and abstracts of the Women and HIV Infection Conference; 1995; Washington, DC. Abstract.

[122] Stevens PE. Lesbians and HIV: clinical, research, and policy issues. *Am Orthopsych Assoc.* 1993;63:289-294.

[123] Einhorn L, Polgar M. HIV risk behavior among lesbian and bisexual women. *AIDS Prev Educ.* 1994;6:514-523.

[124] Young RM, Weissman G, Cohen JB. Assessing risk in the absence of information: HIV risk among women injection-drug users who have sex with woman. *AIDS Public Policy J.* 1992;7:175-183.

[125] Gollub EL, Stein ZA. Commentary: the new female condom - item 1 on a women's AIDS prevention agenda. *Am J Public Health.* 1993;83:498-500.

[126] Stein ZA. More on women and the prevention of HIV infection. *Am J Public Health.* 1995;85:1485-1488.

[127] Freudenberg N. AIDS prevention in the United States: lessons from the first decade. In: Krieger N, Margo G, eds. *AIDS: The Politics of Survival.* Amityville, NY: Baywood Publishing Co.; 1994:61-72.

[128] Krieger N. Overcoming the absence of socioeconomic data in medical records: validation and application of a census-based methodology. *Am J Public Health.* 1992;82:703-710.

[129] Friedman SR, Neigus A, Jose B, Curtis R, et al. Network and sociohistorical approaches to the HIV epidemic among drug injectors. In: Catalan J, Hedge B, Sherr L, ed. [no title] Chur, Switzerland: Harwood Academic Publisher. (in press)

[130] Leslie c, Scientific racism: reflections on peer review, science and ideology. *Sco Sci Med.* 32:891-905.

---

[a] This refers to the biological mechanisms through which women acquire or experienced increase risk for HIV (eg, relative efficiency of viral transmission from men to women, vaginal mucosal immunity, immunological effect of female endocrine levels, and female genital tract inflammation).

[b] This refers to the behavioral and cultural factors that affect health and disease (eg, drug use, prostitution, ethnic customs, and social networks).

[c] This refers to existing behavior change models (eg, Health Belief Model, Theory of Reasoned Action, Social Cognitive Theory, and Stages of Change).

[d] The conflation of "culture" with sociopolitical conditions that force community and individual adaptation to discrimination and dehumanization is not useful. First, it continues to hold accountable the "communities" of African American and Hispanic people for the dangerous conditions in their lives, without mention of how these conditions have been shaped by white Americans of European descent. Second, it reinforces a legacy of scientific racism, promulgated by basic and social scientists, that there are inherent cultural norms that drive the racial/ethnic distribution of HIV as well as other damaging conditions (eg, Rushton and Bogaert's sociobiological account of racial differences in AIDS susceptibility [39] and Leslie's rebuttal [130], addressing both biological and cultural determinism).

[e] We emphasize men inflicting violence against women because research documents that this is the dominant form of interpersonal violence against women. To our knowledge, lesbian interpersonal violence has not been described in relation to HIV [87] in the published literature.

[f] S. Murphy of Prevention Point, a San Francisco needle exchange program, tells this story (personal communication): To improve women's access to clean needles, a San Francisco program created an indoor needle exchange site for women at an existing multiservice women's center. Thus, women attending the site for needles were not identifiable as drug users merely because they came to the center. Still, as one of the organizers of this site noted, women at first were reluctant to use the program. To encourage their attendance, the program offered grocery vouchers. The resulting increased attendance included men who were also hungry for food, for when they learned that this site was giving out grocery vouchers, some dressed as women so that they would be able to feed themselves as well as obtain clean needles.

CHAPTER 7

[1] Wortley PM, Fleming PL. AIDS in women in the United States. *JAMA*. 1997;278:911-916.

[2] Centers for Disease Control and Prevention. Update: trends in AIDS incidence—United States, 1996. *MMWR Morb Mortal Wkly Rep*. 1997;46:861-867.

[3] Centers for Disease Control. Update: acquired immunodeficiency syndrome—United States, 1992. *MMWR Morb Mortal Wkly Rep*. 1993;42:547-551,557.

[4] Wortley PM, Fleming PL. AIDS in women in the United States. *JAMA*. 1997;278:911-916.

[5] Futterman D, Hein K. Medical Care of Adolescents. In: Pizzo P, Wilfert C, eds. *Pediatric AIDS*. 2nd ed. Baltimore, MD: Williams and Wilkins; 1994:757-772.

[6] Merton V. Ethical obstacles to the participation of women in biomedical research. In: Wolf SM. *Feminism and Bioethics: Beyond Reproduction*. New York: Oxford University Press; 1996:216-251.

[7] Healy B. The Yentl syndrome. *N Engl J Med*. 1991:325:274-276.

[8] Rodin J, Ickovics JR. Women's health: review and research agenda as we approach the 21st century. *Am Psychol*. 1990:45:1018-1034.

[9] Anastos K, Charney P, Charon RA, Cohen F, et al. Hypertension in women: what is really known? The Women's Caucus, working group on women's health of the Society of General Internal Medicine. *Ann Int Med*. 1991:115:287-293.

[10] Wenger NK, Speroff L, Packard B. Cardiovascular health and disease in women. *N Engl J Med*. 1993:329:247-256.

[11] Zierler S, Krieger N. Reframing women's risk: social inequalities and HIV infection. *Annu Rev Public Health*. 1997:18:401-436.

[12] Ethier KA, Ickovics JR, Rodin J. For whose benerfit? women and AIDS public policy. In: O'Leary A, Jemmott LS. *Women and AIDS: Coping and Caring*. New York: Plenum Press; 1996.

[13] Rodriguez-Trias H, Marte C. Challenges and possibilities: women, HIV and the health care system in the 1990s. In: Stoller N, Schneider B, eds. *Women as the Key: Leadership in the AIDS Epidemic*. Philadelphia: Temple University Press; 1995.

[14] Anastos K, Marte C. Women—the missing persons in the AIDS epidemic. *Health PAC Bull.* 1989: 19:6-13.

[15] Center for Disease Control and Prevention. *Reports on HIV/AIDS.* 1992 1.Washington, DC: US Dept of Health and Human Services, Center for Disease Control and Prevention; August 1993.

[16] Revision of CDC case definition of acquired immunodeficiency syndrome for national reporting. *MMWR Morb Mortal Wkly Rep.* 1985;34:373-375. Revision of the CDC surveillance case definition for acquired immunodeficiency syndrome. Council of State and Territorial Epidemiologists; AIDS Program, Center for Infectious Diseases. *MMWR Morb Mortal Wkly Rep.* 1987;36(suppl 1):1S-15S.

[17] US Dept of Health and Human Services. *AIDS Public Information Data Set, Public Health Service.* Washington, DC: US Dept of Health and Human Services, Centers for Disease Control, National Center for Infectious Diseases, Division of HIV/AIDS; 1993.

[18] US Dept of Health and Human Services. *AIDS Public Information Data Set, Public Health Service.* Washington, DC: US Dept of Health and Human Services, Centers for Disease Control, National Center for Infectious Diseases, Division of HIV/AIDS; 1993.

[19] US Dept of Health and Human Services. *AIDS Public Information Data Set, Public Health Service.* Washington, DC: US Dept of Health and Human Services, Centers for Disease Control, National Center for Infectious Diseases, Division of HIV/AIDS; 1993. Women who are HIV-positive gradually lose their ability to fight off gynecologic disease and infection. Thus, gynecological infections for these women occur more frequently and with greater severity. Additionally, financially disadvantaged, HIV-infected individuals may suffer bouts of tuberculosis that are more severe. New strains of tuberculosis have been discovered among these individuals. See Chu SY, Buehler JW, Berkelman RL. Impact of the human immunodeficiency virus epidemic on mortality in women of reproductive age. *JAMA.* 1990;264:225-229. See also Daley CL, Small PM, Schecter GF, et al. An outbreak of tuberculosis with accelerated progression among persons infected with the human immunodeficiency virus. An analysis using restriction-fragment-length polymorphisms. *N Engl J Med.* 1992;326:231-235.

[20] Farizo KM, Buehler JW, Chamberland ME, Whyte BM, et al. Spectrum of disease in persons with human immunodeficiency virus infection in the United States. *JAMA.* 1992;267:1798-1805. See also Braun MM, Cote TR, Rabkin CS. Trends in death with tuberculosis during the AIDS era. *JAMA.* 1993;269:2865-2868. See also Gostin LO. Controlling the resurgent tuberculosis epidemic. A 50-state survey of TB statutes and proposals for reform. *JAMA.* 1993;269:255-261. See also Daley CL, Small PM, Schecter GF, et al. An outbreak of tuberculosis with accelerated progression among persons infected with the human immunodeficiency virus. An analysis using restriction-fragment-length polymorphisms. *N Engl J Med.* 1992;326:231-235. See also Braun MM, Truman BI, Maguire B, et al. Increasing incidence of tuberculosis in a prison inmate population. Association with HIV infection. *JAMA.* 1989;261:393-397.

[21] Increase in pneumonia mortality among young adults and the HIV epidemic—New York City, United States. *JAMA.* 1988;260:2181,2185. See also Farizo KM, Buehler JW, Chamberland ME, et al. Spectrum of disease in persons with human immunodeficiency virus infection in the United States. *JAMA.* 1992;267:1798-1805. See also Greenberg AE, Thomas PA, Landesman SH, et al. The spectrum of HIV-1-related disease among outpatients in New York City. *AIDS.* 1992;6:849-859.

[22] Chu SY, Buehler JW, Berkelman RL. Impact of the human immunodeficiency virus epidemic on mortality in women of reproductive age. *JAMA.* 1990;264:225-229. See also Maiman M, et al. Risk for cervical disease in HIV-infected women—New York City. *JAMA.* 1991;265:23-24. See also Maiman M, Fruchter RG, Serur E, Boyce JG. Prevalence of human immunodeficiency virus in a colposcopy clinic. *JAMA.* 1988;260:2214-15. See also Minkoff HL, DeHovitz JA. Care of women infected with the human immunodeficiency virus. *JAMA.* 1991;266:2253-2258.

[23] Wofsy CB. Human immunodeficiency virus infection in women. *JAMA.* 1987;257:2074-2076. See also Grimes DA. Deaths due to sexually transmitted diseases. The forgotten component of reproductive mortality. *JAMA.* 1986;255:1727-1729. See also Washington AE, Cates W Jr, Wasserheit JN. Preventing pelvic inflammatory disease. *JAMA.* 1991;266:2574-2580.

[24] Marte C, Ribble D, Keyes C, Wolbert J, et al. Need for gynecologic protocols in AIDS primary care clinics. In: Program and abstracts from the V International Conference on AIDS; 1989; Montreal, Canada.

[25] Marte C, Kelly P, Cohen M, et al. Pap smear abnormalities in ambulatory care sites for women with the human immunodeficiency virus. *Am J Obstet Gynecol.* 1992:166:1232-1237.

[26] Sullivan, 90 Civ. 6294 (S.D.N.Y.) The plaintiffs were represented by the author, who was lead counsel; Jill A. Boskey of MFY Legal Services; Leslie Salzman and Toby Golick of Cardozo Bet Tzedek Legal Services; Mary Gundrum of the Center for Constitutional Rights and Sandra Lowe, Marian Rosenberg, Michael Isbell and Suzanne Goldberg of Lambda Legal Defense and Education Fund.

[27] These individuals were represented by Nancy Chang, Lauren Shapiro, and Johnson Tyler of Brooklyn Legal Services, Corporation B. Sullivan, 90 Civ. 6294 at 41, 57-59.

[28] This new Listing represents a victory for the plaintiffs in the class-action lawsuit, Sullivan, 90 Civ. 6294 (S.D.N.Y.). The Listing also responds to H.R. 2299, a bill filed by Representative Robert Matsui (D-Calif.), which sought to force the SSA to award benefits to all those disabled by HIV diseases.

[29] Among the conditions are multiple or recurrent bacterial infection, including pelvic inflammatory disease, which requires hospitalization or intravenous antibiotic treatment 3 or more times in 1 year. These conditions also include conditions of the skin or mucous membranes with extensive fungating or ulcerating lesions not responding to treatment, including dermatological conditions such as eczema or psoriasis, vulvovaginal, or other mucosal candida, condyloma, caused by human papilloma virus, genital ulcerative disease, and invasive cervical cancer. 58 *Federal Register* 36008 (1993).

[30] Albert P, Graff L, Schatz B, eds. *AIDS Practice Manual.* 3rd ed. San Francisco: National Gay Rights Advocates, National Lawyers Guild, AIDS Network; 1992:1-17.

[31] Merton V. Ethical obstacles to the participation of women in biomedical research. In: Wolf SM. *Feminism and Bioethics: Beyond Reproduction.* New York: Oxford University Press; 1996:216-251.

[32] McGovern T. Barriers to the inclusion of women in research and clinical trials. In: Goldstein N, Manlowe JL. *The Gender Politics of HIV/AIDS in Women: Perspectives on the Pandemic in the United States.* New York, NY: New York University Press; 1997.

[33] Levine C. Ethics, epidemiology, and women's health. *Ann Epidemiol.* 1994;4:159-165.

[34] Faden R, Kass N, McGraw D. Women as vessels and vectors: lessons from the HIV epidemic. In: Wolf SM. *Feminism and Bioethics: Beyond Reproduction.* New York, NY: Oxford University Press;1996:252-281.

[35] 45 CFR §46.207 (1975).

[36] US Food and Drug Administration. *General Guidelines for the Clinical Evaluation of Drugs.* Washington, DC: US Food and Drug Administration; 1977. 77-3040.

[37] Jones KL, Lacro RV, Johnson KA, Adams J. Pattern of malformations in the children of women treated with carbamazepine during pregnancy. *N Engl J Med.* 1989;320:1661-1666.

[38] Levey BA. Bridging the gender gap in research. *Clin Pharmacol Ther.* 1991;50:641-646. See also Hamilton J, Parry B. Sex related differences in clinical drug response: implications for women's health. *J Am Med Womens Assoc.* 1983;38:129.

[39] *T.N. v FDA*, Case files of HIV Law Project.

[40] The citizen petition was filed on behalf of Mary Lucey, an HIV positive woman who was denied access to clinical trials; ACT UP Women's FDA Working Group; the AIDS Counseling and Education for Women in Transition from Correctional Facilities (ACE OUT); the New Jersey Women and AIDS Network; and Housing Works.

[41] *Federal Register.* 58 Federal Regulations 139.

[42] 1993 guideline at 39409. It is unclear from the 1993 guideline what the criteria are for determining if a disease is serious and affects women. The Public Health Service has issued a report that listed 5 criteria to determine whether a particular disease was a "women's disease": (1) the condition must be unique to women or some subgroup of women; (2) it must be more prevalent in women or some subgroup of women than in men; (3) it must be more serious in women or in some subgroup of women than in men; (4) the condition must be one for which risk factors are different for women or some subgroup of women than in men; (5) it must be

one for which treatment interventions are different for women or some subgroup of women than in men. See US General Accounting Office. *Summary of GAO Testimony by Mark V. Nadel on Problems in Implementing the National Institutes of Health Policy on Women in Study Populations.* Washington, DC: US General Accounting Office; 1990:1. GAO/T-HRD-90-38. The National Institutes of Health Revitalization Act of 1993, Pub L No. 103-43 (to be codified in scattered sections of 42 USC), also defines "women's health conditions" as all diseases, disorders, and conditions (including with respect to mental health): (1) unique to, more serious or more prevalent in women; (2) for which the factors of medical risks or types of medical intervention are different for women; or (3) with respect to which there has been insufficient clinical research involving women as subjects or insufficient clinical research involving women as subjects or insufficient clinical data on women.

[43] Numerous representatives from pharmaceutical companies and independent laboratories, who do not wish to be identified, have confirmed that the FDA is not monitoring this process.

[44] 1993 guideline at 39411.

[45] According to the FDA, the decision to include men of reproductive age should be based upon a risk-benefit analysis of the nature of the abnormalities, the dosage needed to induce them, the consistency of findings in different species, the severity of the illness being treated the potential importance of the drug, the availability of patients of reproductive potential importance of the drug, the availability of alternative treatment and the duration of treatment (1993 guideline at 39411). Where toxicity in animals, the 1993 guideline at 39411.

[46] Male toxic exposures ranging from lead and other heavy metals to dibromochloropropane (DBCP) and chlordecone (Kepone) also have been demonstrated to affect the likelihood both of conception and of spontaneous abortion. See Castleman M. Toxics and male infertility. *Sierra Club Bulletin.* March/April 1985;70:49-52. See also Hemminki K, Kyyronen P, Niemi ML, et al. Spontaneous abortion in an industrialized community in Finland. *Am J Public Health.* 1983;73:32-37.

[47] Uzych L. Teratogenesis and mutagenesis associated with the exposure of human males to lead: a review. *Yale J Biol Med.* 1985;58:9-17. Soyka LF, Joffe JM. Male mediated drug effects on offspring. *Prog Clin Biol Res.* 1980;36:49-66.

[48] Minkoff H, et al. Fetal protection and women's access to clinical trails [sic]. *J Women's Health;* 1;1992:137-140.

[49] Magos L. Paternal exposure to chemicals before conception. *BMJ.* 1993;307:1214. See also Blakeslee S. Research on birth defects shifts to flaws in sperm. *New York Times.* March 27, 1991. See also Brody J. Possible links between babies' health and fathers' habits and working conditions. *New York Times.* December 25, 1991:64.

[50] 1993 guideline at 39411. *Federal Register:* In the introductory section, "C. Current FDA Position on Participation of Women of Childbearing Potential in Clinical Trials," it states, "it is expected that . . . the woman participant is fully informed about the current state of the animal reproduction studies and any other information about the teratogenic potential of the drug" (1993 guideline at 39408). In section G, "Precautions in Clinical Trials Including Women," the 1993 guideline discusses informed consent as stated above.

[51] An informed consent from a large New York City hospital of ACTG study #117 which compares ddI to AZT reads as follows:

> This drug may cause problems to the fetus if you become pregnant or father a child. Women of childbearing age can only be admitted to the study if you are not breast feeding; if you are not pregnant (as determined by a prestudy blood test for pregnancy); if you have been surgically sterilized, or are using effective birth controls.

Another typical informed consent message is exemplified by the language contained in the informed consent form of ACTG #135 conducted in a large New York City hospital. The study tests 5 drugs in the treatment of *Mycobacterium avium* Complex and anticipates the possibility of a woman becoming pregnant during the study. It does not, however, specify policies or procedures for dealing with the pregnant women:

> Pregnancy while you are taking [sic] these drugs may expose your unborn child to significant hazards of deformity. If you are a woman, you are therefore strongly advised not to become pregnant while taking these drugs and, if you are sexually active, you must agree

to use some form of barrier contraception (not the birth control pill) while you participate. If you do become pregnant while on this study, you must agree to immediately
inform the Principal Investigator [name given], at [phone number given].

[52] 21 CFR §50.25(2) requires a description of any reasonably foreseeable risks or discomforts to
the subject. 21 CFR §50.25(b)(1) requires a statement that the particular treatment or procedure
may involve risks to the subject (or to the embryo or fetus, if the subject is or may become
pregnant) which are currently unforseeable. Were the FDA to mandate the completion of
animal reproduction studies prior to human testing, these provisions could be met. Instead,
the 1993 guidelines encourages sponsors to describe discoverable risks as unforseeable.

[53] National Institutes of Health. *NIH Guide to Grants and Contracts*, Vol 15. Washington, DC:
National Institutes of Health; November 28, 1986.

[54] Kirschstein RL. Research on women's health. *Am J Public Health*. 1991;81:291-293.

[55] US General Accounting Office. *National Institutes of Health. Problems in Implementing
Policy on Women in Study Populations*. Washington, DC: US General Accounting Office; 1990.
GAO/T-HRD 90-38.

[56] NIH guidelines on the inclusion of women and minorities as subjects in clinical research.
59 *Federal Register* 46 (1994).

[57] *Mississippi University for Women v Hogan*, 458 US 718, 724 (1982). The FDA's role, through
FDA 77-3040, of authorizing sex discrimination in drug testing constitutes state action sufficient
to violate the equal protection clause of the federal Constitution. See also *West v Atkins*, 487 US
42, 56 (1988). See also *North Georgia Finishing, Inc. v Di-Chem*, 419 US 601 (1975).

[58] In the case of *Frontiero v Richardson*, 411 US 677, 690 (1973).

[59] In the case of *Planned Parenthood v Casey*, 112 S Ct 2791 (1992).

[60] In the case of *Planned Parenthood v Casey*, 112 S Ct 2791 (1992).

[61] The term "drug manufacturers" connotes investigators, sponsors, individuals, partnerships,
corporations, associations, governmental agencies, scientific establishments, or organizational
units thereof, or any other legal entity participating in the manufacture of drugs.

[62] On July 22, 1993, the *Baltimore Sun* reported that the FDA acknowledged that drug companies may have liability concerns about the 1993 guideline. Hoffman-LaRoche's Dr. Stots Reele
stated, "It's not just a liability issue. There is a medical issue. We don't want it to harm the fetus."

[63] Guideline for the study and evaluation of gender differences in the clinical evaluation of
drugs. 58 *Federal Register* 39406-39416 (1993).

[64] Hardy L, ed. Changing demographics of the HIV epidemic: implications for clinical research.
Workshop presented at Institute of Medicine; September 8, 1993; Washington, DC.

[65] US National Research Council Panel on Monitoring the Social Impact of the AIDS Epidemic.
The Social Impact of AIDS in the United States. Washington, DC: National Academy Press; 1993.

[66] US Food and Drug Administration. *General Considerations for the Clinical Evaluation of
Drugs*. Washington, DC; US Food and Drug Administration; 1977. HEW (FDA) 77-3040.

[67] US General Accounting Office. *Women's Health: FDA Needs to Ensure More Study of Gender
Differences in Prescription Drug Testing*. Washington, DC: US General Accounting Office; 1992.
GAO/HRD-93-17.

[68] US Food and Drug Administration. Guideline for the study and evaluation of gender
differences in the clinical evaluation of drugs. 58 *Federal Register* 39406-39416 (1993).

[69] Merkatz RB, Temple R, Subel S, Feiden K, Kessler DA. Women in clinical trials of new drugs:
a change in Food and Drug Administration policy. *N Engl J Med*. 1993;329:292-296.

[70] US General Accounting Office. *Women's Health: FDA Needs to Ensure More Study of Gender
Differences in Prescription Drug Testing*. Washington, DC: US General Accounting Office; 1992.
GAO/HRD-93-17.

[71] Mastroianni AC, Faden R, Federman D, eds. *Women and Health Research: Ethical and Legal
Issues of Including Women in Clinical Studies*. Washington, DC: National Academy Press; 1994.

[72] Merkatz RB, Temple R, Subel S, Feiden K, et al. Women in clinical trials of new drugs: a change in Food and Drug Administration policy. *N Engl J Med.* 1993;329:292-296.

[73] Wathen L, Freimuth W, Cox S, et al. Combination therapy with delavirdine plus zidovudine versus zidovudine alone: demographics, HIV viral load, and CD4 changes in female patients. In: Program and abstracts of the 1st National Conference on Women and HIV; 1997; Pasadena, CA. Abstract 304.4.

[74] Gersten M, Chapman S, Farnsworth A, et al. The safety and efficacy of Viracept (Nelfinavir mesylate) in female patients who participated in pivotal phase II/III double blind randomized controlled trials. In: Program and abstracts of the 1st National Conference on Women and HIV; 1997; Pasadena, CA. Abstract 304.1.

[75] Lucas GM, Chaisson RE, Moore RD. Highly active antiretroviral therapy in a large urban clinic: risk factors for virologic failure and adverse drug reactions. Ann Intern Med 1999;131:81-87.

[76] Halbreich U, Carson SW. Drug studies in women of childbearing age: ethical and method-ological considerations. *J Clin Psychopharmacol.* 1989;9:328-333.

[77] McGovern TM. Mandatory HIV testing and treating of child-bearing women: an unnatural, illegal, and unsound approach. *Columbia Human Rights Law Review.* 1997;28:469-499.

[78] Blanche S, Tardieu M, Rustin P, Slama A, et al. Persistent mitochondrial dysfunction and perinatal exposure to antiretroviral nucleoside analogues. *Lancet.* 1999;354:1084-1089.

[79] Farzadegan HJ, Hoover DR, Astemborski J, et al. Sex differences in HIV-1 viral load and progression to AIDS. *Lancet.* 1998;352:1510-1514.

[80] Junghans C, Ledergerber B, Chan P, Weber R, Egger M [for the Swiss HIV Cohort Study]. Sex differences in HIV-1 viral load and progression to AIDS. *Lancet.* 1999;353:589-591.

[81] Ethier KA, Ickovics JR, Rodin J. For whose benerfit? women and AIDS public policy. In: O'Leary A, Jemmott LS. *Women and AIDS: Coping and Caring.* New York: Plenum Press; 1996.

[82] Rodriguez-Trias H, Marte C. Challenges and possibilities: women, HIV and the health care system in the 1990s. In: Stoller N, Schneider B, eds. *Women as the Key: Leadership in the AIDS Epidemic.* Philadelphia: Temple University Press; 1995.

[83] Rothwell PM. Can overall results of clinical trials be applied to all patients? *Lancet.* 1995;345:1616-1619.

[84] Selwyn P. HIV therapy in the real world. *AIDS.* 1996;10:1591-1593.

[85] Smith M. Zidovudine: does it work for everyone? *JAMA.* 1991;266:2750-2751.

[86] Ickovics JR, Meisler AW. Adherence in AIDS clinical trials: a framework for clinical research and clinical care. *J Clin Epidemiol.* 1997:50:385-391.

[87] Williams A, Friedland G. Adherence, compliance, and HAART. *AIDS Clinical Care.* 1997:9:51-58.

[88] Macklin R, Friedland G. AIDS research: the ethics of clinical trials. *Law Med Health Care.* 1986;14:273-280.

[89] Public Responsibility in Medicine and Research (PRIM&R) and Tufts University School of Medicine. AIDS clinical research and care: meeting the challenges of an epidemic in flux. Paper presented at: October 29-30, 1992.

[90] Hardy L, ed. Changing demographics of the HIV epidemic: implications for clinical research. Workshop presented at Institute of Medicine; September 8, 1993; Washington, DC.

[91] Thomas SB, Quinn SC. The Tuskegee syphilis study, 1932 to 1972: implications for HIV education and AIDS risk education programs in the black community. *Am J Public Health.* 1991;81:1498-1505.

[92] Pharmaceutical Manufacturers Association. *New Medicinces in Development for Women.* Washington, DC: Pharmaceutical Manufacturers Association; 1991.

[93] Cotton DJ, Finkelstein DM, He W, Feinberg J. Determinants of accrual of women to a large, multicenter clinical trials program of human immunodeficiency virus infection. *J Acquir Immune Defic Syndr.* 1993;6:1322-1328.

[94] Faden R, Kass N, McGraw D. Women as vessels and vectors: lessons from the HIV epidemic. In: Wolf SM. *Feminism and Bioethics: Beyond Reproduction*. New York: Oxford University Press; 1996:252-281.

[95] Hardy L, ed. Changing demographics of the HIV epidemic: implications for clinical research. Workshop presented at: Institute of Medicine; September 8, 1993; Washington, DC.

[96] Cotton DJ, Finkelstein DM, He W, Feinberg J. Determinants of accrual of women to a large, multicenter clinical trials program of human immunodeficiency virus infection. *J Acquir Immune Defic Syndr*. 1993;6:1322-1328.

[97] Korvick JA. Trends in federally sponsored clinical trials. In: Kurth A, ed. *Until the Cure: Caring for Women with HIV*. New Haven: Yale University Press; 1993.

[98] National Institute of Allergy and Infectious Diseases; Division of AIDS. Paper presented at: Twenty-third AIDS clinical trials groups meeting; July 19-22, 1997; Washington, DC.

[99] Centers for Disease Contol and Prevention. *HIV/AIDS Surveillance Report*. 1996;8:10-14.

[100] Gostin LO, Ward JW, Baker AC. National HIV case reporting for the United States. A defining moment in the history of the epidemic. *N Engl J Med*. 1997;337:1162-1167.

[101] Goldberg C. Cutting a lifeline to AIDS study: 3 drug-testing programs in New York are eliminated. *New York Times*. January 30, 1996;sect B:1.

[102] Goldberg C. Cutting a lifeline to AIDS study: 3 drug-testing programs in New York are eliminated. *New York Times*. January 30, 1996;sect B:1.

[103] Cotton DJ, Finkelstein DM, He W, Feinberg J. Determinants of accrual of women to a large, multicenter clinical trials program of human immunodeficiency virus infection. *J Acquir Immune Defic Syndr*. 1993;6:1322-1328.

[104] Centers for Disease Control. Update: AIDS among women—United States, 1994. *MMWR Morb Mortal Wkly Rep*. 1995;44:81-84.

[105] Centers for Disease Control. Update: AIDS among women—United States, 1994. *MMWR Morb Mortal Wkly Rep*. 1995;44:81-84.

[106] Geballe S, Gruendel J, Andiman W. *Forgotten Children of the AIDS Epidemic*. New Haven: Yale University Press; 1995.

[107] Levine C. Women as research subjects: new priorities, new questions. In: Blank RH, Bonnicksen AL, eds. *Emerging Issues in Biomedical Policy*. Vol 2. New York: Columbia University Press; 1993:169-188.

[108] Michaels D, Levine C. Estimates of the number of motherless youth orphaned by AIDS in the United States. *JAMA*. 1992;268:3456-3461.

[109] Cunningham WE, Bozzette SA, Hays RD, Kanouse DE, et al. Comparison of health-related quality of life in clinical trial and non-clinical trial HIV infected cohorts. *Med Care*. 1995;33(suppl 4):AS15-25.

[110] Jonson AR, Stryker J, eds. *The Social Impact of AIDS in the United States*. Washingon, DC: National Academy Press; 1993.

[111] Merton V. Ethical obstacles to the participation of women in biomedical esearch. In: Wolf SM. *Feminism and Bioethics: Beyond Reproduction*. New York: Oxford University Press; 1996:216-251.

[112] Besch CL. Compliance in clinical trials. *AIDS*. 1995;9:1-10.

[113] Meisler A, et al. Adherence to clinical trials among women, minorities, and injection drug users. In: Program and abstracts of the IX International Conference in AIDS; 1993; Berlin, Germany.

[114] El-Sadr W, Capps L. The challenge of minority recruitment in clinical trials for AIDS. *JAMA*. 1992;267:954-957.

[115] Cotton DJ, Finkelstein DM, He W, Feinberg J. Determinants of accrual of women to a large, multicenter clinical trials program of human immunodeficiency virus infection. *J Acquir Immune Defic Syndr*. 1993;6:1322-1328.

[116] Lurie N, Slater J, McGovern P, et al. Preventive care for women. Does the sex of the physician matter? *N Engl J Med*. 1993;329:478-482.

[117] Parks VE. Regarding research: HIV+ women consider clinical trials. In: Program and abstracts of the XI International Conference on AIDS; July 7-12, 1996; Vancouver, British Columbia.

CHAPTER 8

[1] Stringer JSA, Vermund SH. Prevention of mother-to-child transmission of HIV-1. *Curr Opin Obstet Gynecol*. 1999:11:427-34.

[2] Constantine NT, Abesamis CG, Dayrit MM. Intervening in bood supply and use systems: HIV testing. In: *Preventing HIV in Developing Countries, Biomedical and Behavioral Approaches*. Gibney L, Di Clemente RJ, Vermund SH, eds. New York: Kluwer Academic/Plenum Publishers; 1999.

[3] Bullough V, Bullough B. *The History of Prostitution*. New Hyde Park, NY: University Books; 1964.

[4] Burnham JC. Medical inspection of prostitutes in America in the nintheenth century: the St. Louis experiment and its sequel. *Bull Hist Med*. 1971; 45(3):203-18.

[5] Brandt AM. *No Magic Bullet: A Social History of Venereal Disease in the United States since 1880*. New York: Oxford University Press; 1985.

[6] Adler MW. The terrible peril: a historical perspective on the venereal diseases. *Br Med J*. 1980;281:206-11.

[7] Dock LL. Hygiene and mortality. *A Manual for Nurses and Others, Giving an Outline of the Medical, Social and Legal Aspect of the Venereal Diseases*. New York: Putnam; 1911.

[8] Haller JS, Haller RM. *The physician and sexuality in Victorian America*. Urbana, IL: University of Illinois Press; 1974.

[9] Selvin, M. Changing medical and societal attitudes towards sexually transmitted diseases: A historical overview. In: Holmes KK, Mardh PA, Sparling PF, Wiesner PJ, eds. *Sexually Transmitted Diseases*. New York, NY: McGraw-Hill Book Co; 1984:3-19.

[10] Vonderlehr RA, Heller JR Jr. *The Control of Venereal Disease*. New York: Reynal & Hitchcock, 1945: 5-8.

[11] Handsfield HH. Sex, science, and society. A look at sexually transmitted diseases. *Postgrad Med*. 1997;101:268-273, 277-278.

[12] Mattelaer JJ. History of venereal diseases. *Acta Urol Belg*. 1993;61:19-28.

[13] Anderson OW. *Syphilis and Society—Problems of Control in the United States, 1912-1964*. Chicago, IL: Center for Health Administration Studies, Health Information Foundation, Research Series 22; 1965.

[14] Amstey MS. The political history of syphilis and its application to the AIDS epidemic. *WHI*. 1994; 4:16-19.

[15] Culter JC, Arnold RC. Venereal disease control by health departments in the past: lessons for the present. *Am J Public Health*. 1988;78:372-76.

[16] Brandt AM. AIDS in historical perspective: four lessons from the history of sexually transmitted diseases. *Am J Public Health*. 1988;78:367-371.

[17] Brandt AM. The syphilis epidemic and its relation to AIDS. *Science*. 1988;239:375-80.

[18] Dritz SK. Medical aspects of homosexuality. *N Engl J Med*. 1980;302:463-464.

[19] Dritz SK, Ainsworth TE, Back A, Boucher LA, et al. Patterns of sexually transmitted enteric diseases in a city. *Lancet*. 1977;2:3-4.

[20] Shilts R. *And the Band Played On: Politics, People, and the AIDS Epidemic*. New York, NY: St. Martin's Press; 1987.

[21] Gao F, Bailes E, Robertson DL, Chen Y, et al. Origin of HIV-1 in the chimpanzee *Pan troglodytes troglodytes*. *Nature*. 1999;397:436-441.

[22] Zhu T, Korber BT, Nahmias AJ, Hooper E, et al. An African HIV-1 sequence from 1959 and implications for the origin of the epidemic. *Nature*.1998;391:594-597.

[23] Nzilambi N, De Cock KM, Forthal DN, Francis H, et al. The prevalence of infection with human immunodeficiency virus over a 10-year period in rural Zaire. *N Engl J Med*. 1988;318:276-279.

[24] Peto J. AIDS and promiscuity. *Lancet*. 1986;2:979.

[25] Greenberg AE, Kadio A, Grant AD, et al. Clinical manifestations of advanced HIV disease using hospital surveillance, clinical and autopsy data in Abidjan, Cote d'Ivoire. Program and abstracts of the XIII International Conference on AIDS; 1998. 2:40(abstract no.12146).

[26] UNAIDS/WHO. *Report on the Global HIV/AIDS Epidemic: June 1998*. Geneva Switzerland: UNAIDS/World Health Organization;1998.

[27] Kaggwa S, Banage DN, Mugisa SM, Kakande VC, et al. Developing family-centred care for HIV/AIDS orphans—a collaboration across disciplines. Program and abstracts of the XIII International Conference on AIDS; 1998. 12:480(abstract no. 24203).

[28] Over M, Piot P. Human immunodeficiency virus infection and other sexually transmitted diseases in developing countries: public health importance and priorities for resource allocation. *J Infect Dis*. 1996;174(suppl 2):S162-S175.

[29] Deschamps MM, Pape JW, Hafner A, Johnson WD Jr. Heterosexual transmission of HIV in Haiti. *Ann Intern Med*. 1996;125:324-30.

[30] Hanenberg RS, Rojanapithayakorn W, Kunasol P, Sokal DC. Impact of Thailand's HIV-control programme as indicated by the decline of sexually transmitted diseases. *Lancet*. 1994;344:243-245.

[31] Nuwagaba D. HIV/AIDS prevention and care among sex workers in Kampala slums: a youth in action approach. Program and abstracts of the XIII International Converence on AIDS; 1998. 12:901(abstract no. 43273).

[32] Mayaud P, Mosha F, Todd J, et al. Improved treatment services significantly reduce the prevalence of sexually transmitted diseases in rural Tanzania: results of a randomized controlled trial. *AIDS*. 1997;11:1873-1880.

[33] Allen S, Serufilira A, Bogaerts J, et al. Confidential HIV testing and condom promotion Africa: impact on HIV and gonorrhea rates. *JAMA*. 1992;268:3338-3343.

[34] Laga M, Alary M, Nzila N, Manoka AT, et al. Condom promotion, sexually transmitted diseases treatment, and declining incidence of HIV-1 infection in female Zairian sex workers. *Lancet*. 1994;344:246-248.

[35] Landis SE, Schoenbach VJ, Weber DJ, Mittal M, et al. Results of a randomized trial of partner notification in cases of HIV infection in North Carolina. *N Engl J Med*. 1992;326:101-106.

[36] Judson F, Cohn D, Douglas J. HIV seroprevalence in heterosexual men and women, Denver metro STD clinic, 1985-1988. Program and abstracts of the IV International Conference on AIDS; 1989. 5:87(abstract no. M.A.P.54).

[37] Gibney L, Di Clemente RJ, Vermund SH, eds. *Preventing HIV in Developing Countries, Biomedical and Behavioral Approaches*. New York, NY: Kluwer Academic/Plenum Publishers; 1999.

[38] Sarkar S, Islam N, Durandin F, Siddiqui N, et al. Low HIV and high STD among commercial sex workers in a brothel in Bangladesh: scope for prevention of larger epidemic. *Int J STD AIDS*. 1998;9:45-47.

[39] Islam N. HIV/AIDS in Bangladesh—an epidemiological mystery. Program and abstracts of the XIII International Conference on AIDS; 1998. 12:958(abstract no. 43568).

[40] Khawaja ZA, Gibney L, Ahmed AL, Vermund SH. HIV/AIDS and its risk factors in Pakistan. *AIDS*. 1997;11:843-848.

[41] Liao SS. HIV in China: epidemiology and risk factors. *AIDS*. 1998;12 (suppl B):S19-S25.

[42] Zhang J. HIV prevalence trends among intravenous drug users in Yunnan Province between 1992-1997. Program and abstracts of the XIII International Conference on AIDS; 1998. 12:935-936(abstract no. 43459).

[43] Schwebke JR, Aira T, Jordan N, Jolly PE, Vermund SH. Sexually transmitted diseases in Ulaanbaatar, Mongolia. *Int J STD AIDS*. 1998;9:354-358.

[44] Purevdawa E, Moon TD, Baigalmaa C, Davaajav K, et al. Rise in sexually transmitted diseases during democratization and economic crisis in Mongolia. *Intl J STD AIDS*. 1997;8:398-401.

[45] Paris M, Gotuzzo E, Goyzueta G, Arambuyu J, et al. Prevalence of gonococcal and chlamydial infections in commercial sex workers in a Peruvian Amazon city. *Sex Transm Dis*. 1999; 26:103-107.

[46] DiClemente R, Funkhouser E, Wingood GM, Fawal H, et al. Russian roulette: are persons being treated with protease inhibitors gambling with high risk sex? Program and abstracts of the XIII International Conference on AIDS; 1998; 12:211(abstract no. 14143).

[47] Rosenberg PS, Biggar RJ. Trends in HIV incidence among young adults in the United States. *JAMA*. 1998;279:1894-1899.

[48] Rogers AS, Futterman DK, Moscicki AB, Wilson CM, et al. The REACH Project of the Adolescent Medicine HIV/AIDS Research Network: design, methods, and selected characteristics of participants. *J Adolesc Health*. 1998;22:300-311.

[49] Christenson B, Stillstrom J. The epidemiology of human immunodeficiency virus and other sexually transmitted diseases in the Stockholm area. *Sex Trans Dis*. 1995;22:281-288.

[50] Cronberg S. The rise and fall of sexually transmitted diseases in Sweden. *Genitourin Med*. 1993;69:184-186.

[51] Cohen MS. Sexually transmitted diseases enhance HIV transmission: no longer a hypothesis. *Lancet*. 1998;351(suppl 3):5-7.

[52] Robinson NJ, Mulder DW, Auvert B, Hayes RJ. Proportion of HIV infections attributable to other sexually transmitted diseases in a rural Ugandan population: simulation model estimates. *Int J Epidemiol*. 1997;26:180-189.

[53] Klouman E, Masenga EJ, Klepp KI, Sam NE, et al. HIV and reproductive tract infections in a total village population in rural Kilimanjaro, Tanzania: women at increased risk. *J Acquir Immune Defic Syndr Hum Retrovirol*. 1997;14:163-168.

[54] Laga M, Manoka A, Kivuvu M, Malele B, et al. Non-ulcerative sexually transmitted diseases as risk factors for HIV-1 transmission in women: results from a cohort study. *AIDS*. 1993;7:95-102.

[55] Cohen MS, Hoffman IF, Royce RA, Kazembe P, et al. Reduction of concentration of HIV-1 in semen after treatment of urethritis: implications for prevention of sexual transmission of HIV-1. AIDSCAP Malawi Research Group. *Lancet*. 1997;349:1868-1873.

[56] Dyer JR, Kazembe P, Vernazza PL, Gilliam BL, et al. High levels of human immunodeficiency virus type 1 in blood and semen of seropositive men in sub-Saharan Africa. *J Infect Dis*. 1998;177:1742-1746.

[57] Rodrigues JJ, Mehendale SM, Shepherd ME, Divekar AD, et al. Risk factors for HIV infection in people attending clinics for sexually transmitted diseases in India. *BMJ*. 1995;311:283-286.

[58] Cleghorn FR, Jack N, Murphy JR, Edward J, et al. HIV-1 prevalence and risk factors among sexually transmitted disease clinic attenders in Trinidad. *AIDS*. 1995;9:389-394.

[59] Coplan PM, Gortmaker S, Hernandez-Avila M, Spiegelman D, et al. Human immunodeficiency virus infection in Mexico City. Rectal bleeding and anal warts as risk factors among men reporting sex with men. *Am J Epidemiol*. 1996;144:817-827.

[60] Vermund SH. Transmission of HIV-1 among adolescents and adults. In: DeVita VT, Hellman S, Rosenberg SA, eds. *AIDS: Etiology, Diagnosis, Treatment and Prevention*. 4th ed. Philadelphia: Lippincott-Raven Publishers, 1996;147-165.

[61] Critchlow CW, Kiviat NB. Detection of human immunodeficiency virus type 1 and type 2 in the female genital tract: implications for the understanding of virus transmission. *Obstet Gynecol Surv*. 1997;52:315-324.

[62] Laga M, Dallabetta G. Sexually transmitted diseases: Treating the whole syndrome. *Lancet*. 1997;350 (suppl 3):25.

[63] Goldenberg RL, Vermund SH, Goepfert AR, Andrews WW. Choriodecidual inflammation: a potentially preventable cause of perinatal HIV-1 transmission? *Lancet*. 1998;352:1927-1930.

[64] Taha TE, Hoover DR, Dallabetta GA, Kumwenda NI, et al. Bacterial vaginosis and disturbances of vaginal flora: association with increased acquisition of HIV. *AIDS.* 1998;12:1699-1706.

[65] Craib KJ, Meddings DR, Strathdee SA, Hogg RS, et al. Rectal gonorrhoea as an independent risk factor for HIV infection in a cohort of homosexual men. *Genitourin Med.* 1995;71:150-154.

[66] Wasserheit JN. Epidemiological synergy: Interrelationships between human immunodeficiency virus infection and other sexually transmitted diseases. *Sex Transm Dis.* 1992;19:61-77.

[67] Hawkins RE, Rickman LS, Vermund SH, Carl M. Association of mycoplasma and human immunodeficiency virus infection: detection of amplified Mycoplasma fermentans DNA in blood. *J Infec Dis.* 1992;165:581-585.

[68] The World Bank. Efficient and equitable strategies for preventing HIV/AIDS. In: *Confronting AIDS: Public Priorities in a Global Epidemic.* New York, NY: Oxford University Press; 1997:103-72.

[69] Gertig DM, Kapiga SH, Shao JF, Hunter DJ. Risk factors for sexually transmitted diseases among women attending family planning clinics in Dar-es-Salaam, Tanzania. *Genitourin Med.* 1997;73:39-43.

[70] Moss GB, Clemetson D, D'Costa L, Plummer FA, et al. Association of cervical ectopy with heterosexual transmission of human immunodeficiency virus: results of a study of couples in Nairobi, Kenya. *J Infec Dis.* 1991;164:588-591.

[71] Adler MW. Sexual health—a Health of the Nation failure. *BMJ.* 1997;314:1743-1747.

[72] Vermund SH. Casual sex and HIV transmission. *Am J Public Health.* 1995;85:1488-1489.

[73] DiClemente RJ. Preventing HIV/AIDS among adolescents.Schools as agents of behavior change. *JAMA.* 1993; 270:760-762.

[74] Prochaska JO, Velicer WF, DiClemente CC, Fava J. Measuring processes of change and decisional balance for twelve problem behaviors. *Health Psychol.* 1994;83:501-503.

[75] Grimley DM, Prochaska GE, Prochaska JO. Condom use adoption and continuation: A Transtheoretical approach. *Health Ed Research: Theory and Practice* 1997;12: 61-75.

[76] Wingood GM, DiClemente RJ. The use of psychosocial models for guiding the design and implementation of HIV prevention interventions: translating theory into practice. In: *Preventing HIV in Developing Countries, Biomedical and Behavioral Approaches.* Gibney L, Di Clemente RJ, Vermund SH, eds. New York, NY: Kluwer Academic/Plenum Publishers; 1999.

[77] Carael M, Cleland J, Deheneffe JC, Ferry B, et al. Sexual behavior in developing countries: implications for HIV control. *AIDS.* 1995;9:1171-1175.

[78] Adhikary SS, Mondal C, Nila M, Sarker PS. Condom promotion success through peer educator: an effective strategy in Faridpur brothels by Shapla Mahila Samity. Program and abstracts of the XIII International Conference on AIDS; 1998. 12:700(abstract no. 33566).

[79] Kalichman SC, Williams E, Nachimson D. Brief behavioural skills building intervention for female controlled methods of STD-HIV prevention: outcomes of a randomized clinical field trial. *Int J STD & AIDS.* 1999; 10:174-181.

[80] Aggleton P, Rivers K. Interventions for Adolescents. In: *Preventing HIV in Developing Countries, Biomedical and Behavioral Approaches.* Gibney L, Di Clemente RJ, Vermund SH, eds. New York, NY: Kluwer Academic/Plenum Publishers; 1999.

[81] Ngugi EN, Branigan E, Jackson DJ. Interventions for commercial sex workers and their clients. In: *Preventing HIV in Developing Countries, Biomedical and Behavioral Approaches.* Gibney L, Di Clemente RJ, Vermund SH, eds. New York, NY: Kluwer Academic/Plenum Publishers; 1999.

[82] Raj A, Mukherjee S, Leviton L. Insights for HIV prevention from industrialized countries experiences. In: *Preventing HIV in Developing Countries, Biomedical and Behavioral Approaches.* Gibney L, Di Clemente RJ, Vermund SH, eds. New York, NY: Kluwer Academic/Plenum Publishers; 1999.

[83] Wiebel W, Jimenez A, Johnson W, Ouellet L, et al. Risk behavior and HIV seroincidence among out-of-treatment injection drug users: a four-year prospective study. *J Acquir ImmuneDefic Syndr Hum Retrovirol.* 1996;12:282-289.

[84] Ickovics JR, Yoshikawa H. Preventive interventions to reduce heterosexual HIV risk for women: current perspectives, future directions. *AIDS*. 1998;12(suppl A):S197-S208.

[85] Des Jarlais DC, Friedman SR. HIV epidemiology and interventions among injecting drug users. *Int J STD AIDS*. 1996;7(suppl 2):57-61.

[86] Celentano DD, Nelson KE, Lyles CM, Beyrer C, et al. Decreasing incidence of HIV and sexually transmitted diseases in young Thai men: evidence for success of the HIV/AIDS control and prevention program. *AIDS*. 1998; 12:F29-F36.

[87] Rugpao S, Tovanabutra S, Beyrer C, Nuntakuang D, et al. Multiple condom use in commercial sex in Lamphun Province, Thailand: a community-generated STD/HIV prevention strategy. *Sex Transm Dis*. 1997;24:546-549.

[88] Gilson L, Mkanje R, Grosskurth H, Mosha F, et al. Cost-effectiveness of improved treatment services for sexually transmitted diseases in preventing HIV-1 infection in Mwanza Region, Tanzania. *Lancet*. 1997; 350:1805-1809.

[89] Hayes R, Wawer M, Gray R, Whitworth J, et al. Randomised trials of STD treatment for HIV prevention: report of an international workshop. HIV/STD Trials Workshop Group. *Genitourin Med*. 1997;73:432-443.

[90] Mabey D, Mosha F, Todd J, et al. Community-randomized trial of a programme to prevent HIV infection and enhance reproductive health among adolescents in rural Tanzania: design of impact evaluation. Program and abstracts of the XIII International Conference on AIDS; 1998. 12:1181 (abstract no. 60993).

[91] Coates TJ, Feldman MD. An overview of HIV prevention in the United States. *J Acquir Immune Defic Syndr Hum Retrovirol*. 1997;14(suppl 2):S13-S16.

[92] Rotheram-Borus MJ, Koopman C, Haignere C, Hunter J, Ehrhardt AA. An effective program for changing sexual risk behaviors of gay male and runaway adolescents. Program and abstracts of the V International Conference on AIDS; 1990. 6:107 (abstract no. S.C.47).

[93] van Ameijden EJ, Coutinho RA. Maximum impact of HIV prevention measures targeted at injecting drug users. *AIDS*. 1998;12:625-633.

[94] Institute of Medicine. Committee on Prevention and Control of Sexually Transmitted Diseases. "Factors That Contribute to the Hidden Epidemic." In: Eng TR, Butler WT, eds. *The Hidden Epidemic: Confronting Sexually Transmitted Diseases*. Washington, DC: National Academy Press; 1997:69-117.

[95] Pinkerton SD, Abramson PR, Turk ME. Updated estimates of condom effectiveness. *J Assoc Nurses AIDS Care*. 1998;9:88-89.

[96] Dallabeta G, Serwadda D, Mugrditchian D. Controlling other sexually transmitted diseases. In: *Preventing HIV in Developing Countries, Biomedical and Behavioral Approaches*. Gibney L, Di Clemente RJ, Vermund SH, eds. New York, NY: Kluwer Academic/Plenum Publishers; 1999.

[97] Karita E. STD/HIV prevention, education and promotion of condom use among military recruits in Rwanda. In: proceedings of the meeting on effective approaches to AIDS prevention. WHO, Geneva, May 1995.

[98] Nagachinta T, Duerr A, Suriyanon V, Nantachit N, et al. Risk factors for HIV-1 transmission from HIV-seropositive male blood donors to their regular female partners in northern Thailand. *AIDS*. 1997;11:1765-1772.

[99] Nopkesorn T, Mock PA, Mastro TD, Sangkharomya S, et al. HIV-1 subtype E incidence and sexually transmitted diseases in a cohort of military conscripts in northern Thailand. *J Acquir Immune Defic Syndr Hum Retrovirol*. 1998;18:372-379.

[100] Rojanapithayakorn W, Hanenberg R. The 100% condom program in Thailand. *AIDS*. 1996;10:1-7.

[101] Ngugi EN, Plummer FA, Simonson JN, Cameron DW, et al. Prevention of transmission of human immunodeficiency virus in Africa: effectiveness of condom promotion and health education among prostitutes. *Lancet*. 1988;2:887-890.

[102] Moses S, Plummer FA, Ngugi EN, Nagelkerke NJ, et al. Controlling HIV in Africa: effectiveness and cost of an intervention in a high-frequency STD transmitter core group. *AIDS*. 1991;5:407-411.

[103] Levine WC, Revollo R, Kaune V, Vega J, et al. Decline in sexually transmitted disease prevalence in female Bolivian sex workers: impact of an HIV prevention project. *AIDS*. 1998;12:1899-1906.

[104] Lawson ML, Katzenstein D, Vermund SH. Emerging Biomedical Interventions. In: *Preventing HIV in Developing Countries, Biomedical and Behavioral Approaches*. Gibney L, Di Clemente RJ, Vermund SH, eds. New York, NY: Kluwer Academic/Plenum Publishers; 1999.

[105] Catania JA, Coates TJ, Stall R, Turner H, et al. Prevalence of AIDS-related risk factors and condom use in the United States. *Science*. 1992;258:1101-1106.

[106] Lusher JM, Operskalski EA, Aledort LM, Dietrich SL. Risk of human immunodeficiency virus type 1 infection among sexual and nonsexual household contacts of persons with congenital clotting disorders. *Pediatrics*. 1991;88:242-249.

[107] Witte SS, el-Bassel N, Wada T, Gray O, et al. Acceptability of female condom use among women exchanging street sex in New York City. *Int J STD AIDS*. 1999;10:162-168.

[108] Heise LL, Elias C. Transforming AIDS prevention to meet women's needs: a focus on developing countries. *Soc Sci Med*. 1995;40:931-943.

[109] Judson FN. Partner notification for HIV control. *Hosp Pract*. 1990;25:63-70,73.

[110] Laga M, De Cock KM, Kaleeba N, Mboup S, et al. HIV/AIDS in Africa: the second decade and beyond. *AIDS*. 1997;11 (suppl B):S1-S3.

[111] Laga M. STD control for HIV prevention—it works! *Lancet*. 1995;346:518-519.

[112] Wawer MJ, Gray RH, Sewankambo NK, Serwadda D, et al. A randomized, community trial of intensive sexually transmitted disease control for AIDS prevention, Rakai, Uganda. *AIDS*. 1998;12:1211-1225.

[113] Hitchcock P, Fransen L. Preventing HIV infection: lessons from Mwanza and Rakai. *Lancet*. 1999;353:513-515.

[114] Mostad SB, Jackson S, Overbaugh J, Reilly M, et al. Cervical and vaginal shedding of human immunodeficiency virus type 1-infected cells throughout the menstrual cycle. *J Infect Dis*. 1998;178:983-991.

[115] McLean AR, Blower SM. Modelling HIV vaccination. *Trends Microbiol*. 1995;3:458-462.

[116] Jackson KA, Rosenbaum SE, Yuen G, Anderson R, et al. Population pharmacokinetic analysis of ViRACEPT (nelfinavir mesylate) in HIV-infected patients enrolled in a phase III clinical trial. Program and abstracts of the XIII International Conference on AIDS; 1998. 12:826-827 (abstract no.42267).

[117] Vermund SH. Rationale for the testing and use of a partially effective HIV vaccine. *AIDS Res Hum Retroviruses*. 1998;14(suppl 3):S321-S323.

CHAPTER 9

[1] Epstein S. *Impure science: AIDS, Activism, and the Politics of Knowledge*. Berkeley: University of California Press; 1996.

[2] Oppenheimer G. In the eye of the storm: the epidemiological construction of AIDS. In: Fee E, Fox D, eds. *AIDS: The Burdens of History*. Berkeley: University of California Press; 1988.

[3] Farmer PE. *AIDS and Accusation: Haiti and the Geography of Blame*. Berkeley: University of California Press; 1992.

[4] Barbacci M, Repke JT, Chaisson RE. Routine prenatal screening for HIV infection. *Lancet*. 1991;337:709-711.

[5] Ward J, Kleinman S, Douglas D, Grindon AJ, et al. Epidemiologic characteristics of blood donors with antibody to human immunodeficiency virus. *Transfusion*. 1988;28:298-301.

[6] Piot P, Plummer F, Mhalu F, Lamboray JL, et al. AIDS: an international perspective. *Science*. 1988;239:573-579.

7 Mann J, Tarantola D, Netter T. *AIDS in the World.* Cambridge, MA.: Harvard University Press; 1992:17.

8 Farmer PE. Social inequalities and emerging infectious diseases. *Emerging Infect Dis.* 1996;2:259-269.

9 Zwi A, Cabral A. Identifying "high risk situations" for preventing AIDS. *BMJ.* 1991;303:1527-1529.

10 McMichael A. The health of persons, populations, and planets: epidemiology comes full circle. *Epidemiology.* 1995; 6:633-636.

11 Connors M. Sex, drugs, and structural violence. In: Farmer P, Connors M, Simmons J, eds. *Women, Poverty, and AIDS: Sex, Drugs, and Structural Violence.* Monroe, Me.: Common Courage Press; 1996.

12 Pearce N. Traditional epidemiology, modern epidemiology, and public health. *Am J Public Health.* 1996;86:678-683.

13 Susser M, Susser E. Choosing a future for epidemiology. I. Eras and paradigms. *Am J Public Health.* 1996;86:668-673.

14 Susser M, Susser E. Choosing a future for epidemiology. II. From black box to Chinese boxes and eco-epidemiology. *Am J Public Health.* 1996;86:674-677.

15 UNAIDS/World Health Organization. *AIDS Epidemic Update: December, 1999.* Geneva, Switzerland: UNAIDS/World Health Organization; 1999.

16 Wasser S, Gwinn M, Fleming P. Urban-nonurban distribution of HIV infection in childbearing women in the United States. *J AIDS.* 1993;6:1035-1042.

17 Centers for Disease Control and Prevention. *HIV/AIDS Surveillance Report.* Vol. 11, No. 1. Atlanta, GA: Centers for Disease Control and Prevention; 1999:1-44.

18 Williams A. *Bridging the Gaps: The World Health Report.* Geneva, Switzerland: World Health Organization; 1995: 32.

19 Centers for Disease Control and Prevention. Update: mortality due to HIV infection among persons aged 25-44 years—United States, 1994. *MMWR Morb Mortal Wkly Rep.* 1996;45:121-124.

20 Green TA, Karon JM, Nwanyanwu OC. Changes in AIDS incidence trends in the United States. *J Acquir Immune Defic Syndr.* 1992;5:547-555.

21 Holmberg S. The estimated prevalence and incidence of HIV in 96 large US metropolitan areas. *Am J Public Health.* 1996;86: 642-654.

22 McQuillan G, Khare M, Ezzati-Rice T, Karon JM, et al. The seroepidemiology of human immunodeficiency virus in the United States household population: NHANES-III, 1988-1991. *J Acquir Immune Defic Syndr.* 1994;7:1195-1201.

23 Center For Disease Control and Prevention. Surveillance for AIDS-defining opportunistic illnesses, 1992-1997. *MMWR Morb Mortal Wkly Rep.* 1999; 48 (SS-2):1-22.

24 de Bruyn M, Jackson H, Wijermars M, et al. *Facing the Challenges of HIV, AIDS, and STDs: A Gender-Based Response.* Geneva, Switzerland: World Health Organization; 1995.

25 Barongo L, Borgdorff M, Mosha F, Nicoll A, et al. The epidemiology of HIV-1 infection in urban areas, roadside settlements, and rural villages in Mwanza Region, Tanzania. *AIDS.* 1992;6:1521-1528.

26 Berkley S, Naamara W, Okware S, Downing R, et al. AIDS and HIV infection in women in Uganda—are women more infected than males? *AIDS.* 1990;4:1237-1242.

27 Kimball A, Berkley S, Ngugi E, Gayle H. International aspects of the AIDS/HIV epidemic. *Annu Rev Public Health.* 1995;16:253-282.

28 Simmons J, Farmer P, Schoepf B. A global perspective. In: Farmer P, Connors M, Simmons J, eds. *Women, Poverty, and AIDS: Sex, Drugs and Structural Violence.* Monroe, Me.: Common Courage Press; 1996.

29 In Kinshasa, Zaire, 35% of sex workers were found to be HIV positive (Nzila N, Laga M, Thiam A, Mayimona K, et al. HIV and other sexually transmitted diseases among female prostitutes in Kinshasa. *AIDS.* 1991;5: 715-721). Rates of 58% were found among commercial sex

workers in Burkina Faso (Lankoandé S, Meda N, Sangaré L, Compaore I, et al. Prevalence and risk of HIV infection among female sex workers in Burkina Faso. *Int J STD AIDS*. 1998;9:146-150). In 1995, nearly 80% of sex workers in Abidjan, Côte d'Ivoire were infected with HIV (Ghys DP, Dialo OM, Ettiègne-Traoré V, et al. Genital ulcers associated with human immunodeficiency virus-related immunosuppression in female sex workers in Abidjan, Ivory Coast. *J Infect Dis*. 1995;172:1-4). Rates of seropositivity have been reported as high as 88% among sex workers in Butare, Rwanda (Hunt CW. Migrant labor and sexually transmitted disease: AIDS in Africa. *J Health Soc Behav*. 1989;30:353-373).

[30] Bwayo J, Plummer F, Omari M, Mutere A, et al. Human immunodeficiency virus infection in long-distance truck drivers in East Africa. *Arch Intern Med*. 1994;154:1391-1396.

[31] Fisher P, Toko R. HIV seroprevalence in healthy blood donors in Northeastern Zaire. *Int J STD AIDS*. 1995;6:284-286.

[32] Berkley S, Naamara W, Okware S, et al. The epidemiology of AIDS and HIV infection in women in Uganda. Paper presented at: Fourth International Conference on AIDS and Associated Cancers in Africa; October 1989; Marseilles, France.

[33] Soto-Ramirez L, Renjifo B, McLane M, Marlink R, et al. HIV-1 Langerhans' cell tropism associated with heterosexual transmission of HIV. *Science*. 1996;271:1291-1293.

[34] Brown JE, Okako BA, Brown RC. Dry and tight: Sexual practices and potential risk in Zaire. *Soc Sci Med*. 1993;37:989-994.

[35] Farmer P. Women, poverty, and AIDS. In: Farmer P, Connors M, Simmons J, eds. *Women, Poverty, and AIDS: Sex, Drugs and Structural Violence*. Monroe, Me.: Common Courage Press; 1996.

[36] Lurie P, Hintzen P, Lowe RA. Socioeconomic obstacles to HIV prevention and treatment in developing countries: the roles of the International Monetary Fund and the World Bank. *AIDS*. 1995;9:539-546.

[37] Allen S, Lindan C, Serufilira A, Van de Perre P, et al. Human immunodeficiency virus infection in urban Rwanda. *JAMA*. 1991;266:1657-1663.

[38] Serwadda D, Mugerwa RD, Sewankambo NK, Lwegaba A, et al. Slim disease: a new disease in Uganda and its association with HTLV-III infection. *Lancet*. 1985;2:849-852.

[39] Lucas SB, De Cock KM, Hounnou A, Peacock C, et al. Contribution of tuberculosis to slim disease in Africa. *BMJ*. 1994;308:1531-1533.

[40] Desvarieux M, Pape J. HIV and AIDS in Haiti: Recent developments. *AIDS Care*. 1991;3:271-279.

[41] Cortes E, Silva J, Vilela A, et al. Changes in transmission patterns in 12 years of the AIDS epidemic in Brazil. Presented at: VIII International Conference on AIDS; July 1996; Amsterdam, The Netherlands.

[42] UNAIDS/World Health Organization. *Epidemiological Fact Sheet on HIV/AIDS and Sexually Transmitted Diseases: Brazil*. Geneva, Switzerland: UNAIDS/World Health Organization; 1998.

[43] Liautaud B, et al. Preliminary data on STDs in Haiti. In: Program and Abstacts of the VIII International Conference on AIDS/III STD World Congress; July 19-24, 1992; Amsterdam, The Netherlands. Abstract C4302.

[44] Mellon RL, Liautaud B, Pape JW, Johnston WD Jr. Association of HIV and STDs in Haiti: implications for blood banks and vaccine trials. *J Acquir Immune Defic Syndr Hum Retrovirol*. 1995;8(2):214.

[45] Pape J, Johnson WD Jr. AIDS in Haiti: 1982-1992. *Clin Infect Dis* 1993;17(Suppl 2):S341-S345.

[46] Guérin J, Malebranche R, Elie R, Laroche AC, et al. Acquired immune deficiency syndrome: specific aspects of the disease in Haiti. *Ann NY Acad Sci*. 1984;437:254-261.

[47] Johnson WD Jr, Pape JW. AIDS in Haiti. *Immunol Ser*. 1989;44:65-78.

[48] Farmer PE. *Infections and Inequalities: The Modern Plagues*. Berkeley: University of California Press; 1999.

[49] Pape J, Johnson W. "Epidemiology of AIDS in the Caribbean." *Baillière's Clin Trop Med and Commun Dis* 1988;3(1): 31-42.

[50] During the past decade, political violence has hampered research on HIV in Haiti. No large seroprevalence surveys have been conducted since 1992, when seroprevalence was 10% in urban areas, and approximately 5% in rural areas (Pape J, Johnson WD Jr. AIDS in Haiti: 1982-1992. *Clin Infect Dis.* 1993;17(Suppl 2):S341-S345). The urban predominance will likely wane with time. Among total AIDS cases registered in Haiti, the percentage from rural areas more than tripled between 1979 and 1990. Recent estimates place the percentage of AIDS cases from rural areas at 35% (Pape JW, Deschamps MM, Verdier RI, Jean S, et al. The urge for an AIDS vaccine: perspectives from a developing country. *AIDS Research and Human Retroviruses.* 1992;8:1535-1537).

[51] Farmer P. Culture, poverty, and the dynamics of HIV transmission in rural Haiti. In: Brummelhuis H, Herdt G, eds. *Culture and Sexual Risk: Anthropological Perspectives on AIDS.* New York, NY: Gordon and Breach; 1995.

[52] Surasiengsunk S, Kiranandana S, Wongboonsin K, Garnett GP, et al. Demographic impact of the HIV epidemic. *AIDS.* 1998;12:775-784.

[53] These estimates are made in the context of the "100% condom program," a program built on a robust preexisting infrastructure of STD surveillance (see also Chapter 8 for details). The program, implemented in 1991, was designed to promote the use of condoms by all prostitutes and their clients. Prevalence of condom use was reported to increase from 14% in 1989 to 94% in 1993 (Hanenberg RS, Rojanapithayakorn W, Kunasol P, Sokal DC. Impact of Thailand's HIV-control programme as indicated by the decline of sexually transmitted diseases. *Lancet.* 1994;344:243-245). Studies of military conscripts, major vectors of HIV infection inside Thailand, found decreasing rates of infection, from an incidence of 3 per 100 person-years in 1993 to 0.3 per 100 person-years in 1995 (Carr JK, Sirisopana N, Torugsa K, Jugsudee A, et al. Incidence of HIV-1 infection among young men in Thailand. *J Acquir Immune Defic Syndr.* 1994;7:1270-1275; Celentano DD, Nelson KE, Suprasert S, Eiumtrakul S, et al. Risk factors for HIV-1 seroconversion among young men in northern Thailand. *JAMA.* 1996;275:122-127). Additionally, Nelson and colleagues found increasing rates of condom use among military conscripts, from 61% in 1991 to 92% in 1995 (Nelson KE, Celentano DD, Eiumtrakol S, Hoover DR, et al. Changes in sexual behavior and a decline in HIV infection among young men in Thailand. *N Engl J Med.* 1996;335:297-303). The program has its limitations, however, and recent surveys suggest ongoing transmission among commercial sex workers (Kilmarx PH, Palanuvej D, Chitvarakorn A, St Louis ME, et al. Seroprevalence of HIV among female sex workers in Bangkok: evidence of ongoing infection risk after the "100% condom program" was implemented. *J Acquir Immune Defic Syndr.* 1999;21:313-316). The relevance of the Thai experience to sub-Saharan African countries has been questioned, since the GNP of Thailand—almost $3000 per year—is an order of magnitude higher than many countries in which HIV is endemic (World Bank. *World Development Indicators,* 1999. Washington, DC:World Bank; 1999).

[54] UNAIDS/World Health Organization. *Epidemiological Fact Sheet on HIV/AIDS and Sexually Transmitted dDiseases: India.* Geneva, Switzerland: UNAIDS/World Health Organization; 1998.

[55] Jain M, John T, Keusch G. Epidemiology of HIV and AIDS in India. *AIDS.* 1994;8(S2): S61-S75.

[56] Jain M, John T, Keusch G. A review of human immunodeficiency virus infection in India. *J Acquir Immune Defic Syndr.* 1994;7:1185-1194.

[57] Gangakhedkar R, Bentley M, Rompalo A, et al. STDs and HIV infection among female noncommercial sex workers attending STD clinics in Pune, India. In: Program and abstracts of the XI International Conference on AIDS. July 7-12, 1996; Vancouver, British Columbia. Abstract C.226.

[58] Weniger B, Limpakarnjanarat K, Ungchusak K, Thanprasertsuk S, et al. The epidemiology of HIV infection and AIDS in Thailand. *AIDS.* 1991;5(Suppl 2): S71-S85.

[59] Zheng X, Zhang J, Tian C, Cheng HH, et al. Cohort study of HIV infection among drug users in Ruili, Longchuan, and Luxi of Yunnan Province, China. *Biomed Environ Sci.* 1993;6:348-351.

[60] Singh S, Crofts D, Gertig D. HIV infections among IDUs in North East Malaysia. Presented at: IX International Conference on AID; 1993; Berlin, Germany.

[61] Ministry of Health, P R China, and UN Theme Group on HIV/AIDS in China. *China Responds to AIDS: HIV/AIDS Situation and Needs Assessment Report, 1997.* Geneva, Switzerland: World Health Organization; 1997.

[62] Padrian NS, Shiboski SC, Jewell NP. Female to male transmission of HIV. *JAMA.* 1991;266:1664-1667.

[63] Cameron DW, Simonson JN, D'Costa LJ, Ronald AR, et al. Female to male transmission of human immunodeficiency virus type 1: risk factors for seroconversion in men. *Lancet* 1989;2:403-407.

[64] Chakraborty A, Jana S, Das A, Khodakevich L, et al. Community based survey of STD/HIV infection among commercial sex workers in Calcutta (India). Part I: Some social features of commercial sex workers. *J Commun Dis.* 1994;26:161-167.

[65] Das S. *AIDS in India: An Ethnography of HIV/AIDS Amongst Bombay's Commercial Sex Workers.* Cambridge, Mass.: Harvard University Press; 1995.

[66] Quinn T, Mann J, Curran J, Piot P. AIDS in Africa: an epidemiological paradigm. *Science.* 1986;234:955-963.

[67] Elvin K, Lumbwe C, Luo N, Bjorkman A, et al. *Pneumocystis carinii* is not a major cause of pneumonia in HIV-infected patients in Lusaka, Zambia. *Trans R Soc Trop Med Hyg.* 1989;83:553-555.

[68] McLeod D, Neill P, Robertson V, Latiff AS, et al. Pulmonary diseases in patients infected with the human immunodeficiency virus in Zimbabwe, Central Africa. *Trans R Soc Trop Med Hyg.* 1989;83:694-697.

[69] Lucas S, Hounnou A, Peacock C, Beaumel A, et al. The mortality and pathology of HIV infection in a West African city. *AIDS.* 1993;7:1569-1579.

[70] Batungwanayo J, Taelman H, Lucas S, Bogaerts J, et al. Pulmonary disease associated with the human immunodeficiency virus in Kigali, Rwanda. *Am J Respir Crit Care Med.* 1994;149:1591-1596.

[71] Russian D, Kovacs J. *Pneumocystis carinii* in Africa: An emerging pathogen? *Lancet.* 1995;346:1242-1243.

[72] Malin A, Gwanzura L, Klein S, Robertson VJ, et al. *Pneumocystis carinii* pneumonia in Zimbabwe. *Lancet.* 1995;346:1258-1261.

[73] Sudre P, ten Dam G, Kochi A. Tuberculosis: a global overview of the situation today. *Bull World Health Organ.* 1992;70: 149-159.

[74] Collins, FM. The immunology of tuberculosis. *Am Rev Resp Dis.* 1982;125:42-49.

[75] Dye C, Scheele S, Dolin P, Pathania V, et al. Consensus statement. Global burden of tuberculosis: Estimated incidence, prevalence, and mortality by country. WHO Global Surveillance and Monitoring Project. *JAMA.* 1999;282:677-686.

[76] Farmer P. Letter from Haiti. *AIDS Clin Care.* 1997;9:83-85.

[77] Johnson W, Pape J. AIDS in Haiti. In: Levy J, ed. *AIDS: Pathogenesis and Treatment.* New York, NY: Marcel Dekker; 1989.

[78] Farmer P, Robin S, Ramilus S, Kim JY. Tuberculosis, poverty, and 'compliance:' lessons from rural Haiti." *Semin Respir Infect.* 1991;6:254-260.

[79] Mohar A, Romo J, Salido F, Jessurun J, et al. The spectrum of clinical and pathological manifestations of AIDS in a consecutive series of autopsied patients in Mexico. *AIDS* 1992;6:467-473.

[80] Moreira E, Silva N, Brites C, Carvlho EM, et al. Characteristics of the acquired immune deficiency syndrome in Brazil. *Am J Trop Med Hyg.* 1993;48:687-692.

[81] Fleming P, Ciesielski C, Byers R, et al. Gender differences in reported AIDS-indicative diagnoses. *J Infect Dis.* 1993;68: 61-71.

[82] Klatt E, Nichols L, Noguchi T. Evolving trends revealed by autopsies of patients with the acquired immune deficiency syndrome. *Arch Pathol Lab Med.* 1994;118: 884-890.

[83] Minkoff H, DeHovitz J. Care of women with the human immunodeficiency virus. *JAMA.* 1991;266:2253-2258.

[84] Mackie I. AIDS, the female patient, and the family physician. *Can Fam Physican.* 1993;39:1600-1607.

[85] Sha BE, Benson CA, Pottage JC, Urbanski PA, et al. HIV infection in women: an observational study of clinical characteristics, disease progression and survival for a cohort of women in Chicago. *J Acquir Immune Defic Syndr.* 1995;8:486-495.

[86] Khalsa AM, Currier J. Women and HIV. A review of current epidemiology, gynecologic manifestations, and perinatal transmission. *Prim Care*. 1997;24: 617-641.

[87] Des Jarlais D, Stoneburner R, Thomas P. Declines in the proportion of Kaposi's sarcoma among cases of AIDS in multiple risk groups in New York City. *Lancet*. 1987;2:1024-1025.

[88] Rutherford GW, Schwarcz S, Lemp G, Barnhart JL, et al. The epidemiology of AIDS-related Kaposi's sarcoma in San Francisco. *J Infect Dis*. 1989;159:569-572.

[89] Rates of pneumococcal bacteremia are estimated to be as much as 100-fold higher in patients with AIDS compared with seronegative controls (Redd SC, Rutherford GW, Sande M, Lifson AR, et al. The role of HIV infection in pneumococcal bacteraemia in San Francisco residents. *J Infect Dis*. 1990;162:1012-1017). Similarly, HIV-positive individuals have been shown to be 20 times more likely to acquire salmonella infections than seronegative controls; bacteremia is 100 times more prevalent in HIV-positive patients (Gruenewald R, Blum S, Chan J. Relationship between human immunodeficiency virus infection and salmonellosis in 20- to 59-year-old residents of New York City. *Clin Infect Dis*. 1994;18:358-363).

[90] Tumbarello M, Tacconelli E, Caponera S, Cauda R, et al. The impact of bacteremia on HIV infection. Nine years experience in a large Italian university hospital. *J Infect*. 1995;31:123-131.

[91] Celum C, Chaisson R, Rutherford G, Barnhart JL, et al. Incidence of salmonellosis in patients with AIDS. *J Infect Dis*. 1987;156:998-1002.

[92] Selwyn P, Feingold A, Hartel D, Schoenbaum EE, et al. Increased risk of bacterial pneumonia in HIV-infected drug users without AIDS. *AIDS*. 1988;2:267-272.

[93] Krieger N, Rowley D, Herman A, Avery B, et al. Racism, sexism, and social class: implications for studies of health, disease, and well-being. *Am J Prev Med*. 1993;9(6 Suppl): 82-122.

[94] Navarro V. Race or class versus race and class: mortality differentials in the United States. *Lancet*. 1990;336:1238-1240.

[95] Marmot M. Social differentials in health within and between populations. *Daedalus*. 1994;123:197-216.

[96] Hogg R, Strathdee S, Craib K, O'Shaughnessy MV, et al. Lower socioeconomic status and shorter survival following infection with HIV. *Lancet*. 1994;344:1120-1124.

[97] Horner P, McBride M, Coker R, Crowley S, et al. Outpatient follow-up in women with HIV infection in Parkside Health Authority. *Genitourin Med*. 1993;69:370-372.

[98] Loue S, Slymen D, Morgenstern H, Whalen C. Health insurance and utilization in *Pneumocystis carinii* pneumonia. *J Gen Intern Med*. 1995;10:461-463.

[99] Although the HER study found, that among women with CD4 counts less than 200 per mm^3, 87.8% reported a history of antiretroviral therapy, less than half of them were receiving such treatment at the time of the interview (Solomon L, Stein M, Flynn C, Schuman P, et al. Health services use by urban women with or at risk for HIV-1 infection: the HIV epidemiology research study (HERS). *J Acquir Immune Defic Syndr Hum Retrovirol*. 1998;17:253-261).

[100] Weiss P, Kennedy C, Wallace M, Nguyen MT, et al. Medication costs associated with the care of HIV infected patients. *Clin Ther*. 1993;15:912-916.

[101] Perdue BE, Weidle PJ, Everson-Mays RE, Bozek PS. Evaluating the cost of medications for ambulatory HIV-infected persons in association with landmark changes in antiretroviral therapy. *J Acquir Immune Defic Syndr Hum Retrovirol*. 1998;17:354-360.

[102] Moore RD, Bartlett JG. Combination antiretroviral therapy in HIV infection. *Pharmacoeconomics*. 1996;10:109-113.

[103] Turner B, Markson L, McKee L, Houchens R, et al. Health care delivery, zidovudine use and survival of women and men with AIDS. *J Acquir Immune Defic Syndr*. 1994;7:1250-1262.

[104] Moore R, Hidalgo J, Sugland B, Chaisson RE. Zidovudine and the natural history of acquired immune deficiency syndrome. *N Engl J Med*. 1991;324:1412-1416.

[105] Stein M, Leibman B, Wachtel T, Carpenter CC, et al. HIV positive women: reasons they are tested for HIV and their clinical characteristics on entry into the health care system. *J Gen Intern Med*. 1991;6:286-289.

[106] Solomon L, Stein M, Flynn C, Schuman P, et al. Health services use by urban women with or at risk for HIV-1 infection: The HIV epidemiology research study (HERS). *J Acquir Immune Defic Syndr Hum Retrovirol.* 1998;17:253-261.

[107] Friedland G, Saltzman B, Vileno J, Freeman K, et al. Survival differences in patients with AIDS. *J Acquir Immune Defic Syndr.* 1991;4:144-153.

[108] Lemp G, Hirozawa A, Cohen J, Derish PA, et al. Survival for women and men with AIDS. *J Infect Dis.* 1992;166:74-79.

[109] Rothernberg R, Woelfel M, Stoneburner R, Milberg J, et al. Survival with acquired immune deficiency syndrome: experience with 5833 cases in New York City. *N Engl J Med.* 1987;317:1297-1302.

[110] Mocroft A, Johnson M, Phillip A. Factors affecting survival in patients with AIDS. *AIDS.* 1996;10:1057-1065.

[111] Santoro-Lopes G, Harrison LH, Moulton LH, Lima LA, et al. Gender and survival after AIDS in Rio de Janeiro, Brazil. *J Acquir Immune Defic Syndr Hum Retrovirol.* 1998;19:403-407.

[112] Des Jarlais D, Padian N, Winkelstein W Jr. Targeted HIV prevention programs. *N Engl J Med.* 1994;331:1451-1453.

[113] World Health Organization. *The Global AIDS Strategy.* Geneva, Switzerland: World Health Organization; 1992:14.

[114] Bacellar H, Munoz A, Hoover D, Phair JP, et al. Incidence of clinical AIDS conditions in a cohort of homosexual men with CD4+ counts < 100/mm^3. *J Infect Dis.* 1994;170:1284-87.

[115] In a study comparing the efficacy of PCP prophylaxis, Antinori and colleagues found that, among patients given trimethoprim-sulfamethoxazole, incidence of PCP was as low as 2 per 100 person-years (Antinori A, Murri R, Ammassari A, De Luca A, et al. Aerosolized pentamide, cotrimoxazole and dapsone-pyrimethamine for primary prophylaxis of *Pneumocystis carinii* pneumonia and toxoplasmic encephalitis. *AIDS* 1995;9:1343-1350).

[116] Shoenbaum EE, Webber MP. The underrecognition of HIV infection in women in an inner-city emergency room. *Am J Publ Health.* 1993;83:363-368.

[117] Ferguson K, Stapleton J, and Helms C. Physicians' effectiveness in assessing risk for human immunodeficiency virus infection. *Arch Inter Med.* 1991;151:561-564.

[118] Schappert SM. *The National Ambulatory Medical Care Survey: 1990 Summary.* Hyattsville, Md.: U.S. Department of Health and Human Services, Public Health Service, Centers for Disease Control, National Center for Health Statistics; 1992.

[119] Gerbert B, Maguire BT, Huley SB, Coates TJ. Physicians and acquired immune deficiency syndrome. *JAMA* 1989; 262:1969-1972.

[120] Kitahata M, Koepsell T, Deyo R, Maxwell CL, et al. Physicians' experience with the acquired immunodeficiency syndrome as a factor in patients' survival. *N Engl J Med.* 1996;334:701-706.

[121] Stepherson J. Survival of patients with AIDS depends on physicians' experience with treating the disease. *JAMA.* 1996;275:745-746.

[122] Van Bergen I. The role of the general practitioner in prevention of sexually transmitted infections in the Netherlands. Preliminary results of a peer-centered continuous education programme. In: Program and abstracts of the XI International Conference on AIDS; July 7-12, 1996; Vancouver, British Columbia. Abstract Number Lb.B.6018.

[123] Moore R, Hidalgo J, Sugland B, Chaisson RE. Zidovudine and the natural history of acquired immune deficiency syndrome. *N Engl J Med.* 1991;324:1412-1416.

[124] Easterbrook P, Keruly J, Creagh-Kirk T, Richman DD, et al. Racial and ethnic differences in outcome in zidovudine-treated patients with advanced HIV disease. *JAMA.* 1991;266:2713-2718.

[125] Chaisson R, Keruly J, Moore R. Race, sex, drug use and progression of human immunodeficiency virus disease. *N Engl J Med.* 1995;333:751-756.

248   *The Emergence of AIDS*

CHAPTER 10

[1] Bayer R. *Private Acts, Social Consequences: AIDS and the Politics of Public Health.* New York: Free Press; 1989.

[2] American Association of Physicians for Human Rights. *Newsletter.* November 12, 1985.

[3] *AIDS and Civil Liberties.* San Francisco: Northern California Branch, American Civil Liberties Union. March 1986.

[4] Bayer R, Levine C, Wolf SM. HIV antibody screening: an ethical framework for evaluating proposed programs. *JAMA.* 1986;256:1768-1774.

[5] Association of State Territorial Health Officials. *ASTHO Guide to Public Health Practice: HTLV III Antibody Testing and Community Approaches.* Washington, DC: Public Health Foundations; 1985.

[6] American Medical Association. *Report of the Council on Ethical and Judicial Affairs: Ethical Issues Involved in the Growing AIDS Crisis.* Chicago, Ill: American Medical Association; 1987.

[7] Colombotos J, Messeri P, McConnell M, et al. Physicians, nurses and AIDS: findings from a national study. (unpublished manuscript)

[8] Jones L. HIV infection labeled as STD: board to clarify testing policy. *Am Med News.* December 14, 1990:28.

[9] Heagarty MC. AIDS, IV drug use and children. In: Rogers DE, Ginzberg E, eds. *The AIDS Patient: An Action Agenda.* Boulder, Colo: Westview Press; 1988.

[10] Bayer R. Public health policy and the AIDS epidemic: an end to HIV exceptionalism. *N Engl J Med.* 1991; 324:1500-1504.

[11] Institute of Medicine. *HIV Screening of Pregnant Women and Newborns.* Washington, DC: National Academy Press; 1991.

[12] Working Group on PCP Prophylaxis in Children. Guidelines for prophylaxis against *Pneumocystis carinii* pneumonia for children infected with human immunodeficiency virus. *MMWR Morb Mortal Wkly Rep.* 1991;40(RR-2):1-13.

[13] Garret L. Treatment benefitting AIDS babies. *New York Newsday.* April 3, 1991:7.

[14] American Academy of Pediatrics Task force on Pediatrics AIDS: Perinatal human immunodeficiency virus (HIV) testing. *Pediatrics.* 1992;89(4 pt 2):791-794.

[15] *News from Assemblywoman Nettie Mayersohn.* July 1993. (newsletter)

[16] It's OK to tell: parents should know HIV results. [editorial] *New York Newsday.* May 27, 1993:64.

[17] Navarro M. Testing newborns for AIDS virus raises issue of mother's privacy. *New York Times.* August 8, 1993:1.

[18] AIDS babies pay the price. [editorial] *New York Times.* August 13, 1993:A26.

[19] New York Governor's Program, Bill No. 123 (1996).

[20] New York State Association of County Health Officials. *Memorandum.* March 15, 1995.

[21] 1996 NY Laws, Ch 220.

[22] Bateman DA, Cooper A, Abrams EJ. Newborn human immunodeficiency virus testing in New York: a legislative quandary. *Arch Pediatr Adolesc Med.* 1995;149:581-582.

[23] Connor EM, Sperling RS, Gelber R, Kiselev P, et al. Reduction of maternal-infant transmission of human immunodeficiency virus type 1 with zidovudine treatment. *N Engl J Med.* 1994; 331:1173-1180.

[24] Rovner J. U.S. specialists object to AMA's call for mandatory HIV testing. *Lancet.* 1996; 348:330.

[25] Segel AI. Physicians' attitudes towards human immunodeficiency virus testing in pregnancy. *Am J Obstet Gynecol.* 1996;174:1750-1755.

[26] Minkoff H, Willoughby A. Pediatric HIV disease, zidovudine in pregnancy, and unblinding heelstick surveys. *JAMA.* 1995;274:1165-1168.

[27] Carusi D, Learman LA, Posner SF. Human immunodeficiency virus test refusal in pregnancy: a challenge to voluntary testing. *Obstet Gynecol.* 1998;91:540-545.

[28] Institute of Medicine. *Reducing the Odds: Preventing Perinatal Transmission of HIV in the United States.* Washington, DC: National Academy Press; 1998.

[29] Shelton DL. Delegates push mandatory HIV testing for pregnant women, American Medical Association House of Delegates vote. Annual Meeting News. *Am Med News* 1996;31:1.

[30] Centers for Disease Control and Prevention. *HIV Testing: Straud Document.* Atlanta, Ga: Centers for Disease Control and Prevention; 1999 (unpublished). AIDS Policy Center Brief, May 22, 1996. (unpublished)

[31] *AAPHR Newsletter.* July 1983.

[32] Thomas Vernon. November 14, 1986; Denver, Colorado. (interview R.B.)

[33] *Amendment to the Rules and Regulations Pertaining to Communicable Disease Control to Require the Reporting of HTLVIII Antibody Tests.* Submitted to: Colorado Board of Health; August 21, 1985.

[34] James Mason. Letter to State and Territorial Health Officials. December 6, 1985. (unpublished)

[35] Presidential Commission on the Human Immunodeficiency Virus Epidemic. *Report.* June 1998:76.

[36] Joseph SC. Remarks made to: V International Conference on AIDS; June 5, 1989; Montreal, Canada.

[37] *New York Times.* January 19, 1990:B-1.

[38] *Newark Star Ledger.* January 5, 1990.

[39] Intergovernmental Health Policy Project. HIV reporting in the states. *Intergovernmental AIDS Reports* Nov-Dec 1989.

[40] Centers for Disease Control and Prevention. Update: Public health surveillance for HIV infection—United States, 1989 and 1990. *MMWR Morb Mortal Wkly Rep.* 1990;39:853,859-861.

[41] Centers for Disease Control and Prevention. *HIV/AIDS Surveillance Rep.* 1998;8(1).

[42] Centers for Disease Control and Prevention. Evaluation of HIV case surveillance through the use of non-name unique identifiers: Maryland and Texas, 1994-1996. *MMWR Morb Mortal Wkly Rep.* 1998;46:1254-1258,1271.

[43] Gostin LO, Ward JW, Baker AC. National HIV case reporting for the United States: a defining moment in the history of the epidemic. *N Engl J Med.* 1997;337:1162-1167.

[44] National Minority AIDS Council. *Memorandum.* (unpublished, ND)

CHAPTER 11

[1] Centers for Disease Control and Prevention (CDC). *Supplemental guidance on HIV prevention community planning for noncompeting continuation of cooperative agreements for HIV prevention projects.* Atlanta, GA: Centers for Disease Control and Prevention; 1993.

[2] Though many of these changes have affected public health practice worldwide, this article will focus exclusively on experiences in the United States.

[3] To verify that states are complying with the representation requirement, CDC obligates jurisdictions to complete planning group profiles and resource allocation tables that show alignment with local and regional HIV epidemiology.

[4] Valdiserri R, Aultman T, Curran J. Community planning: a national strategy to improve HIV prevention programs. *J Community Health.* 1995;20:87-100.

[5] The Ryan White Comprehensive AIDS Resources Emergency Act (CARE Act) was enacted into law by Congress in 1990 as P.L. No. 101-381. Through multiple funding streams, it provides clinical and social support services for people with HIV/AIDS through directly funded community-

based organizations and through city and state structures. Title I and Title II of the Act both require community planning processes.

[6] In 1989, the NIH created the AIDS Clinical Trials Group Community Advisory Board, the first of a multitude of official innovations that obligated diverse, participatory processes in HIV/AIDS research development, implementation and oversight.

[7] Centers for Disease Control and Prevention. Pneumocystis Pneumonia. *MMWR Morbidity and Morta Wkly Rep.* 1981;30:305-308.

[8] See, for example: Shilts R. *And the Band Played On: Politics, People and the AIDS Epidemic.* New York, NY: St. Martin's Press; 1987; D'Emilio J. *Making Trouble: Essays on Gay History, Politics and the University.* New York, NY: Routledge; 1992; and Duberman M. *Stonewall.* New York, NY: Penguin Books; 1993.

[9] As a modest reflection of that, the American Public Health Association by 1980 included over 25 practice sections reflective of public health arenas as diverse as epidemiology, medical care, public health nursing, laboratory sciences, and social work.

[10] The discovery of the HIV virus in 1984 and the subsequent availability of ELISA and confirmatory Western Blot antibody testing ushered in an era where viral detection, potentially well in advance of disease manifestation, became a reality. The late 1980s were marked by active policy debates and community resistance regarding the utility and potential risks of diagnosing a stigmatized fatal disease.

[11] AIDS vaccine development provides one interesting vantage point from which to view this disciplinary diversity. Among those who have contributed to the vaccine preparedness projects and evolving literature are virologists, infectious disease practitioners, psychologists, anthropologists, educators, and sociologists.

[12] See, for example, Shilts (ref.8); Arno P, Feiden K. *Against the Odds: The Story of AIDS Drug Development, Politics, and Profits.* New York, NY: Harper Collins; 1992; Burkett E. *The Gravest Show on Earth: America in the Age of AIDS.* Boston, MA: Houghton Mifflin; 1995.

[13] Perhaps the most remarkably diverse HIV-related policy collaboration occurred during the 1990 passage of both the Ryan White CARE Act and the Americans with Disabilities Act. The national organizations that supported these efforts included the American Hospital Association, the American Medical Association, the National Gay and Lesbian Task Force, the Child Welfare League, the US Catholic Conference, and the American Psychological Association—among many, many others.

[14] John James, editor of *AIDS Treatment News;* Mark Harrington, a MacArthur award winner, and his colleagues at the Treatment Action Group; Martin Delaney from Project Inform; and David Barr and other colleagues from Gay Men's Health Crisis all contributed substantially to both the front line activism and the thoughtful negotiations that led to such drug development changes as expanded and parallel track preapproval access; increased surrogate marker utilization for efficacy trials; and accelerated Phase II and III trial processes.

[15] See Spector M, Kitsuse J. *Constructing Social Problems.* Menlo Park, CA: Cummings Publishing; 1977; Hoffman L. *The Politics of Knowledge: Activist Movements in Medicine and Planning.* Albany, NY: State University of New York Press; 1989; Larana E, Johnston H, Gusfield J, eds. *New Social Movements: From Ideology to Identity.* Philadelphia, PA: Temple University Press; 1994.

[16] By the mid 1980s, consumer-based disability organizations like People First, the Independent Living Centers, Paralyzed Veterans, the National Alliance of the Mentally Ill, and the Disability Rights Education and Defense Fund, among others, had become critical participants in federal statutory and regulatory developments related to building and housing accessibility, educational and vocational training access, medical treatment coverage, and civil rights protections.

[17] Disability organizations articulated a broad range of clinical, educational, and social services considered necessary for meaningful habilitation. They successfully acquired program reimbursement for many of these services under Medicaid and certain federal discretionary programs. Equally as important, the disability community framed ethical and legal requirements for the rendering of these services in the least restrictive environments, assuring the development of continuums of care in community-based settings.

[18] Schneider B, Stoller N, eds. *Women Resisting AIDS: Feminist Strategies of Empowerment.* Philadelphia, PA: Temple University Press; 1995.

[19] See: Fee E. *Women and Health: The Politics of Sex in Medicine.* Farmingdale, NY: Baywood Publishing Company; 1982. See also: Aday L. *At Risk in America: The Health and Health Care Needs of Vulnerable Populations in the United States.* San Francisco, CA: Jossey-Bass Publishers; 1993. See also: Jones W, Rice M. *Health Care Issues in Black America.* New York, NY: Greenwood Press; 1987.

[20] Sodomy continues to be illegal in a majority of states; sex work and drug paraphernalia possession are illegal virtually everywhere.

[21] On June 24, 1988, the Presidential Commission issued a comprehensive report and a national plan often referred to as the "Watkins Report." The background testimony and research provides an excellent compilation of the expanding terrain of discrimination then being experienced by people with HIV/AIDS. See also: Hunter N, Rubenstein W, eds. *AIDS Agenda: Emerging Issues in Civil Rights.* New York, NY: The New Press; 1992.

[22] Regarding the impact of discrimination and fear on affected African Americans communities, see: Thomas S, Quinn S. The Tuskegee Syphilis Study, 1932-1972: Implications for HIV education and AIDS risk education programs in the black community. *Am J Public Health.* 1991;81:1498-1505. For an early assessment of the impact of antidiscrimination and other health care system policies on care access and professional responses, see: Gostin L, ed. *AIDS and the Health Care System.* New Haven, CT: Yale University Press; 1990.

[23] In particular, evolving right to HIV treatment challenges under the Americans with Disabilities Act offer potential opportunities for claims by individuals with other infectious diseases and chronic disabilities.

[24] Berridge V. Histories of harm reduction: illicit drugs, tobacco, and nicotine. *Subst Use Misuse.* 1999;34:35-47.

[25] See, for example: Warner KE. Bags, buckles, and belts: the debate over mandatory passive restraints in automobiles. *J Health Polit Policy Law.* 1983;8:44-75. See also: Weiss B. Preventing bicycle-related head injuries. *New York State Journal of Medicine.* 1987;87:319-20. See also: Giesbrecht N. Reducing risks associated with drinking among young adults: promoting knowledge-based perspectives and harm reduction strategies. *Addiction.* 1999; 94:353-355.

[26] Wallace R, Fullilove MT, Flisher AJ. AIDS, violence and behavioral coding: information theory, risk behavior and dynamic process on core-group sociogeographic networks. *Soc Sci Med.* 1996;43:339-352.

[27] See, for example: McKusick L, Horstman W, Coates T. AIDS and sexual behavior reported by gay men in San Francisco. *Am J Public Health.* 1985;75:493-6. See also: Greenwood J. Creating a new drug service in Edinburgh. *BMJ.* 1990;300:587-589. See also: Friedman S, Des Jarlais D. Re: "The harm reduction approach and risk factors for human immunodeficiency virus (HIV) seroconversion in injecting drug users, Amsterdam". *Am J Epidemiol.* 1993;138:768-771. See also: Wodak A. Harm reduction: Australia as a case study. *Bull NY Acad Med.* 1995;72:339-347.

[28] See: Stein Z, Saez H, el-Sadr W, Healton C, et al. Safer sex strategies for women: the hierarchical model in methadone treatment clinics. *J Urban Health.* 1999;76:62-72. See also: Sikkema K, Kelly J, Winett R, Solomon L, et al. Outcomes of a randomized community-level HIV prevention intervention for women living in 18 low-income housing developments. *Am J Public Health.* 2000;90:57-63.

[29] See: Hein K. Aligning science with politics and policy in HIV prevention. *Science.* 1998;280:1905-1906. See also: Fortenberry JD. Condom availability in high schools. *Adolesc Med.* 1997;8:449-454. See also: Stryker J, Coates TJ, DeCarlo P, Haynes-Sanstad K, et al. Prevention of HIV infection. Looking back, looking ahead. *JAMA.* 1995;273:1143-1148.

[30] Lurie P. When science and politics collide: the federal response to needle-exchange programs. *Bull N Y Acad Med.* 1995;72:380-396. See also: Friedman S, Des Jarlais D. *Am Epidemiol.* 138(9):768-771;1993.

[31] In 1998, the Secretary of HHS issued a determination that needle exchange was a scientifically proven HIV prevention intervention but kept in place the ongoing federal ban against funding needle exchange programs. Among the ongoing federally funded assessments of

efficacy of this intervention was the following article by David Holtgrave, now of the CDC: Holtgrave DR, Pinkerton SD, Jones TS, Lurie P, et al. Cost and cost-effectiveness of increasing access to sterile syringes and needles as an HIV prevention intervention in the United States. *J Acquir Immune Defic Syndr Hum Retrovirol.* 1998;18 Suppl 1:S133-138.

[32] Berkley SF, Widy-Wirski R, Okware SI, et al. Risk factors associated with HIV infection in Uganda. *J Infect Dis.* 1989;160:22-30. See also: Barongo LR, Borgdorff MW, Mosha FF, Nicoll A, et al. The epidemiology of HIV-1 infection in urban areas, roadside settlements and rural villages in Mwanza Region, Tanzania. *AIDS.* 1992;6:1521-1528. See also: Campbell C. Selling sex in the time of AIDS: the psycho-social context of condom use by sex workers on a Southern African mine. *Soc Sci Med.* 2000;50:479-494.

[33] Nelson KE, Celentano DD, Suprasert S, Wright N, et al. Risk factors for HIV infection among young adult men in northern Thailand. *JAMA.* 1993;270:955-960.

[34] Fullilove RE, Fullilove MT, Northridge ME, Ganz ML, et al. Risk factors for excess mortality in Harlem. Findings from the Harlem Household Survey. *Am J Prev Med.* 1999;3 Suppl:22-28.

[35] For background on empowerment strategies, see: Wallerstein N. Introduction to community empowerment, participatory education, and health. *Health Educ Q.* 1994;21:141-148. See also: MacKenzie JE, Hobfoll SE, Ennis N, Kay J, et al. Reducing AIDS risk among inner-city women: a review of the Collectivist Empowerment AIDS Prevention (CE-AP) Program. *J Eur Acad Dermatol Venereol.* 1999;13:166-174.

[36] For empowerment model evaluation recommendations, see: Wallerstein N, Bernstein E. Empowerment education: Freire's ideas adapted to health education. *Health Educ Q.* 1988; 15:379-394. Additionally, the August, 1999 HIV Prevention Conference conducted by the Centers for Disease Control and Prevention featured several program implementation research efforts focused on empowerment strategies.

[37] "Least restrictive environment (LRE)" evolved as a legal concept most notably in the 1974 federal Education for the Handicapped Act. It has been reflected in numerous national disability-related education, health care access, deinstitutionalization, and vocational rehabilitation policy and program developments over the course of the ensuing 25 years. Along with the concept of "reasonable accommodation," developed under Section 504 of the 1973 Rehabilitation Act, LRE requirements have envisioned an integrated, community-based world of opportunities for people with disabilities and chronic illnesses. For an excellent assessment of national disability integration policies, see: Minow M. *Making All the Difference: Inclusion, Exclusion, and American Law.* Ithaca, NY: Cornell University Press; 1990.

[38] O'Neill JF, Alexander CS. Palliative medicine and HIV/AIDS. *Prim Care.* 1997;24:607-615.

[39] Most recently, in FY1999, HRSA struggled with guidance for Ryan White CARE Act funding for acupuncture and other complementary and alternative therapies.

[40] A recent discussion in Massachusetts is indicative of other current perspectives. In broad community-based discussions regarding the reauthorization of the Ryan White CARE Act in 2000, representatives of communities of color challenged the increasing emphasis on primary care and related reimbursement through the Act, arguing that the reauthorization should not eclipse the prior availability of nonallopathic supports that they felt their communities had yet to access fully.

[41] For a review of compliance literature prior to the onset of HIV, see: Koltun A, Stone GC. Past and current trends in patient noncompliance research: focus on diseases, regimens, programs, and provider disciplines. *J Compliance Health Care.* 1986;1:21-32. For discussions by authors who have attempted to revisit patient adherence and assess drug delivery and other compliance considerations, see: Steiner JF, Fihn SD, Blair B, Inut TS. Appropriate reductions in compliance among well-controlled hypertensive patients. *J Clin Epidemiol.* 1991;44:1361-1371. See also: Langer N. Culturally competent professionals in therapeutic alliances enhance patient compliance. *J Health Care Poor Underserved.* 1999;10:19-26. See also: Cochrane MG, Bala MV, Downs KE, Mauskopf J, et al. Inhaled corticosteroids for asthma therapy: patient compliance, devices, and inhalation technique. *Chest.* 2000;117:542-550.

[42] Shilts, R. (ref.8); Arno P and Feiden K. (ref.12); Epstein S. *Impure Science: AIDS Activism, and the Politics of Knowledge.* Berkeley: University of California Press; 1996.

[43] See: Brandt A. *No Magic Bullet: A Social History of Venereal Disease in the United States Since 1880*. New York, NY: Oxford University Press. 1985.

[44] Most recently, the state of Colorado's legislature sought to acquire its Department of Public Health's AIDS surveillance data for cross-matching with criminal records information.

[45] For an early historical perspective on the evolution of HIV surveillance, reporting, confidentiality, and other public health measures, see: Parmet W. AIDS and quarantine: the revival of an archaic doctrine. *Hofstra Law Review*. 1985;14(53). See also: Clark ME. AIDS prevention: legislative options. *Am J Law Med*. 1990;16:107-153; Gostin L, Curran W. Legal control measures for AIDS: reporting requirements, surveillance, quarantine, and regulation of public meeting places. *Am J Public Health*. 1987;77:214-218. See also: Gostin L, Porter H. AIDS Litigation Project: a national review of court and human rights decisions. *US Public Health Service*. 1990. For more recent discussions, see: Gostin LO, Hadley J. Health services research: public benefits, personal privacy, and proprietary interests. *Ann Intern Med*. 1998;129:833-835.

[46] Among these changes have been, increased preapproval drug access through expanded compassionate use and treatment IND regulatory changes, and through parallel track structures for Phase III testing. Additionally, advocates helped shaped geographically diverse AIDS clinical testing sites, including through community-based research mechanisms.

[47] In fact, this was the approval of aerosolized pentamidine for prophylactic use against PCP constituted the first time the FDA had issued a drug approval solely on the basis of community research data. For further discussion, see: Epstein S. (ref. 42); Nussbaum B. *Good Intentions: How Big Business and the Medical Establishment are Corrupting the Fight Against AIDS*. New York, NY: The Atlantic Monthly Press; 1990.

[48] In 1988, Congress provided, through the HHS appropriation process, its first directives to the NIH and HRSA to collaborate through their respective research and care programs in the delivery of clinical trials to people with HIV/AIDS. During that same year, it provided the first funding for the NIH Community Program in Clinical Research on AIDS, another mechanism intended to make trials available in clinical care sites. In 1990, the passage of the Ryan White CARE Act, assured clinical trial linkages through Title IIIb early intervention programs and through Title IV pediatric services. The following year, in response to yet another Congressional mandate, HRSA and NIH formalized an interagency clinical trial access coordination agreement, targeting, in particular, the participation of women and people of color. In 1992, NIH moved to requiring all of its extramural HIV clinical research sites to increase participation of women and minorities, spurring further collaborations with HIV primary care settings.

[49] See: McGuire J. *Research=Care: A Critique of the Right to Research Claim*. [Unpublished PhD dissertation]. Waltham, MA: Brandeis University; 1996. See also: Kass NE, Sugarman J, Faden R, Schoch-Spana M. Trust, The fragile foundation of contemporary biomedical research. *Hastings Cent Rep*. 1996;26:25-29.

[50] For example, collaborations between the National Association of Community Health Centers and the National Heart, Lung, and Blood Institute resulted in a recently completed multisite study of comparative anti-hypertensive treatments in over 50 000 enrollees.

[51] Other federal agencies contributing considerably smaller HIV prevention and care funding to states include: other segments of the Department of Health and Human Services, including the Developmental Disabilities Administration, the Office of Minority Health, and the Substance Abuse and Mental Health Administration. Beyond HHS, other federal agencies involved in state-based HIV-related support are the Department of Housing and Urban Development and the Department of Education.

[52] State health agencies are organized in many different ways, with a typical bifurcation occurring between programs that receive discretionary state and federal funding, such as CDC prevention and HRSA care resources, and agencies that manage entitlement resources such as Medicaid and, until recently, welfare. Furthermore, many of them have sub-agency divisions that often result in considerable administrative distance between HIV surveillance, prevention and care efforts.

[53] Two recent developments further illustrate this reality. For the first time in several years, HRSA, in early 2000, hosted a cross-title conference for all the Ryan White grantees, obligating each grantee to give at least one of its conference slots to a participating consumer. Similarly, consumer activity reporting requirements are a part of contract compliance for all Ryan White

funded programs. The CDC has both struggled with the framework of who constitutes a "consumer" of prevention and with its process for verifying the participation of those individuals. In spite of its community planning requirements established in 1994, in 1996-1997, the CDC found itself on the defensive for underrepresentation of people from communities of color. The resulting Congressional Black Caucus actions of 1998-1999 have forced new resource allocation and planning processes intended to improve representation in HIV prevention efforts.

[54] As an ongoing example of the program delivery and funding effects of these fissures, HRSA continues to disallow the financing of HIV counseling and testing efforts through Ryan White Title I and II, characterizing these activities to more appropriately belong in the domain of prevention.

[55] The availability of more effective therapies has raised questions about the goals and the appropriate focus of long-term prevention behavior change efforts; on the care side, the efficacy of social and emotional support systems has come into question.

[56] In 1999, several federal initiatives gave evidence of new integration efforts. They included: combined HIV, STD, hepatitis C, and substance abuse related program requirements under the CDC's and SAMHSA's Congressional Black Caucus HIV-related activities; joint funding and management by HRSA and CDC of a multiyear, multisite HIV demonstration project in jails and prisons; and increased service integration reporting requirements for state and local cooperative agreements from both CDC and HRSA.

[57] In 1998, CDC issued new partner referral and support guidelines; in early 2000, they issued updated HIV counseling and testing guidelines; and they and HRSA have been revising STD and substance abuse integration requirements. All of these speak to new and evolving prevention and care connections.

[58] As noted earlier, state grants and cooperative agreements increasingly include specific verification of STD integration activities.

[59] Among other arenas in which prevention and care integration are evolving are teen sexual health, education, and pregnancy prevention programs; tobacco cessation and other alcohol and drug treatment integration; adult hypertension wellness, preventive care, and clinical treatment services.

[60] Intermediate care facilities for people with mental retardation (ICF/MR) were developed under Medicaid during the early 1980s in response to increasing pressures to deinstitutionalize people with developmental disabilities. This became a reimbursement mechanism for community based care alternatives for disabled individuals. Among the achievements of this program was the development of consumer and consumer advocate input into the treatment planning process. It both reflected, and became a model for, growing efforts in the broader disability independent living and right to treatment movements.

[61] The 1983 meeting resulted in the creation of what would become 3 national organizations. The AIDS Action Council was specifically established to undertake federal policy development. The National AIDS Network, a member service organization for the fledgling AIDS groups that were slowly developing, NAN closed its doors in 1991.The National Association for People with AIDS (NAPWA), which continues to represent the interests of consumers and peer groups across the country.

[62] Epstein S. (ref.42); Burkett E. (ref.12).

[63] A notable indication of the growing visibility and credibility of this part of the public health work force is the inclusion of community health workers as a section now within the American Public Health Association.

[64] For an early discussion of volunteer commitment and support, see: Velentgas P, Bynum C, Zierler S. The buddy volunteer commitment in AIDS care. *Am J Public Health*. 1990;80:1378-1380.

[65] The San Francisco model, often cited in the early HIV literature, was a coordinated system of social supports, acute and palliative clinical care, deeply dependent on integrated emotional support structures and extensive volunteers. It was adapted in many jurisdictions and provided the basis for the coordinated care model envisioned in the Ryan White CARE Act. What most distinguished San Francisco—and later Seattle—from other coordinated systems of clinical and social support was the integrated role the acute care setting, San Francisco General, played.

[66] McKinney MM. Consortium approaches to the delivery of HIV services under the Ryan White CARE Act. *AIDS Pub Pol*. 1993; 8:115-125; Marconi K, Rundall T, Genry D, et al. The organization and availability of HIV-related services in Baltimore, Maryland, and Oakland, California. *AIDS Pub Pol*. 1994;9:173-181. See also: Holtgrave D. Priority setting and HIV prevention community planning. *AIDS Pub Pol J;* 1996: 11.

[67] See, for example, Kieler BW, Rundall TG, Saporta I, Sussman PC, et al. Challenges faced by the HIV Health Services Planning Council in Oakland, California, 1991-1994. *Am J Prev Med*. 1996;12(4 suppl):26-32.

[68] As noted earlier, lack of congruency between state and local CDC cooperative agreement funding and HIV epidemiologic profiles has led to redirection of funding initiatives by the CDC.

[69] Marmor T, Morone J. Representing consumer interests: imbalanced markets, health planning, and the HSAs. *Milbank Mem Fund Q Health Soc*. 1980;58:125-165.

[70] Butterfoss FD, Goodman RM, Wandersman A. Community coalitions for prevention and health promotion. *Health Educ Res*. 1993;8:315-330.

INDEX